2013
YEAR BOOK OF
ORTHOPEDICS®

The 2013 Year Book Series

Year Book of Critical Care Medicine®: Drs Dries, Zanotti-Cavazzoni, Latenser, Martinez, Rincon, and Zwank

Year Book of Emergency Medicine®: Drs Hamilton, Bruno, Handly, Minczak, Quintana, and Ramoska

Year Book of Endocrinology®: Drs Schott, Apovian, Clarke, Eugster, Meikle, Oetgen, Ovalle, Schteingart, and Toth

Year Book of Hand and Upper Limb Surgery®: Drs Yao, Adams, Isaacs, and Rizzo

Year Book of Medicine®: Drs Barker, Garrick, Gersh, Khardori, LeRoith, Panush, Talley, and Thigpen

Year Book of Neonatal and Perinatal Medicine®: Drs Fanaroff, Benitz, Donn, Neu, Papile, and Van Marter

Year Book of Neurology and Neurosurgery®: Drs Klimo, Minagar, Gandhi, Liu, Panagariya, Rezania, Riel-Romero, Riesenburger, Robottom, Schwendimann, Shafazand, and Yang

Year Book of Obstetrics, Gynecology, and Women's Health®: Drs Dungan and Shulman

Year Book of Oncology®: Drs Arceci, Bauer, Chiorean, Gordon, Lawton, Murphy, Thigpen, and Tsao

Year Book of Ophthalmology®: Drs Rapuano, Cohen, Flanders, Hammersmith, Milman, Myers, Nagra, Nelson, Penne, Pyfer, Sergott, Shields, Talekar, and Vander

Year Book of Orthopedics®: Drs Morrey, Huddleston, Rose, Swiontkowski, and Trigg

Year Book of Otolaryngology-Head and Neck Surgery®: Drs Sindwani, Balough, Franco, Gapany, and Mitchell

Year Book of Pathology and Laboratory Medicine®: Drs Raab and Bissell

Year Book of Pediatrics®: Dr Stockman

Year Book of Plastic and Aesthetic Surgery™: Drs Miller, Boehmler, Gosman, Gutowski, Ruberg, Salisbury, and Smith

Year Book of Psychiatry and Applied Mental Health®: Drs Talbott, Ballenger, Buckley, Frances, Krupnick, and Mack

Year Book of Pulmonary Disease®: Drs Barker, Jones, Maurer, Spradley, Tanoue, and Willsie

Year Book of Sports Medicine®: Drs Shephard, Cantu, Feldman, Galea, Jankowski, Janssen, Lebrun, and Nieman

2013

The Year Book of ORTHOPEDICS®

Editor-in-Chief

Bernard F. Morrey, MD

Professor of Orthopedics, Mayo Graduate School of Medicine; Professor of Orthopedics, University of Texas, Health Science Center, San Antonio, Texas

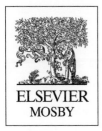

ELSEVIER
MOSBY

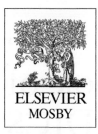

ELSEVIER
MOSBY

Senior Vice President, Content: Linda Belfus
Developmental Editor: Jennifer Flynn-Briggs
Production Supervisor, Electronic Year Books: Donna M. Skelton
Electronic Article Manager: Mike Sheets
Illustrations and Permissions Coordinator: Dawn Vohsen

2013 EDITION
Copyright 2013, Mosby, Inc. All rights reserved.

Composition by TNQ Books and Journals Pvt Ltd, India

Editorial Office:
Elsevier, Inc.
Suite 1800
1600 John F. Kennedy Blvd
Philadelphia, PA 19103-2899

International Standard Serial Number: 0276-1092
International Standard Book Number: 978-1-4557-7283-4

Printed and bound by CPI Group (UK) Ltd, Croydon, CR0 4YY

Transferred to digital print 2012

Editorial Board

Table of Contents

Journals Represented

Journals represented in this YEAR BOOK are listed below.

Acta Orthopaedica
AJR American Journal of Roentgenology
American Journal of Sports Medicine
American Journal of Surgical Pathology
Anesthesiology
Annals of Plastic Surgery
Annals of the Rheumatic Diseases
Archives of Physical Medicine and Rehabilitation
Arthritis & Rheumatism
Arthroscopy
Bone and Joint Journal
British Journal of Sports Medicine
British Medical Journal
Clinical Biomechanics
Clinical Orthopaedics and Related Research
European Journal of Pain
European Journal of Plastic Surgery
European Journal of Radiology
Foot & Ankle International
Injury
JAMA Internal Medicine
Journal of Bone and Joint Surgery (American)
Journal of Bone and Joint Surgery (British)
Journal of Bone Mineral Research
Journal of Clinical Endocrinology & Metabolism
Journal of Clinical Oncology
Journal of Diabetic Complications
Journal of Hand Surgery
Journal of Neurosurgery Spine
Journal of Orthopaedic Research
Journal of Orthopaedic Trauma
Journal of Pediatric Orthopedics
Journal of Plastic, Reconstructive & Aesthetic Surgery
Journal of Surgical Oncology
Journal of the American Medical Association
Journal of Trauma and Acute Care Surgery
Journal of Vascular Surgery
Medical Care
Microsurgery
Neurology
Neurosurgery
Orthopedics
Pediatric Emergency Care
Plastic and Reconstructive Surgery
Sarcoma
Skeletal Radiology
Spine

Spine Journal
Sports Medicine
Surgical Oncology
Wound Repair and Regeneration

STANDARD ABBREVIATIONS

The following terms are abbreviated in this edition: acquired immunodeficiency syndrome (AIDS), anterior cruciate ligament (ACL), anteroposterior (AP), avascular necrosis (AVN), cardiopulmonary resuscitation (CPR), central nervous system (CNS), cerebrospinal fluid (CSF), computed tomography (CT), deoxyribonucleic acid (DNA), electrocardiography (ECG), health maintenance organization (HMO), human immunodeficiency virus (HIV), intensive care unit (ICU), intramuscular (IM), intravenous (IV), magnetic resonance (MR) imaging (MRI), range of motion (ROM), ribonucleic acid (RNA), total hip arthroplasty (THA), total knee arthroplasty (TKA), ultrasound (US), and ultraviolet (UV).

NOTE

The YEAR BOOK OF ORTHOPEDICS® is a literature survey service providing abstracts of articles published in the professional literature. Every effort is made to assure the accuracy of the information presented in these pages. Neither the editors nor the publisher of the YEAR BOOK OF ORTHOPEDICS® can be responsible for errors in the original materials. The editors' comments are their own opinions. Mention of specific products within this publication does not constitute endorsement.

To facilitate the use of the YEAR BOOK OF ORTHOPEDICS® as a reference tool, all illustrations and tables included in this publication are now identified as they appear in the original article. This change is meant to help the reader recognize that any illustration or table appearing in the YEAR BOOK OF ORTHOPEDICS® may be only one of many in the original article. For this reason, figure and table numbers will often appear to be out of sequence within the YEAR BOOK OF ORTHOPEDICS®.

Introduction

As in previous years, the continuing challenges facing our specialty are reflected in this year's volume. These challenges largely relate to the pressures of external influence demanding greater "evidence-based and cost-effective orthopedic solutions." We have focused on the higher level evidence studies in this year's selections even more so than in the past. While this requirement seems to be driven by external forces, we have long been aware that this is the appropriate direction for our specialty specifically, but also for medicine in general. We must behave in a more responsible manner reflected by clinical decisions based on the simple formula:

"Evidence-based cost-effective" procedures. Given this, there continues to be exciting advances in this profession as reflected in a better understanding of hip impingement as a cause of osteoarthritis in the young, the ever-increasing application of growth factors in the clinical practice, and enhanced use of analytical reviews of the literature to clarify the knowledge base of controversial issues. These advances have been documented to improve patient outcomes and enhance the functional result of intervention. As in the past, I have recognized the significant personal benefit, as the privilege of serving as editor of the YEAR BOOK and reviewing several sections allows me to maintain a personal awareness of the exciting events in the specialty. It is my sincere hope that this volume, which focuses on individuals with a general orthopedic practice, will benefit the reader as much as I and the other editors have benefited from selecting and reviewing the spectrum of topics.

Bernard F. Morrey, MD

1 Basic Science

Introduction

The themes expressed in the basic science section have not changed dramatically. We continue to try to develop the ongoing application of growth factors in orthopedic and its various tissue applications: cartilage, bone, and tendon. The complementary advances in the engineered, biodegradable scaffolding also hold great promise in managing structural defects. The basic science selection reflects these trends. In addition, there is a growing body of basic health science research that is reflected principally in the meta-analysis and analytical reviews of the literature. The selection of these articles has been strengthened in the appropriate section rather than sequestered in the section of basic research. It is hoped that the reader will appreciate the scientific basis of our clinical practice, the emerging trends, and exciting future prospects for improved patient management through basic and health science research.

Bernard F. Morrey, MD

Does prior sustained compression make cartilage-on-bone more vulnerable to trauma?

Kim W, Thambyah A, Broom N (Univ of Auckland, New Zealand)
Clin Biomech 27:637-645, 2012

Background.—This study investigated how varying levels of prior creep deformation in cartilage-on-bone samples influences their mechanical response and vulnerability to structural damage following a single traumatic impact.

Methods.—Bovine patellae were subjected to varying intervals of prior creep loading at a constant stress of 4 MPa. Immediately following removal of this stress the samples were impacted with a pendulum indenter system at a fixed energy of 2.2 J.

Findings.—With increasing prior creep, the peak force on impact rose, the duration of impact and time to reach peak force both decreased, and both the energy dissipated during impact and the magnitude of impulse were both unchanged by the level of prior creep. With increasing prior creep, the severity of impact-induced osteochondral damage increased: articular cartilage cracks penetrated to a greater depth, extending to the calcified cartilage layer resulting in hairline fractures or articular cartilage delamination and associated secondary damage to the vascular channels in the subchondral bone.

Interpretation.—The study shows that exposure of the cartilage-on-bone system to prior creep can significantly influence its response to subsequent impact, namely force attenuation and severity of damage to the articular cartilage, calcified cartilage and vascular channel network in the subchondral bone.

▶ This interesting study is reviewed because it has direct clinical relevance. Whenever we attempt to mobilize a stiff joint, there is of necessity increased compressive and probably shear force across the joint. If prolonged, this force will induce creep in the articular cartilage. Although some have hypothesized that this can create degenerative changes, this experiment clearly reveals increased vulnerability to single-impact trauma. This would seem to have implications in the remobilization and turn to activity after brace or splint therapy for joint ankylosis.

B. F. Morrey, MD

Altered Loading in the Injured Knee After ACL Rupture

Gardinier ES, Manal K, Buchanan TS, et al (Univ of Delaware, Newark)
J Orthop Res 31:458-464, 2013

Articular loading is an important factor in the joint degenerative process for individuals with anterior cruciate ligament (ACL) rupture. Evaluation of loading for a population that exhibits neuromuscular compensation for injury requires an approach which can incorporate individual muscle activation strategies in its estimation of muscle forces. The purpose of this study was to evaluate knee joint contact forces for patients with ACL deficiency using an EMG-driven modeling approach to estimate muscle forces. Thirty athletes with acute, unilateral ACL rupture underwent gait analysis after resolving range of motion, effusion, pain, and obvious gait impairments. Electromyography was recorded bilaterally from 14 lower extremity muscles and input to a musculoskeletal model for estimation of muscle forces and joint contact forces. Gait mechanics were consistent with previous reports for individuals with ACL-deficiency. Our major finding was that joint loading was altered in the injured limb after acute ACL injury; patients walked with decreased contact force on their injured knee compared to their uninjured knee. Both medial and lateral compartment forces were reduced without a significant change in the distribution of tibiofemoral load between compartments. This is the first study to estimate medial and lateral compartment contact forces in patients with acute ACL rupture using an approach which is sensitive to individual muscle activation patterns. Further work is needed to determine whether this early

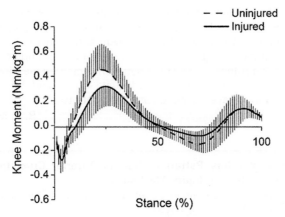

FIGURE 2.—Sagittal plane knee moments for the stance phase of gait. Positive values represent external knee flexion moments. Whiskers are standard deviations. (Reprinted from Gardinier ES, Manal K, Buchanan TS, et al. Altered loading in the injured knee after ACL rupture. *J Orthop Res.* 2013;31:458-464, with permission from Journal of Orthopaedic Research and John Wiley and Sons, www.interscience.wiley.com.)

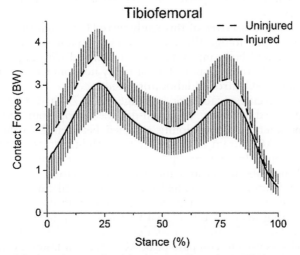

FIGURE 4.—Tibiofemoral contact forces for the stance phase of gait. Whiskers are standard deviations. (Reprinted from Gardinier ES, Manal K, Buchanan TS, et al. Altered loading in the injured knee after ACL rupture. *J Orthop Res.* 2013;31:458-464, with permission from Journal of Orthopaedic Research and John Wiley and Sons, www.interscience.wiley.com.)

decreased loading of the injured limb is involved in the development of osteoarthritis in these patients (Figs 2 and 4).

▶ This is an important study because it seeks to better understand the ultimate consequence of the anterior cruciate ligament deficient knee: osteoarthritis. The methodology is sophisticated and, although some limitations exist and are recognized by the authors, the main findings are valid and interesting. The injured knee exhibits a lower moment in the sagittal plane (Fig 2) as well as decreased contact stresses (Fig 4). These observations surprised me, because I would have expected the opposite (ie, greater moment and greater contact stresses). We don't know if this changes with longer follow-up; this study was less than 7 months. Also, the authors should have better characterized the clinical features of the sample—noncopers is not quite adequate in my mind. Specifically, did these patients all truly have a symptomatic pivot shift test?

B. F. Morrey, MD

Clinically Relevant Injury Patterns After an Anterior Cruciate Ligament Injury Provide Insight into Injury Mechanisms

Levine JW, Kiapour AM, Quatman CE, et al (The Univ of Toledo, OH; et al)
Am J Sports Med 41:385-395, 2013

Background.—The functional disability and high costs of treating anterior cruciate ligament (ACL) injuries have generated a great deal of interest in understanding the mechanism of noncontact ACL injuries. Secondary bone bruises have been reported in over 80% of partial and complete ACL ruptures.

Purpose.—The objectives of this study were (1) to quantify ACL strain under a range of physiologically relevant loading conditions and (2) to evaluate soft tissue and bony injury patterns associated with applied loading conditions thought to be responsible for many noncontact ACL injuries.

Study Design.—Controlled laboratory study.

Methods.—Seventeen cadaveric legs (age, 45 ± 7 years; 9 female and 8 male) were tested utilizing a custom-designed drop stand to simulate landing. Specimens were randomly assigned between 2 loading groups that evaluated ACL strain under either knee abduction or internal tibial rotation moments. In each group, combinations of anterior tibial shear force, and knee abduction and internal tibial rotation moments under axial impact loading were applied sequentially until failure. Specimens were tested at 25° of flexion under simulated 1200-N quadriceps and 800-N hamstring loads. A differential variable reluctance transducer was used to calculate ACL strain across the anteromedial bundle. A general linear model was used to compare peak ACL strain at failure. Correlations between simulated knee injury patterns and loading conditions were evaluated by the χ^2 test for independence.

Results.—Anterior cruciate ligament failure was generated in 15 of 17 specimens (88%). A clinically relevant distribution of failure patterns was observed including medial collateral ligament tears and damage to the menisci, cartilage, and subchondral bone. Only abduction significantly contributed to calculated peak ACL strain at failure ($P = .002$). While ACL disruption patterns were independent of the loading mechanism, tibial plateau injury patterns (locations) were significantly ($P = .002$) dependent on the applied loading conditions. Damage to the articular cartilage along with depression of the midlateral tibial plateau was primarily associated with knee abduction moments, while cartilage damage with depression of the posterolateral tibial plateau was primarily associated with internal tibial rotation moments.

Conclusion.—The current findings demonstrate the relationship between the location of the tibial plateau injury and ACL injury mechanisms. The resultant injury locations were similar to the clinically observed bone bruises across the tibial plateau during a noncontact ACL injury. These findings indicate that abduction combined with other modes of loading (multiplanar loading) may act to produce ACL injuries.

Clinical Relevance.—A better understanding of ACL injury mechanisms and associated risk factors may improve current preventive, surgical, and rehabilitation strategies and limit the risk of ACL and secondary injuries, which may in turn minimize the future development of posttraumatic osteoarthritis of the knee.

▶ For me, the most important issue of anterior cruciate ligament (ACL) injury is when it has to be repaired. Hence studies that clarify the injury pattern are of great value. This is a rather elaborate study employing simulated muscle loading as well as angular loading moments to create ACL failure. There is no surprise that the ACL fails in abduction. The finding of posterior medial tibial bruising being associated with concurrent internal tibial rotation may be useful clinically. Obtaining such a history of injury mechanism will enhance concern of this associated injury to the medial tibial cartilage.

B. F. Morrey, MD

Effects of platelet-rich plasma (PRP) on the healing of Achilles tendons of rats
Kaux J-F, Drion PV, Colige A, et al (Univ of Liége, Belgium; et al)
Wound Repair Regen 20:748-756, 2012

Platelet-rich plasma (PRP) contains growth factors involved in the tissular healing process. The aim of the study was to determine if an injection of PRP could improve the healing of sectioned Achilles tendons of rats. After surgery, rats received an injection of PRP ($n = 60$) or a physiological solution ($n = 60$) in situ. After 5, 15, and 30 days, 20 rats of both groups were euthanized and 15 collected tendons were submitted to a biomechanical test using cryo-jaws before performing transcriptomic analyses. Histological and biochemical analyses were performed on the five remaining tendons in each group. Tendons in the PRP group were more resistant to rupture at 15 and 30 days. The mechanical stress was significantly increased in tendons of the PRP group at day 30. Histological analysis showed a precocious deposition of fibrillar collagen at day 5 confirmed by a biochemical measurement. The expression of tenomodulin was significantly higher at day 5. The messenger RNA levels of type III collagen, matrix metalloproteinases 2, 3, and 9, were similar in the two groups at all time points, whereas type I collagen was significantly increased at day 30 in the PRP group. In conclusion, an injection of

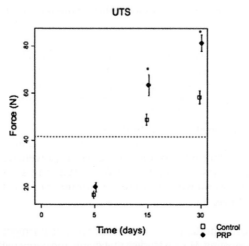

UTS

FIGURE 3.—(A) Breaking strength expressed in newton (N) recorded in control groups ($n = 15$ at each time point) and PRP groups ($n = 15$ at each time point) (mean ± SD) at increasing time after surgery (5, 15, and 30 days). The dotted line represents the mean value measuring for healthy Achilles tendons of rats (42 N, $n = 10$). A significant increase of UTS occurred in both groups with time, the PRP group showing significantly higher values than the control group at day 15 and 30. *p-value < 0.05. (Reprinted from Kaux J-F, Drion PV, Colige A, et al. Effects of platelet-rich plasma (PRP) on the healing of Achilles tendons of rats. *Wound Repair Regen.* 2012;20:748-756, with permission from Wound Repair and Regeneration and John Wiley and Sons, www.interscience.wiley.com.)

PRP in sectioned rat Achilles tendon influences the early phase of tendon healing and results in an ultimately stronger mechanical resistance (Fig 3A).

▶ As the debate and clinical uncertainty rages regarding platelet-rich plasma (PRP), it is useful to turn to the basic science investigations of the topic. Simply put, this particular preparation of PRP, and there are many, did enhance tensile strength at 30 days (Fig 3A). Most likely this is because of the advanced expression of type 1 collagen, as the authors surmise. Regardless, this is encouraging. The problem remains in the clinical setting; what is the phase of the diseased tendon being treated, and what are the active elements of the PRP preparation? Although the experiment involves the rabbit Achilles tendon, it is likely the findings can be extrapolated to other tendon systems.

B. F. Morrey, MD

Adipose-derived stem cells enhance primary tendon repair: Biomechanical and immunohistochemical evaluation

Uysal CA, Tobita M, Hyakusoku H, et al (Baskent Univ Faculty of Medicine, Ankara, Turkey; Nippon Med School, Tokyo, Japan)

J Plast Reconstr Aesthetic Surg 65:1712-1719, 2012

Background.—Primary tendon repair aims at increased tensile strength at the time of mobilisation. Tendon repair and regeneration using mesenchymal stem cells have been described in different studies; however, adipose-derived stem cell (ASC) use for tendon regeneration and repair has recently been taken into consideration. In this study, we sought to determine whether ASCs would be beneficial in primary tendon healing.

Materials and Methods.—Both the Achilles tendons of rabbits ($n = 6$) were incised and consequently repaired. To the left side was applied platelet-rich plasma (PRP) gel and to the right side autologous ASC-mixed PRP. The tensile strength was measured on the 4th week. The samples were taken for immunohistochemical evaluation of collagen type I, transforming growth factor beta (TGF-β) 1, 2, 3, fibroblast growth factor (FGF) and vascular endothelial growth factor (VEGF).

Results.—The tensile strengths in control and experimental groups were found out to be 29.46 ± 3.66 and 43.06 ± 3.80 kgf. Collagen type I, FGF and VEGF levels were statistically higher, whereas TGF-β1, 2, 3 were lower in the experimental group.

Conclusion.—ASCs enhance primary tendon healing; however, the complex interaction and the cascades by which ASCs could increase collagen type I, FGF and VEGF and decrease TGF-β levels should further be investigated.

▶ This study is reviewed for several reasons. First and foremost, to introduce the evolving interest and line of research involving adipose-derived stem cells (ASC). Second, to portray the complexity of not only the experiment but of the analysis and of the subject matter. This is not the kind of article most practicing orthopedic surgeons would wish to read. But it does reveal the level of sophistication in which the research that supports our practice is engaged. As the authors point out, whereas the strength of the ACS tendons is stronger, this occurred with increased measurements of collagen I, fibroblast growth factor, and of vascular endothelial growth factor; however, assays of transforming growth factor beta were decreased! The conclusions are further obscured by the recognition that platelet-rich plasma was used not only on the control tendon, but also along with ASC tendon.

B. F. Morrey, MD

Comparison of Mesenchymal Stem Cells (Osteoprogenitors) Harvested From Proximal Humerus and Distal Femur During Arthroscopic Surgery
Beitzel K, McCarthy MBR, Cote MP, et al (Univ of Connecticut Health Ctr, Farmington)
Arthroscopy 29:301-308, 2013

Purpose.—The aim of this study was to examine the relations between age, gender, and number of viable mesenchymal stem cells (MSCs) in concentrated bone marrow (BM) obtained from the proximal humerus and distal femur during arthroscopic surgery.

Methods.—BM was aspirated from either the proximal humerus ($n = 55$) or distal femur ($n = 29$) during arthroscopic surgery in 84 patients

(51.3 ± 11.6 years). MSCs were obtained from fractionated bone marrow after a 5-minute spin at 1,500 rpm. Volume of BM and number of nucleated cells (NCs) were calculated, and samples were cultured for 6 days, after which point colony-forming units (CFUs) were quantified and fluorescence-activated cell sorting (FACS) analysis was performed. Simple linear regression was used to explore relations between age, gender, volume of aspirated BM, and MSCs per milliliter.

Results.—BM aspirations yielded a mean quantity of 22.6 ± 12.3 mL. After centrifugation, $30.0 ± 16.7 × 10^6$ nucleated cells/mL of concentrated BM were harvested. The proximal humerus provided $38.7 ± 52.6 × 10^6$, and the distal femur, $25.9 ± 14.3 × 10^6$, for an overall 766.3 ± 545.3 MSCs/mL of concentrated BM (proximal humerus: 883.9 ± 577.6, distal femur: 551.3 ± 408.1). Values did not significantly differ by age, gender, or donor site.

Conclusions.—Arthroscopic aspiration of bone marrow from the proximal humerus and distal femur is a reproducible technique and yields reliable concentrations of MSCs. The use of an intraoperative concentration method resulted in consistent amounts of MSCs in all clinically relevant age groups without a significant drop of the number of isolated MSCs.

Clinical Relevance.—Human MSCs derived from concentrated bone marrow aspirate are a promising biological addition that may have practical use in the future of soft tissue augmentation. Arthroscopic techniques for bone marrow aspiration that do not require an additional surgical site for aspiration (e.g., iliac crest) or a second operative procedure may facilitate future use of MSCs in arthroscopic surgery.

▶ I'm not sure this is the most earth shaking article I've seen. However, it does proffer 2 points that I think are of value to the reader. The first is to emphasize the increasing potential value of stem cells in our practice. The concept is here to stay. The technique will vary. It is of some value to know that the stem cell does not differ in its apparent functional potential whether harvested from proximal humerus or distal femur. That's about it.

B. F. Morrey, MD

Failed Healing of Rotator Cuff Repair Correlates With Altered Collagenase and Gelatinase in Supraspinatus and Subscapularis Tendons
Robertson CM, Chen CT, Shindle MK, et al (The Hosp for Special Surgery, NY; Univ of Texas Southwestern Med Ctr, Dallas)
Am J Sports Med 40:1993-2001, 2012

Background.—Despite improvements in arthroscopic rotator cuff repair technique and technology, a significant rate of failed tendon healing persists. Improving the biology of rotator cuff repairs may be an important focus to decrease this failure rate. The objective of this study was to determine the mRNA biomarkers and histological characteristics of repaired

TABLE 2.—Levels of mRNA Expression in Subscapularis Tendon (Sub), Supraspinatus Tendon (Sup), Bursal Tissue (Bur), and Synovium (Syn)[a]

	Subscapularis Tendon Healing	Subscapularis Tendon Defect	Supraspinatus Tendon Healing	Supraspinatus Tendon Defect	P Value (t Test) Sub	P Value (t Test) Sup
IL-1β*1000	0.39 ± 0.11	0.25 ± 0.08	0.48 ± 0.20	4.09 ± 2.64	.466	.073[c]
IL-6*100	0.44 ± 0.13	0.28 ± 0.08	0.86 ± 0.22	0.36 ± 0.07	.422	.164
TNF-α*1000	0.33 ± 0.13	0.45 ± 0.21	0.26 ± 0.10	0.46 ± 0.13	.597	.273
iNOS*1000	0.25 ± 0.08	0.27 ± 0.16	0.20 ± 0.06	0.27 ± 0.12	.899	.598
COX-2	0.50 ± 0.16	0.37 ± 0.11	0.31 ± 0.15	0.90 ± 0.24	.630	.054[c]
VEGF*10	0.06 ± 0.03	0.05 ± 0.01	0.98 ± 0.33	0.13 ± 0.03	.832	.123
MMP-9*100	0.46 ± 0.17	1.92 ± 0.41	0.39 ± 0.14	1.38 ± 0.55	.001[b]	.021[b]
MMP-1*100	0.38 ± 0.14	1.16 ± 0.62	0.40 ± 0.15	2.47 ± 1.06	.090[c]	.006[b]
MMP-13*100	0.24 ± 0.10	0.26 ± 0.11	1.64 ± 1.49	6.61 ± 4.42	.886	.183
TIMP1	0.30 ± 0.12	0.15 ± 0.03	0.29 ± 0.09	0.35 ± 0.10	.496	.700
COL1A1*10	0.94 ± 0.38	1.86 ± 0.56	3.36 ± 1.46	7.88 ± 1.90	.225	.095[c]
COL3A1	1.02 ± 0.34	1.28 ± 0.27	4.70 ± 1.34	1.04 ± 0.34	.662	.098[c]
SMA*10	1.39 ± 0.57	1.04 ± 0.26	0.80 ± 0.31	1.13 ± 0.37	.725	.547
Biglycan	0.68 ± 0.16	1.04 ± 0.39	1.91 ± 0.42	0.53 ± 0.07	.340	.045[b]
COL1/COL3	1.13 ± 0.76	0.26 ± 0.11	0.32 ± 0.11	1.10 ± 0.43	.502	.023[b]

	Bursa Healing	Bursa Defect	Synovium Healing	Synovium Defect	P Value (t Test) Bur	P Value (t Test) Syn
IL-1β*1000	0.81 ± 0.35	0.82 ± 0.32	1.90 ± 0.75	0.77 ± 0.28	.988	.357
IL-6*100	0.60 ± 0.21	0.46 ± 0.01	0.87 ± 0.41	1.02 ± 0.34	.705	.817
TNF*1000	0.33 ± 0.12	0.09 ± 0.03	2.01 ± 0.53	1.39 ± 0.41	.263	.475
iNOS*1000	0.19 ± 0.12	0.06 ± 0.02	0.63 ± 0.19	1.03 ± 0.40	.545	.302
COX-2*10	1.09 ± 0.23	2.36 ± 0.02	0.31 ± 0.16	0.04 ± 0.01	.005[b]	.307
VEGF*10	0.08 ± 0.03	0.01 ± 0.00	0.17 ± 0.08	0.01 ± 0.00	.123	.219
MMP-9*100	1.81 ± 1.26	0.05 ± 0.00	0.86 ± 0.20	0.89 ± 0.48	.434	.943
MMP-1*100	1.14 ± 0.52	0.11 ± 0.03	39.95 ± 13.1	6.50 ± 1.18	.217	.219
MMP-13*100	0.55 ± 0.28	0.90 ± 0.33	0.42 ± 0.09	0.14 ± 0.02	.496	.104
TIMP1	0.15 ± 0.04	0.04 ± 0.01	2.34 ± 0.65	0.38 ± 0.10	.108	.083[c]
COL1*10	0.68 ± 0.28	0.34 ± 0.07	2.08 ± 0.51	0.34 ± 0.05	.440	.078[c]
COL3	0.37 ± 0.20	0.02 ± 0.00	2.25 ± 0.46	2.04 ± 0.73	.285	.814
SMA*10	0.77 ± 0.22	0.13 ± 0.03	6.53 ± 3.19	1.40 ± 0.37	.087[c]	.356
Biglycan	0.29 ± 0.13	0.02 ± 0.00	1.28 ± 0.28	0.78 ± 0.28	.196	.346
COL1/COL3	0.84 ± 0.57	1.96 ± 0.39	0.18 ± 0.06	0.14 ± 0.13	.235	.808

[a]All expressions were normalized to a housekeeping gene (GAPDH). Values are shown as mean ± standard error of the mean. Statistics comparison between the healed and defect groups was performed using the Student t test.
[b]$P < .05$.
[c]$.05 < P < .10$.

rotator cuffs that healed or developed persistent defects as determined by postoperative ultrasound.

Hypothesis.—Increased synovial inflammation and tendon degeneration at the time of surgery are correlated with the failed healing of rotator cuff tendons.

Study Design.—Case-control study; Level of evidence, 3.

Methods.—Biopsy specimens from the subscapularis tendon, supraspinatus tendon, glenohumeral synovium, and subacromial bursa of 35 patients undergoing arthroscopic rotator cuff repair were taken at the time of surgery. Expression of proinflammatory cytokines, tissue remodeling genes, and angiogenesis factors was evaluated by quantitative real-time polymerase chain reaction. Histological characteristics of the affected tissue were also assessed. Postoperative (>6 months) ultrasound was used to evaluate the healing of the rotator cuff. General linear modeling with selected mRNA biomarkers was used to predict rotator cuff healing.

Results.—Thirty patients completed all analyses, of which 7 patients (23%) had failed healing of the rotator cuff. No differences in demographic data were found between the defect and healed groups. American Shoulder and Elbow Surgeons shoulder scores collected at baseline and follow-up showed improvement in both groups, but there was no significant difference between groups. Increased expression of matrix metalloproteinase 1 (MMP-1) and MMP-9 was found in the supraspinatus tendon in the defect group versus the healed group ($P = .006$ and .02, respectively). Similar upregulation of MMP-9 was also found in the subscapularis tendon of the defect group ($P = .001$), which was consistent with the loss of collagen organization as determined by histological examination. From a general linear model, the upregulation of MMP-1 and MMP-9 was highly correlated with failed healing of the rotator cuff ($R^2 = .656$).

Conclusion.—The upregulation of tissue remodeling genes in the torn rotator cuff at the time of surgery provides a snapshot of the biological environment surrounding the torn rotator cuff that is closely related to the healing of repaired rotator cuffs (Table 2).

▶ I think this is an important study for the orthopedic community, and for the Year Book. The authors introduce us to the future of investigating the genetic expression of cuff tissue and its propensity to heal based on the genetic expression of the pathologic tissue. One of my sons is involved in similar cutting edge research under the direction of Professor Carr at Oxford. The concept is intriguing and the implications expansive. We have long been perplexed as to why some patients do so well after cuff repair and others do not heal. In general, we therefore recognize the concepts of host variation (Table 2). This study shows the complexity and the ability to identify those up- and down-regulated genes that are associated with, if not responsible for, the variation we witness clinically.

B. F. Morrey, MD

Concomitant Evolution of Wear and Squeaking in Dual-Severity, Lubricated Wear Testing of Ceramic-on-Ceramic Hip Prostheses
Sanders A, Tibbitts I, Brannon R (Univ of Utah; Salt Lake City)
J Orthop Res 30:1377-1383, 2012

Ceramic-on-ceramic (CoC) hip bearings were tested in short-term wear tests with a systematically varied contact force. Continuous vibration and intermittent surface roughness measurements were obtained to elucidate potential causes of in vivo hip joint squeaking. The three-phase test comprised alternating cycles of edge loading (EL) and concentric articulation (CA), always using ample serum lubricant. A 50,000-cycle wear trial in which the contact force during CA was distant from the head's wear patch yielded no squeaking and practically no liner roughening. In 10-cycle trials

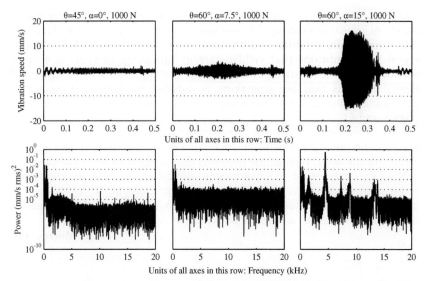

FIGURE 5.—Vibrations during three VQ trials. Top row: Vibration signals; Bottom row: Respective power spectra. Left: Minimal vibration; Middle: Increased vibration without squeak; Right: Audible squeak. (Reprinted from Sanders A, Tibbitts I, Brannon R. Concomitant evolution of wear and squeaking in dual-severity, lubricated wear testing of ceramic-on-ceramic hip prostheses. *J Orthop Res.* 2012;30:1377-1383, with permission from Journal of Orthopaedic Research and John Wiley and Sons, www.interscience.wiley.com.)

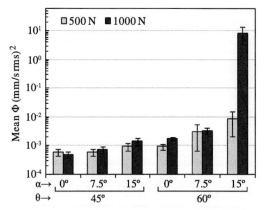

FIGURE 6.—Mean squeaking power (Φ) from 10-cycle trials in VQ phase. Error bars are ± 1 std. dev., except 60°/15° where they are ± ½ std. dev. (Reprinted from Sanders A, Tibbitts I, Brannon R. Concomitant evolution of wear and squeaking in dual-severity, lubricated wear testing of ceramic-on-ceramic hip prostheses. *J Orthop Res.* 2012;30:1377-1383, with permission from Journal of Orthopaedic Research and John Wiley and Sons, www.interscience.wiley.com.)

of an edge-worn head coupled with a pristine liner, the contact force was varied in magnitude and point of application; immediate, recurrent squeaking occurred only when the contact force exceeded a critical threshold value and was centered upon the head's wear patch. In a 27,000-cycle wear trial with the contact force applied near the margin of the head's wear patch, recurrent squeaking emerged progressively as the liner's inner surface was roughened via its articulation with the worn portion of the head. The results reveal key conditions that yield recurrent squeaking in vitro in various scenarios without resorting to implausible dry conditions. A fundamental theory explains that hip squeaking is induced by myriad stress waves emanating from asperity collisions; yet, the root cause is edge loading (Figs 5 and 6).

▶ This is a nicely done experiment addressing the central issue of joint replacement: articular wear. With all the problems emanating from the metal-on-metal bearing, the ceramic bearing is being reconsidered by some. This study addresses and answers a major concern with ceramic bearings: squeaking. This elegant study confirms the source of squeaking is edge loading that comes about from increasing loads being imparted to a poorly oriented acetabular socket (Fig 6). QED.

B. F. Morrey, MD

2 General Orthopedics

Introduction

In some way, general orthopedics might be considered a more difficult area since virtually all of orthopedics seems to be subdivided into anatomic parts or surgical procedures. However, as is evidenced by this section, there are quite a number of topics that relate to the orthopedic practice in general and not a specific pathologic condition or type of intervention. These have been included in this section and have been selected based on their broad-based relevance to the practice, both surgical and nonsurgical. As in the past, I have found the section on general orthopedics to be one of the most interesting, and I'm confident it will also be of interest and value to the reader.

Bernard F. Morrey, MD

Availability of Consumer Prices From US Hospitals for a Common Surgical Procedure
Rosenthal JA, Lu X, Cram P (Univ of Iowa Carver College of Medicine, Iowa City)
JAMA Intern Med 173:427-432, 2013

Importance.—Many proposals for health care reform incentivize patients to play a more active role in selecting health care providers on the basis of quality and price. While data on quality are increasingly available, availability of pricing data is uncertain.

Objective.—To examine whether we could obtain pricing data for a common elective surgical procedure, total hip arthroplasty (THA).

Design.—We randomly selected 2 hospitals from each state (plus Washington, DC) that perform THA, as well as the 20 top-ranked orthopedic hospitals according to *US News and World Report* rankings. We contacted each hospital by telephone between May 2011 and July 2012. Using a standardized script, we requested from each hospital the lowest complete "bundled price" (hospital plus physician fees) for an elective THA that was required by one of the author's 62-year-old grandmother. In our scenario, the grandmother did not have insurance but had the means to pay out of pocket. We explained that we were seeking the lowest complete price for the procedure. When we encountered hospitals that could provide the hospital fee only, we contacted a random hospital affiliated orthopedic surgery practice to obtain the physician fee. Each hospital was contacted up to 5 times in efforts to obtain pricing information.

Setting/Participants.—All top-ranked and a sample of non–top-ranked US hospitals performing THA.

Main Outcome Measures.—Percentage of hospitals able to provide a complete price estimate for THA (physician and hospital fee) for top-ranked and non–top-ranked hospitals and range of prices quoted by each group.

Results.—Nine top-ranked hospitals (45%) and 10 non–top-ranked hospitals (10%) were able to provide a complete bundled price ($P < .001$). We were able to obtain a complete price estimate from an additional 3 top-ranked hospitals (15%) and 54 non–top-ranked hospitals (53%) ($P = .002$) by contacting the hospital and physician separately. The range of complete prices was wide for both top-ranked ($12 500-$105 000) and non–top-ranked hospitals ($11 100-$125 798).

Conclusions and Relevance.—We found it difficult to obtain price information for THA and observed wide variation in the prices that were quoted. Many health care providers cannot provide reasonable price estimates. Patients seeking elective THA may find considerable price savings through comparison shopping.

▶ This topic is a little unusual. But this article is reviewed here because it is clearly a signal of things to come. Who would have even thought of this question several years ago? But it is a relevant issue, if for no other reason than to recognize that total hip arthroplasty is one of the most commonly performed procedures, and it accounts for a considerable amount of the total health dollars spent annually in the United States. What is most striking is the dramatic difference in total costs—a factor of times 10!

Note that this is true for both top-tier and lower-tier hospitals. This cannot and will not continue. I hope that, as a profession, we have not lost the right to participate in the ongoing discussion.

B. F. Morrey, MD

American Academy of Orthopaedic Surgeons Clinical Practice Guideline on: Preventing Venous Thromboembolic Disease in Patients Undergoing Elective Hip and Knee Arthroplasty
Jacobs JJ, Mont MA, Bozic KJ, et al
J Bone Joint Surg Am 94:746-747, 2012

Background.—The American Academy of Orthopaedic Surgeons has published a clinical practice guideline concerning prevention of venous thromboembolic disease in patients who are having elective hip and knee arthroplasty. The recommendations are not intended to stand alone but should be used as guidelines and combined with an understanding of all the circumstances peculiar to the specific patient. Mutual communication between patient, physician, and other healthcare providers is essential in determining the optimal course of action.

Recommendations.—Routine postoperative duplex ultrasonographic screening of patients who have elective hip or knee arthroplasty is not recommended. Because these patients are already at high risk for venous thromboembolism, physicians may choose to assess the individual's specific risk by determining whether he or she has had a venous thromboembolism previously. Evidence does not clearly indicate which other factors might increase the patient's risk level. However, bleeding and other bleeding-associated complications are more likely in patients having elective hip or knee arthroplasty, so patients should be assessed for known bleeding disorders such as hemophilia and for active liver disease, which can increase bleeding and bleeding complication risk. Antiplatelet agents should be discontinued before surgery. However, pharmacologic agents and/or mechanical compressive devices to prevent venous thromboembolism for these patients are advised. The specific strategy or strategies that are optimal remain to be identified. The duration of this prophylactic approach should be determined by the patient and physician. For patients who have had a previous venous thromboembolism and are now undergoing elective hip or knee arthroplasty, pharmacologic prophylaxis and mechanical compressive devices are advised. For patients who have a known bleeding disorder and/or active liver disease, mechanical compressive devices are also advised to prevent venous thromboembolism. Neuraxial anesthesia is advised for patients having elective hip or knee arthroplasty to limit blood loss. Evidence does not link this anesthetic approach to venous thromboembolic disease. Current evidence does not indicate whether inferior vena cava filters prevent pulmonary embolism in patients who undergo arthroplasty and have a contraindication to chemoprophylaxis and/or known residual venous thromboembolic disease. After surgery, patients should be mobilized early. This low-cost intervention is consistent with current practice and offers minimal risk of complications to the patient.

Conclusions.—The quality of evidence currently available to support these recommendations varies. In many cases the recommendations are based on consensus of the work group. Physicians are advised to read the full guidelines and evidence report to evaluate these recommendations.

▶ This report is included in the YEAR BOOK to encourage the reader to read the entire 10-point summary. It is comprehensive and very clear regarding the strength of the evidence that supports a recommendation. Most of what is included is known. Two points to emphasize: In spite of literally hundreds of articles on various prophylactic pharmacologic agents, there is no strong evidence to make a specific recommendation of one over the other. Use of anticoagulants is known to cause serious, sometimes life-threatening, complications. They should never be administered "just in case."

B. F. Morrey, MD

Do Workers With Chronic Nonspecific Musculoskeletal Pain, With and Without Sick Leave, Have Lower Functional Capacity Compared With Healthy Workers?

Soer R, de Vries HJ, Brouwer S, et al (Univ of Groningen, The Netherlands)
Arch Phys Med Rehabil 93:2216-2222, 2012

Objectives.—(1) To analyze whether functional capacity (FC) of sick listed workers with chronic nonspecific musculoskeletal pain (CMP) referred for rehabilitation (SL-Rehab group) and workers with CMP who stay at work (SAW group) differ from the FC of healthy workers (HW group). (2) To analyze if FC of workers with CMP is insufficient to meet work demands, and to assess factors associated with insufficient FC.

Design.—A 3-group cross-sectional comparison.

Setting.—Rehabilitation center.

Participants.—Workers (N = 942) were included (SL-Rehab group: n = 122, SAW group: n = 119, and HW group: n = 701).

Interventions.—All subjects performed a short Functional Capacity Evaluation (FCE) and completed questionnaires assessing demographics, personal, and work characteristics.

Main Outcome Measure.—FCE performances. Participants' FC was insufficient to meet their work demands when their FC was lower than the 5th percentile of the HW group's FC.

Results.—Both the SL-Rehab and SAW groups had significantly lower FC compared with the HW group; 15% to 71% demonstrated insufficient FC. Insufficient FC was associated with group status (SL Rehab group: odds ratio [OR] = 6.5; SAW group: OR = 7.2), having physically high demanding work (OR = 35.1), being a woman (OR = 35.7), higher age (OR = 1.2), and lower effort level during FCE (OR = 1.9). Among subjects with CMP, kinesiophobia, physical health, and perceived disability were associated with having an insufficient FC for work.

Conclusions.—Workers in the SL-Rehab group have lower FC than their working counterparts. Many workers in both groups with CMP demonstrated insufficient FC. Not the pain itself, but personal and work-related factors are related to insufficient FC.

▶ This sophisticated analysis provides objective evidence of what we have observed in our clinical practice. Specifically, the impact of being off work, for whatever reason, is complex and extends well beyond the objective functional parameters. The very act of being out of work influences functional capacity, regardless of other factors. For me the most interesting finding was the documentation that the functional deficiency of those with nonspecific pain was related to factors other than the pain itself. Conclusion: The societal problem of worker's compensation goes beyond the treating orthopedic surgeon.

B. F. Morrey, MD

Associations between serum levels of inflammatory markers and change in knee pain over 5 years in older adults: a prospective cohort study

Stannus OP, Jones G, Blizzard L, et al (Univ of Tasmania, Hobart, Australia; et al)

Ann Rheum Dis 72:535-540, 2013

Objective.—To determine the association between inflammatory markers and change in knee pain over 5 years.

Methods.—A total of 149 randomly selected subjects (mean 63 years, range 52—78; 46% female) was studied. Serum levels of high sensitivity C-reactive protein (hs-CRP), tumour necrosis factor alpha (TNF—α) and interleukin (IL)-6 were measured at baseline and 2.7 years later. Knee pain was recorded using the Western Ontario and McMasters osteoarthritis index questionnaire at baseline and 5 years later. Knee radiographic osteoarthritis of both knees was assessed at baseline, and knee bone marrow lesions, joint effusion and cartilage defects were determined using T1 or T2-weighted fat saturated MRI.

Results.—After adjustment for confounding variables, baseline hs-CRP was positively associated with change in total knee pain ($\beta = 0.33$ per mg/l, $p = 0.032$), as well as change in the pain at night in bed ($\beta = 0.12$ per ml/pg, $p = 0.010$) and while sitting/lying ($\beta = 0.12$ per ml/pg, $p = 0.002$). Change in hs-CRP was also associated with change in knee pain at night and when sitting/lying (both $p < 0.05$). Baseline TNFα and IL-6 were associated with change in pain while standing ($\beta = 0.06$ per ml/pg,

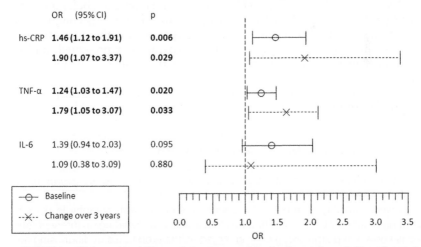

FIGURE 2.—OR for multivariable associations between either baseline or change in biomarkers and increase (change ≥3) in Western Ontario and McMasters osteoarthritis index total knee pain. Adjusted for age, sex, body mass index, baseline pain, current smoking, asthma, bronchitis, diabetes, heart disease and steps per day. Bars denote CI. Bold denotes significant association. hs-CRP, high-sensitivity C-reactive protein; IL-6, interleukin 6; TNFα, tumour necrosis factor alpha. (Reprinted from Stannus OP, Jones G, Blizzard L, et al. Associations between serum levels of inflammatory markers and change in knee pain over 5 years in older adults: a prospective cohort study. *Ann Rheum Dis*. 2013;72:535-540, with permission from the BMJ Publishing Group Ltd.)

$p = 0.033$; $\beta = 0.16$ per ml/pg, $p = 0.035$, respectively), and change in TNFα was positively associated with change in total knee pain ($\beta = 0.66$ ml/pg, $p = 0.020$) and change in pain while standing ($\beta = 0.26$ ml/pg, $p = 0.002$). Adjustment for radiographic osteoarthritis or MRI-detected structural abnormalities led to no or minor attenuation of these associations.

Conclusion.—Systemic inflammation is an independent predictor of worsening knee pain over 5 years (Fig 2).

▶ This is a really interesting study. The authors demonstrate a statistically significant association between the inflammatory markers of high sensitivity C-reactive protein and tissue necrosis factor-α and the progression of knee pain over time (Fig 2). This would suggest the process of degenerative arthritis, as a cause of knee pain alters the serum inflammatory indicators and has an inflammatory etiology. One might speculate whether this information might not be useful in detecting the cause of unexplained pain after joint arthroplasty.

B. F. Morrey, MD

Conventional 3-T MRI and 1.5-T MR Arthrography of Femoroacetabular Impingement
Robinson P (Chapel Allerton Hosp, Leeds, UK)
AJR Am J Roentgenol 199:509-515, 2012

Objective.—This article provides a review of femoroacetabular impingement (FAI) and the role MRI is attempting to fulfill in this complex and sometimes controversial condition. A perspective on the current status and on the advantages of 1.5-T MR arthrography is presented, and its usefulness in this setting is compared with the potential of nonarthrographic 3-T MRI.

Conclusion.—With its increasing availability, 3-T MRI has the potential to provide routine, less invasive assessment of the hip for FAI.

▶ This is a very comprehensive and detailed article from the radiology discipline. We have included it here because it does underscore an important point regarding femoral-acetabular impingement. Just as the orthopedic community is not completely clear on the significance and indications for intervention, the value of imaging is also in flux. This paper makes this point and documents the improved reliability of the 1.5 T magnetic resonance arthrography in demonstrating what may be relevant findings that assist us in deciding on interventions. As is known, hip arthroscopy has emerged as the workhorse in diagnosing and now in treating this condition. However, as is pointed out by the authors, there is a high percent of the normal population with evidence of "impingement" with no symptoms. So, we will continue to monitor this issue as it evolves, awaiting better outcome data correlated with the indications for the intervention.

B. F. Morrey, MD

Femoroacetabular Impingement: Current Clinical Evidence

Sink EL, Kim Y-J (Hosp for Special Surgery, NY; Children's Hosp Boston, MA)

J Pediatr Orthop 32:S166-S171, 2012

Femoroacetabular impingement (FAI) is a recognized cause of hip pain in adolescents and is an etiologic factor in progressive hip osteoarthritis (OA). Optimum care includes early and accurate diagnosis to impede cartilage delamination and progression to OA. Here, we present the current perspectives and spectrum of data pertaining to the association of hip deformity and OA. Management of FAI is reviewed, and the need for efficacy studies is underscored. Further, this paper considers existing (short-term to mid-term) study results and highlights the importance of strengthening data quality and developing a standardized method of reporting outcomes data in surgical treatment for FAI. For the purposes of illustration, outcomes of surgical dislocation of the hip and arthroscopic technique are taken into account; results of surgical management of FAI in athletes are also explored. Through numerous examples from the literature, we demonstrate that current outcome studies of surgical correction for FAI are variable in their

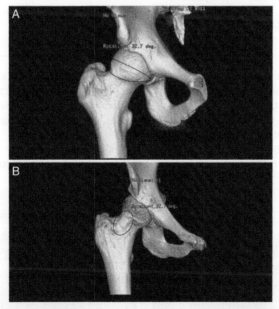

FIGURE 1.—Three-dimensional computed tomography of male and female hips showing different morphologic abnormalities of the proximal femur at the head and neck junctions that result in impingement. A, A Cam lesion in a 16-year-old male. The region of the prominent head and neck offset bony morphology is circled. B, A more subtle impingement with the deficient offset at the head/neck junction circled in a 28-yearold female. The femoral neck is slightly longer and narrower than the male hip and the anterior/lateral aspect of the acetabulum covers less of the femoral head. The outlined region on the images has abnormal contact with the acetabular rim in positions of hip flexion. (Reprinted from Sink EL, Kim Y-J. Femoroacetabular impingement: current clinical evidence. *J Pediatr Orthop.* 2012;32:S166-S171, with permission from Lippincott Williams & Wilkins.)

description and measurement of disease characteristics, type of surgical procedure, and documentation of complications. A standardized method of data collection and reporting is a fundamental step toward understanding the effects of surgical intervention on the natural history of FAI. Together with a future diagnostic standard and long-term study data, we will be better equipped to provide first-rate operative care for this population of patients (Fig 1).

▶ I am aware of my predilection for articles relating to femoroacetabular impingement. The reason is it is a relatively new insight, and is so important to ultimately be able to avoid hip replacement if properly managed. Although the clinical characteristics of the 2 varieties—cam (Fig 1) and pincer—are well known, this nice review highlights a real deficiency. Specifically, the current orthopedic literature is not adequate to truly understand the best type or timing of intervention to alter the natural history of the disease. If we ever needed a good, legitimate, prospective, randomized study of a topic, this is it!

B. F. Morrey, MD

Femoroacetabular impingement
Anderson SE, Siebenrock KA, Tannast M (The Univ of Notre Dame Australia, New South Wales, Sydney; Univ of Bern, Switzerland)
Eur J Radiol 81:3740-3744, 2012

Femoroacetabular impingement (FAI) is a pathomechanical concept describing the early and painful contact of morphological changes of the hip joint, both on the acetabular, and femoral head sides. These can lead clinically to symptoms of hip and groin pain, and a limited range of motion with labral, chondral and bony lesions.

Pincer impingement generally involves the acetabular side of the joint where there is excessive coverage of the acetabulum, which may be focal

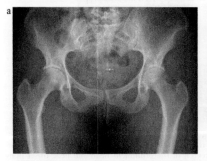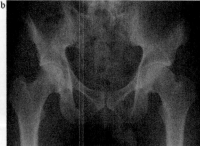

FIGURE 1.—(a) Radiographic examples of a *Pincer form* of FAI, with bilateral acetabular overcoverage in a female patient, 4th decade. (b) *Cam form* of FAI with left sided pistol grip deformity of the femoral head, aspheric left femoral head, in a male patient, 3rd decade. Note is made of circumferential femoral head osteophytes. (Reprinted from the European Journal of Radiology. Anderson SE, Siebenrock KA, Tannast M. Femoroacetabular impingement. *Eur J Radiol.* 2012;81:3740-3744, Copyright 2012, with permission from Elsevier.)

or more diffuse. There is linear contact of the acetabulum with the head/ neck junction. *Cam impingement* involves the femoral head side of the joint where the head is associated with bony excrescences and is aspheric. The aspheric femoral head jams into the acetabulum. Imaging appearances are reviewed below. This type is evident in young males in the second and third decades. The main features of FAI are described (Fig 1).

▶ I have had a tendency to select topics that relate to femoral acetabular impingement (FAI) since it was introduced by Ganz more than a decade ago. This article's main goal is to describe the features of the process as confirmed by magnetic resonance imaging. However, the main goal for selecting this is to reaffirm the 2 types: pincer, mainly an acetabular coverage issue, and cam, primarily a femoral head/neck pathology (Fig 1). In both instances, the essential pathology is a variable, but often mild dysplasia. Also, of importance, the diagnosis is suspected by history, reinforced by examination, and confirmed by imaging—usually plain films suffice.

B. F. Morrey, MD

Arthroscopic Labral Repair Versus Selective Labral Debridement in Female Patients With Femoroacetabular Impingement: A Prospective Randomized Study
Krych AJ, Thompson M, Knutson Z, et al (Mayo Clinic, Rochester, MN; Drisko, Fee & Parkins Orthopedics, Independence, MO; Oklahoma Sports and Orthopedics Inst, Norman; et al)
Arthroscopy 29:46-53, 2013

Purpose.—The purpose of this prospective randomized study was to compare the outcomes of arthroscopic labral repair and selective labral debridement in female patients undergoing arthroscopy for the treatment of pincer-type or combined pincer- and cam-type femoroacetabular impingement.

Methods.—Between June 2007 and June 2009, 36 female patients undergoing arthroscopic hip treatment for pincer- or combined-type femoroacetabular impingement were randomized to 2 treatment groups at the time of surgery: labral repair or labral debridement. The repair group comprised 18 patients with a mean age of 38; the debridement group comprised 18 patients with a mean age of 39. All patients underwent the same rehabilitation protocol postoperatively. At a minimum of 1 year, all patients were assessed using a validated Hip Outcome Score (HOS) to determine hip function, and also completed a simple subjective outcome measure.

Results.—All 36 patients were available for follow-up at an average time of 32 months (range, 12 to 48). In both groups, HOSs for activities of daily living (ADL) and sports improved significantly from before surgery to the final follow-up (P < .05). The postoperative ADL HOS was significantly better in the repair group (91.2; range, 73 to 100) compared with the debridement group (80.9; range, 42.6 to 100; P < .05). Similarly, the

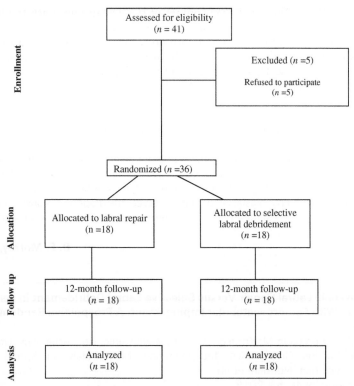

Enrollment

Allocation

Follow up

Analysis

FIGURE 1.—CONSORT diagram showing the flow of participants through each stage of this randomized trial. (Reprinted from Arthroscopy: The Journal of Arthroscopic and Related Surgery. Krych AJ, Thompson M, Knutson Z, et al. Arthroscopic labral repair versus selective labral debridement in female patients with femoroacetabular impingement: a prospective randomized study. *Arthroscopy*. 2013;29:46-53, Copyright 2013, with permission from the Arthroscopy Association of North America.)

postoperative sports HOS was significantly greater in the repair group (88.7; range, 28.6 to 100) than in the debridement group (76.3; range, 28.6 to 100; $P < .05$). Additionally, patient subjective outcome was significantly better in the labral repair group ($P = .046$).

Conclusions.—Arthroscopic treatment of femoroacetabular impingement with labral repair in female patients resulted in superior improvement in hip functional outcomes compared with labral debridement. In addition, a greater number of patients in the repair group subjectively rated their hip function as normal or nearly normal after surgery compared with the labral debridement group.

Level of Evidence.—Level I, prospective randomized study (Fig 1).

▶ The topic of femoroacetabular impingement is so important as a means of understanding coxarthrosis in the young patient. Hence, I find myself drawn to those studies that clarify the management of this condition. This study has several merits, in addition to the clear conclusion: It is prospective and randomized

(Fig 1), it is focused on the female population, and it compares 2 accepted treatment options. I am surprised that the repair group did better and am impressed that our colleagues have developed the expertise to become so good in performing a difficult procedure. The key now is to see what happens long term. Does it really matter?

B. F. Morrey, MD

A Biomechanical Comparison of Repair Techniques for Complete Gluteus Medius Tears

Dishkin-Paset JG, Salata MJ, Gross CE, et al (Rush Univ Med Ctr, Chicago, IL)
Arthroscopy 28:1410-1416, 2012

Purpose.—The purpose of this study was to compare the biomechanical fixation stability conferred by 2 specific arthroscopic repair techniques for complete gluteus medius tendon tears.

Methods.—Twelve fresh-frozen human cadaveric hemi-pelves were tested. Six received double-row repair with massive cuff stitches (DR-MCS), whereas the remaining 6 underwent double-row repair with knotless lateral anchors (DR-KLA). Constructs were preloaded to 10 N, tested from 10 N to 125 N at 90 N/s for 150 cycles, and then loaded to failure at 1 mm/s. Markers were placed on the tissue for video tracking.

Results.—No significant differences in cyclic outcomes were observed. The DR-KLA construct showed a significantly higher normalized yield load than the DR-MCS construct. Post-yield extension for the DR-MCS construct was significantly higher than that for the DR-KLA construct. At yield load, the optically measured soft-tissue elongation of the DR-KLA construct was significantly higher than that of the DR-MCS construct.

Conclusions.—This study strongly suggests that the biomechanical stability conferred by DR-MCS and DR-KLA constructs for gluteus medius tendon repair is similar. Because the failure load of the DR-KLA construct is strongly correlated to bone mineral density (BMD), clinical considerations of bone quality may be particularly important for gluteus medius repairs.

Clinical Relevance.—Maximum load was strongly correlated to BMD in the DR-KLA group. On the basis of this analysis, BMD should be considered during surgical planning.

▶ This study was reviewed primarily to highlight the existence of the gluteal medius muscle tear and to present some of the effort being taken to study the optimum treatment. I have some issues with this study as not being very realistic. The pathology involves degenerated tissue that is retracted, like a rotator cuff. This or any cadaver study cannot truly replicate the pathology, hence the conclusions are in my opinion of limited value. A conclusion that documents that the effectiveness of suture anchors is a function of the quality of bone is not surprising and has been shown many times before. My major concern is that I have had to revise arthroscopic "medius repair" that revealed some random sutures and no repair of the pathologic process whatsoever. Hence, I applaud those performing such investigations and pushing the envelope. But for me, at this time, the appropriate repair of this lesion is with an open procedure.

B. F. Morrey, MD

Do Patients Lose Weight After Joint Arthroplasty Surgery? A Systematic Review

Inacio MCS, Kritz-Silverstein D, Paxton EW, et al (San Diego State Univ/Univ of California; Univ of California San Diego School of Medicine; Kaiser Permanente, San Diego, CA; et al)
Clin Orthop Relat Res 471:291-298, 2013

Background.—The ability of patients with a total joint arthroplasty (TJA) to lose weight after surgery has been investigated in a few studies with inconsistent results.

Questions/Purposes.—We asked: (1) What is the quality of evidence of current published literature on postoperative weight trends for patients who have had a TJA? (2) Do patients lose any weight after TJA? (3) Do patients lose a clinically meaningful amount of weight after TJA?

Methods.—We conducted a systematic review of PubMed and the Cochrane Library. Studies were summarized according to the Preferred Reporting Items for Systematic Reviews and Meta-analyses Statement. Studies were reviewed for quality of evidence and limitations according to the Grading of Recommendations Assessment, Development, and Evaluation (GRADE) criteria. Twelve studies were identified, one case-cohort study and 11 case series. Most studies were from single-surgeon or single-hospital series. Five studies included THAs and TKAs, four only THAs, and three only TKAs. We determined study type, level of evidence, inclusion criteria, procedures, proportion of patients who changed weight, body composition assessment, time of composition assessment, statistical analysis performed, and subgroup analysis conducted.

Results.—Owing to the observational nature of the studies and the serious limitations identified, all were considered very low quality according to GRADE criteria. Studies reported 14% to 49% of patients had some weight loss at least 1 year postoperatively.

Conclusions.—We found no conclusive evidence that weight or body composition increases, decreases, or remains the same after TJA (Table 2).

▶ I read this article with a bias to accept because I am interested in the topic and methodology. When I read the conclusions, I didn't know whether to laugh or cry. As a surgeon, a conclusion such as offered here just isn't acceptable. After a careful review of the extensive data on this subject, the conclusion is: We know nothing (Table 2).

I really don't think this is good enough. I take several insights from this article. The orthopedic literature is woefully inadequate by the standards applied here. Unless the formal standards of appropriate research are met, any conclusions are discounted. The reality expressed here is typical of virtually every orthopedic

TABLE 2.—Summary of Study Limitations Using the GRADE Criteria

Study	Failure to Develop and Apply Appropriate Eligibility Criteria (Selection Bias)	Flawed Measurement of Exposure and Outcome (Detection Bias) Exposure (Joint Arthroplasty)	Risk of Bias Outcome (Weight Assessment)	Failure to Adequately Control Confounding	Incomplete Followup (Attrition Bias) (Loss to Followup)
Stets et al. [34]	High	Low	High	High	Low (0%)
Woodruff and Stone [36]	High	Low	Unclear	High	Low (0%)
Heisel et al. [17]	High	Low	Unclear	High	Low (0%)
Abu-Rajab et al. [1]	High	Low	Low	Low	Low (0%)
Donovan et al. [10]	Unclear	Low	Unclear	High	High (27%)
Aderinto et al. [2]	Unclear	Low	Unclear	High	Low (2.1%)
Middleton and Boardman [26]	Unclear	Low	Unclear	High	Low (0%)
Jain et al. [18]	Low	Low	High	High	High (20%)
Dowsey et al. [11]	Low	Low	Low	High	Low (1.5%)
Dowsey et al. [12]	Low	Low	Low	High	Low (1.5%)
Lachiewicz and Lachiewicz [22]	Moderate	Low	Low	Moderate	High (19%)
Zeni and Snyder-Mackler [37]	High	Low	Low	High	Low (0%)

Editor's Note: Please refer to original journal article for full references.
GRADE = Grading of Recommendations Assessment, Development, and Evaluation.

question subjected to this methodology: We know nothing! Solution? Two things: We must develop better orthopedic research studies, and we must as a speciality define what is legitimate research for our speciality.

B. F. Morrey, MD

A Systematic Review and Meta-Analysis Comparing Complications Following Total Joint Arthroplasty for Rheumatoid Arthritis Versus for Osteoarthritis

Ravi B, Escott B, Shah PS, et al (Univ of Toronto, Ontario, Canada; et al)
Arthritis Rheum 64:3839-3849, 2012

Objective.—Most of the evidence regarding complications following total hip arthroplasty (THA) and total knee arthroplasty (TKA) is based on studies of patients with osteoarthritis (OA), with little being known about outcomes in patients with rheumatoid arthritis (RA). The objective of the present study was to review the current evidence regarding rates of THA/TKA complications in RA versus OA.

Methods.—Data sources used were Medline, EMBase, Cinahl, Web of Science, and reference lists of articles. We included reports published between 1990 and 2011 that described studies of primary total joint arthroplasty of the hip or knee and contained information on outcomes in ≥200 RA and OA joints. Outcomes of interest included revision, hip dislocation, infection, 90-day mortality, and venous thromboembolic events. Two reviewers independently assessed each study for quality and extracted data. Where appropriate, meta-analysis was performed; if this was not possible, the level of evidence was assessed qualitatively.

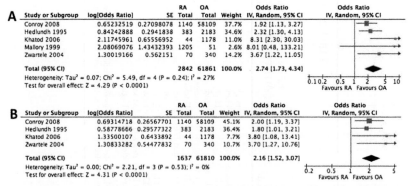

FIGURE 2.—Analysis of the likelihood of dislocation of the index hip within 5 years of hip arthroplasty in patients with rheumatoid arthritis (RA) versus patients with osteoarthritis (OA), without (A) and with (B) adjustment for confounders. 95% CI = 95% confidence interval. (Reprinted from Ravi B, Escott B, Shah PS, et al. A systematic review and meta-analysis comparing complications following total joint arthroplasty for rheumatoid arthritis versus for osteoarthritis. *Arthritis Rheum.* 2012;64:3839-3849, with permission from American College of Rheumatology.)

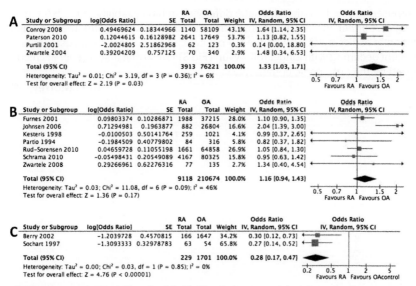

FIGURE 3.—Analysis (unadjusted) of the likelihood of revision of the index arthroplasty in patients with RA versus patients with OA, within 5 years of total hip arthroplasty (A), 6—10 years after total hip arthroplasty (B), and >10 years after total hip arthroplasty (C). See Figure 2 for definitions. (Reprinted from Ravi B, Escott B, Shah PS, et al. A systematic review and meta-analysis comparing complications following total joint arthroplasty for rheumatoid arthritis versus for osteoarthritis. *Arthritis Rheum.* 2012;64:3839-3849, with permission from American College of Rheumatology.)

Results.—Forty studies were included in this review. The results indicated that patients with RA are at increased risk of dislocation following THA (adjusted odds ratio 2.16 [95% confidence interval 1.52–3.07]). There was fair evidence to support the notion that risk of infection and risk of early revision following TKA are increased in RA versus OA. There was no evidence of any differences in rates of revision at later time points, 90-day mortality, or rates of venous thromboembolic events following THA or TKA in patients with RA versus OA. RA was explicitly defined in only 3 studies (7.5%), and only 11 studies (27.5%) included adjustment for covariates (e.g., age, sex, and comorbidity).

Conclusion.—The findings of this literature review and meta-analysis indicate that, compared to patients with OA, patients with RA are at higher risk of dislocation following THA and higher risk of infection following TKA (Figs 2 and 3).

▶ The simplicity of the title belies the complexity of the analysis. As I reviewed this article I was struck and disappointed, again, by the relative lack of quality in orthopedic literature. Considering the thousands of articles written on these subjects, the conclusions were drawn from a small handful of quality studies. One could possibly, therefore, wonder if the conclusions are valid in spite of the sophisticated methodology. Regardless, the observation of a greater infection rate in the rheumatoid arthritis (RA) patient comes as no surprise. I, however, was surprised to see the rather dramatic difference in hip instability in the RA patient (Fig 2). Further, in spite of the observation of similar revision rates, the documentation of earlier revisions with the RA patient and revisions with the osteoarthritis patient occurring with longer follow-up (Fig 3) is also one that is generally recognized by the orthopedic community.

B. F. Morrey, MD

3 Forearm, Wrist, and Hand

Introduction

As in previous years, the spectrum of contributions in the area of the hand and wrist has been significant. This year I have made special effort to try to comment on the contributions that best reflect this diverse spectrum of pathology from the elbow to the fingers. In this context I have also attempted to blend articles that I found interesting from a diagnostic perspective as well as from a therapeutic standpoint. The selections this year, as in the past, do therefore include a cross section of an upper-extremity practice with a bit more emphasis on proximal pathology, such as medial epicondylitis and forearm osteotomy. Advances in basic and clinical research are also included specifically when it is felt that they have clinical relevance, as in the genetic basis of Dupuytren's contracture. Just as I have enjoyed reviewing and selecting these articles, I hope this section will be both useful and enjoyable to the reader.

Bernard F. Morrey, MD

Evaluation and Diagnosis

Pulse Oximetry Measurements in the Evaluation of Patients With Possible Thoracic Outlet Syndrome
Braun RM, Rechnic M, Shah KN (Univ of California, San Diego; Univ of California, Irvine)
J Hand Surg 37A:2564-2569, 2012

Purpose.—We present our experience in using pulse oximetry as an aid in the diagnosis of thoracic outlet syndrome (TOS). Our attention was given to those symptomatic patients without objective confirmatory data on imaging or electrodiagnostic evaluation.

Methods.—Using a pulse oximeter, we measured the oxygen saturation and the pulse rate during a provocative extremity abduction stress test exercise maneuver in 18 patients with symptoms and signs consistent with a diagnosis of nonspecific neurogenic TOS. The oxygen saturation and pulse rates in 18 asymptomatic subjects were used as a control.

Results.—Resting oxygen saturation above 97% was present in both groups initially. After the provocative exercise maneuver, there was a significant reduction in the oxygen saturation levels, which dropped to 86% in the symptomatic TOS group compared with 94% in the control group. There was a significant increase in pulse rate in those subjects suspected of having TOS compared with a minimal increase in pulse rate in control subjects.

Conclusions.—Pulse oximetry produced objective confirmatory measurements, which support a hypothesis that hypoperfusion in the upper limb during provocative activities or exercise may cause disabling symptoms associated with nonspecific neurogenic TOS. This method may be a useful, noninvasive, rapid, and inexpensive clinical tool in the diagnosis of TOS, a condition frequently lacking in objective, confirmatory diagnostic data.

▶ The diagnosis of thoracic outlet syndrome is largely made from clinical diagnosis and reported symptoms, because no single reference, objective vascular, imaging, or neurophysiological test is considered confirmatory. Likewise, the clinical diagnosis is generally incremental and requires several positive provocative tests, most notably the Adson test—finger pallor of the digits following rapid gripping with the arms elevated, and pulse diminishment with arm abduction. Many patients are misdiagnosed with other disorders, including fibromyalgia, and delays in treatment are all too frequent. Moreover, my experience is that too many first rib resections and scalene releases are performed without objective preoperative evaluation. This study is important on several fronts. It is simple to perform and uses commonly available digit pulse oximetry devices. Their findings of hypoperfusion with drops in oxygen saturation as measured by pulse oximetry, pain, and increases in heart rate provide objective data to help sort out patients suspected of having thoracic outlet syndrome from other patients with complaints of diffuse or nonspecific upper extremity symptoms.

S. D. Trigg, MD

The Effect of Osteoporosis on Outcomes of Operatively Treated Distal Radius Fractures

Fitzpatrick SK, Casemyr NE, Zurakowski D, et al (Harvard Med School, Boston, MA; Boston Children's Hosp, MA)
J Hand Surg 37A:2027-2034, 2012

Purpose.—We hypothesized that postmenopausal osteoporotic women with distal radius fractures treated with open reduction internal fixation had worse functional outcomes than women without osteoporosis sustaining similar injuries.

Methods.—We retrospectively reviewed prospectively collected data for 64 postmenopausal women treated with open reduction internal fixation for distal radius fractures between 2006 and 2010 with known bone mineral density measured by dual-energy x-ray absorptiometry at the time of injury (osteopenia, n = 44; osteoporosis, n = 20). Data collected included age, mechanism of injury, fracture severity, and associated comorbidities. Outcomes included range of motion, Disabilities of the Arm, Shoulder, and Hand (DASH) scores, and radiographic parameters of fracture reduction. We calculated patients' Charlson Comorbidity Index and tabulated complications. The primary outcome was DASH score at 12 months after injury. We applied multiple linear regression to determine whether bone mineral density status was predictive of functional outcomes 12 months after injury. We used logistic regression analysis to identify factors independently associated with poor outcomes and applied likelihood estimation to determine predictors of a high DASH score at 12 months.

Results.—At 1 year postoperatively, women with osteoporosis had average DASH scores 15 points higher than those with osteopenia. Both osteoporosis and the Charlson Comorbidity Index were strong positive independent predictors of higher DASH scores (ie, poorer functional outcomes). There were no significant differences in range of motion or radiographic data between groups. Patients with osteoporosis had a higher rate of major complications.

Conclusions.—Osteoporosis had a negative impact on functional outcomes for women with distal radius fractures treated with open reduction internal fixation. Surgeons should identify high-risk patients, ensure close monitoring, and initiate appropriate preventative measures in this patient population.

Type of Study/Level of Evidence.—Prognostic II.

▶ The recent acceleration of research directed toward women's health in orthopedic surgery, bone physiology, and gender-specific implant design is long overdue. Perhaps no other topic in this area of research is more important than the negative effects of osteoporosis on fracture frequency, complexity, treatment complications, and outcomes. It is now generally well known that osteoporosis-related fractures of the distal radius are more common in perimenopausal women and occur earlier than osteoporosis-related fractures of the hip and spine. In one sense then, distal radius fractures in women 50 years and older should be clearly recognized as an important bellwether for an increased probability of more debilitating hip and spine fractures for any given individual. The rapid pace of development and use of locking distal radius plates for treatment of distal radius fractures is undoubtedly one of the most important treatment advances in the last quarter century. Despite the explosive growth in the use of volar locking plates for osteoporosis-related fractures, only a few studies have investigated the relationship of degree of osteoporosis with functional and radiographic outcomes. It should come as no surprise that outcome data from this study mirror the negative association for treatment outcomes from open reduction and internal fixation of osteoporosis-related fractures of the spine and intertrochanteric fractures of the hip.

S. D. Trigg, MD

Concordance of qualitative bone scintigraphy results with presence of clinical complex regional pain syndrome 1: Meta-analysis of test accuracy studies

Ringer R, Wertli M, Bachmann LM, et al (Balgrist Univ Hosp, Zurich, Switzerland; Univ of Zurich, Switzerland)
Eur J Pain 16:1347-1356, 2012

Background.—To date, no attempt has been made to investigate the agreement between qualitative bone scintigraphy (BS) and the presence of complex regional pain syndrome 1 (CRPS 1) and the agreement between a negative BS in the absence of CRPS 1.

Aims.—To summarize the existing evidence quantifying the concordance of qualitative BS in the presence or absence of clinical CRPS 1.

Data Sources.—We searched Medline, Embase, Dare and the Cochrane Library and screened bibliographies of all included studies.

Study Eligibility Criteria.—We selected diagnostic studies investigating the association between qualitative BS results and the clinical diagnosis of CRPS 1. The minimum requirement for inclusion was enough information to fill the two-by-two tables.

Results.—Twelve studies met our inclusion criteria and were included in the meta-analysis. The pooled mean sensitivity of 12 two-by-two tables was 0.87 (95% CI, 0.68–0.97) and specificity was 0.69 (95% CI, 0.47–0.85). The pooled mean sensitivity for the subgroup with clearly defined diagnostic criteria (seven two-by-two tables) was 0.80 (95% CI, 0.44–0.95) and specificity was 0.73 (95% CI, 0.40–0.91).

Conclusions.—Based on this study, clinicians must be advised that a positive BS is not necessarily concordant with presence of absence or CRPS 1. Given the moderate level of concordance between a positive BS in the absence of clinical CRPS 1, discordant results potentially impede the diagnosis of CRPS 1.

▶ Complex regional pain syndrome (CRPS), formerly commonly referred to as *reflex sympathetic dystrophy* and *causalgia*, is a neuropathic and systemic process, the etiology of which is likely multifactorial. CRPS frequently affects the upper extremity. The diagnosis of CRPS is by clinical criteria; however, early associated plain x-ray abnormalities (periarticular patchy osteopenia) were recognized and became by default common diagnostic tools. Bone scintigraphy historically has gained popularity as a diagnostic tool, but as the authors of this study have shown, there is little level 1 evidence that proves concordance between bone scintigraphy and the presence or absence of CRPS. This is an important study and has relevant clinical and diagnostic information with obvious economic impact in management of this challenging condition.

S. D. Trigg, MD

Dupuytren Diathesis and Genetic Risk

Dolmans GH, de Bock GH, Werker PM (Univ Med Ctr Groningen and Univ of Groningen, the Netherlands)
J Hand Surg 37A:2106-2111, 2012

Purpose.—Dupuytren disease (DD) is a benign fibrosing disorder of the hand and fingers. Recently, we identified 9 single nucleotide polymorphisms (SNPs) associated with DD in a genome-wide association study. These SNPs can be used to calculate a genetic risk score for DD. The aim of this study was to test whether certain clinical characteristics (including the DD diathesis features) of patients with DD are associated with a high genetic risk score.

Methods.—Between 2007 and 2010, we prospectively invited all DD patients (1,120 in total) to participate. Clinical characteristics were noted using patient- and doctor-completed questionnaires, and blood was obtained for DNA analysis. We analyzed a total of 933 subjects with genetic and clinical data. The 9 previously identified DD SNPs were used to calculate a weighted genetic risk score. Patients were categorized into high and low genetic risk score groups, according to their weighted genetic risk score. Logistic regression was performed to study the association of clinical characteristics with a high genetic risk score.

Results.—In a univariate regression model, patients with an age of onset of DD younger than 50 years, a family history positive for DD, knuckle pads, and Ledderhose disease were statistically significantly associated with a high genetic risk score. In an additional analysis using high and low genetic risk groups that deviate further from the median, Ledderhose disease was no longer significantly associated with DD.

Conclusions.—Patients with DD who present with these diathesis features, and predominantly patients with knuckle pads, are more likely to carry more risk alleles for the discovered DD SNPs than patients without these diathesis features.

Clinical Relevance.—These markers may prove useful in predicting disease progression or recurrence.

▶ Progression of Dupuytren's disease is individually variable and changes over time. The term *Dupuytren's diathesis* has been used to delineate certain clinical findings that are assumed to be associated with a more aggressive course of the disease. Classically, bilateral hand involvement, positive family history, early onset (age younger than 50), knuckle pads, male sex, Peyronie disease, and Ledderhose disease were considered to be evidence of diathesis. The presence of Dupuytren's diathesis has often been used as a basis for clinical decision making without a complete understanding of what attributes of diathesis are more significant. In recent years, genetic testing of Dupuytren's disease has found that it is a complex genetic disorder and can be affected by many environmental and newly identified risk genotyping. This study is important to the clinician on several fronts, as it clarifies what attributes of diathesis are associated with a higher genetic risk score and will no doubt serve as a basis for understanding of future combined genetic and clinical research of Dupuytren's disease.

S. D. Trigg, MD

Incidence of subsequent hip fractures is significantly increased within the first month after distal radius fracture in patients older than 60 years
Chen C-W, Huang T-L, Su L-T, et al (China Med Univ Hosp, Taichung, Taiwan; China Med Univ, Taichung, Taiwan; et al)
J Trauma Acute Care Surg 74:317-321, 2013

Background.—Distal radius fracture is recognized as an osteoporosis-related fracture in aged population. If another osteoporosis-related fracture occurs in a short period, it represents a prolonged hospitalization and a considerable economic burden to the society. We evaluated the relationship between distal radius fracture and subsequent hip fracture within 1 year, especially in the critical time and age.

Methods.—We identified newly diagnosed distal radius fracture patients in 2000 to 2006 as an exposed cohort (N = 9,986). A comparison cohort (N = 81,227) was randomly selected from patients without distal radius fracture in the same year of exposed cohort. The subjects were followed up for 1 year since the recruited date. We compared the sociodemographic factors between two cohorts. Furthermore, the time interval following the previous distal radial fracture and the incidence of subsequent hip fracture was studied in detail.

Results.—The incidence of hip fracture within 1 year increased with age in both cohorts. The risk was 5.67 times (84.6 vs. 14.9 per 10,000 person-years) greater in the distal radial fracture cohort than in the comparison cohort. The multivariate Cox proportional hazard regression analyses showed the hazard ratios of hip fracture in relation to distal radial fracture

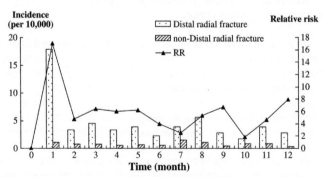

FIGURE 2.—Incidence rates of hip fracture in cohorts with and without distal radius fracture and relative risk by follow-up month. (Reprinted from Chen C-W, Huang T-L, Su L-T, et al. Incidence of subsequent hip fractures is significantly increased within the first month after distal radius fracture in patients older than 60 years. *J Trauma Acute Care Surg.* 2013;74:317-321, with permission from Lippincott Williams & Wilkins.)

was 3.45 (95% confidence interval = 2.59−4.61). The highest incidence was within the first month after distal radial fracture, 17-fold higher than the comparison cohort (17.9 vs. 1.05 per 10,000). Among comorbidities, age > 60 years was also a significant factor associated with hip fracture (hazard ratio = 8.67, 95% confidence interval = 4.51−16.7).

Conclusions.—Patients with distal radius fracture and age > 60 years will significantly increase the incidence of subsequent hip fracture, especially within the first month.

Level of Evidence.—Prognostic/epidemiologic study, level II (Fig 2).

▶ Fractures of the hip and distal radius are among the most common fractures in older patients and are a worldwide health problem. Treatment of these fractures is associated with significant economic expenditures and prolonged morbidity, decreases in quality of life, and, in the case of hip fractures, with increased mortality. Common denominators for the occurrence of these fractures include age older than 50, sex (women greater than men), and osteoporosis. There is emerging evidence that any osteoporotic fracture increases the risk for future fractures. It may seem initially counterintuitive that a distal radius fracture would be an associated risk factor for subsequent hip fracture, but both types of fracture are frequently associated with a trip and fall from a standing height. The information from this study is important and should be shared with the patient, particularly the increased risk of hip fracture in the early treatment period after their distal radius fracture.

S. D. Trigg, MD

Forearm and Wrist

Scapholunate Instability: Current Concepts in Diagnosis and Management
Kitay A, Wolfe SW (Hosp for Special Surgery, NY)
J Hand Surg 37A:2175-2196, 2012

Injuries to the scapholunate joint are the most frequent cause of carpal instability and account for a considerable degree of wrist dysfunction, lost time from work, and interference with activities. Although it is insufficient to cause abnormal carpal posture or collapse on static radiographs, an isolated injury to the scapholunate interosseous ligament may be the harbinger of a relentless progression to abnormal joint mechanics, cartilage wear, and degenerative changes. Intervention for scapholunate instability is aimed at arresting the degenerative process by restoring ligament continuity and normalizing carpal kinematics. In this review, we discuss the anatomy, kinematics, and biomechanical properties of the scapholunate articulation and provide a foundation for understanding the spectrum of scapholunate ligament instability. We propose an algorithm for treatment based on the stage of injury and the degree of secondary ligamentous damage and arthritic change.

▶ I generally do not select current concepts reviews for your consideration, but this article in my view is one of the most succinct and complete discussions yet published on this difficult injury. The authors' proposed treatment algorithm, based on the stage of carpal instability and arthritic sequelae, is novel with respect to its organization and clarification of terms of radiographic and clinical diagnosis. In short, this is a must read for 2013.

S. D. Trigg, MD

Biomechanical Analysis of a Volar Variable-Angle Locking Plate: The Effect of Capturing a Distal Radial Styloid Fragment
Stanbury SJ, Salo A, Elfar JC (Univ of Rochester, NY)
J Hand Surg 37A:2488-2494, 2012

Purpose.—Variable-angle volar locked constructs for distal radius fractures are a recent treatment addition. This study sought to biomechanically evaluate a variable-angle volar locking plate as compared with a fixed-angle construct.

Methods.—We created 2 different AO-C3 osteotomies in fourth-generation synthetic composite distal radiuses and labeled them proximal and distal. The distal osteotomy consisted of a smaller radial styloid fragment. We then fixed both sets of specimens with either a fixed-angle or variable-angle volar locking construct. We tested samples in axial compression with regard to cyclical loading and load to failure. Articular step-off, stiffness, and load to failure data were then analyzed.

Results.—Neither the proximal nor the distal osteotomy groups showed articular failure after cyclic loading, significant loss of stiffness over cycling, or superior stiffness compared with the other. After load to failure in the proximal osteotomy, 1 of 8 fixed-angle and none of 8 variable-angle constructs had articular failure, whereas in the distal osteotomy, all 8 fixed-angle and none of 8 variable-angle constructs had articular failure.

Conclusions.—Variable-angle and fixed-angle volar locked fixation of unstable intra-articular distal radius fractures in fourth-generation composite radii provide mechanically sound constructs with high load to failure values and no loss of stiffness over testing. The variable-angle construct exhibited excellent resistance to articular stepoff at load to failure and no loss of stiffness throughout cyclic loading, and did not exhibit significantly less overall stiffness compared with fixed-angle constructs. The variable-angle fixation exhibited a distinct mechanical advantage over fixed-angle fixation in the setting of a smaller radial styloid fragment.

Clinical Relevance.—Variable-angle constructs could be expected to hold up to standard loads in the postoperative period as well as traditional fixed-angle devices. The additional cost associated with variable-angle constructs may be warranted when treating distal radius fractures with radial styloid fragments, owing to the fragment-specific fixation allowed by customized screw placement.

▶ Lateral epicondylitis is a common yet frustrating problem to treat. The condition most frequently involves patients in their mid-40s to early 60s. Lateral epicondylitis can be significantly disabling both in the workplace and on the playing fields. Several studies have found that most affected patients will improve within one year no matter what nonoperative treatment is administered. There is very little level-1 evidence that any physiotherapeutic modalities or regimens are optimum or speed resolution, and yet, undoubtedly untold millions of dollars are spent annually in physical therapy. The condition is described as an overuse-related injury (although many affected patients have no criteria to establish overuse) with resultant angiofibroblastic degeneration of the common extensor origin most notably the extensor carpi radialis brevis. The Nirschl procedure, resection of the degenerative common extensor origin, is the most frequently performed surgical procedure, but treatment failures are known despite generally favorable results. Several researchers, including the senior author of this article, contend that the pain from lateral epicondylitis is multifactorial and specifically stems from microneuromata (tearing) of the sensory afferent nerve branches, which innervate the lateral epicondyle. This article should be considered preliminary but is certainly ripe for a prospective randomized study. The patient selection, anatomic details, and results are noteworthy, and I think this article warrants your review.

S. D. Trigg, MD

Computer-Assisted Corrective Osteotomy for Malunited Diaphyseal Forearm Fractures
Miyake J, Murase T, Oka K, et al (Osaka Univ Graduate School of Medicine, Japan)
J Bone Joint Surg Am 94:e150.1-e150.11, 2012

Background.—Corrective osteotomy for malunited diaphyseal forearm fractures remains a challenging procedure. We developed a computer-assisted system for corrective surgery, including a three-dimensional simulation program and a custom-made osteotomy template, and investigated the results of corrective surgery for malunited diaphyseal forearm fractures with use of this technology.

Methods.—Twenty patients (fifteen male patients and five female patients) with malunited diaphyseal forearm fractures were managed with three-dimensional corrective osteotomy with a custom-made osteotomy template based on computer simulation. We performed osteotomy of both radius and ulna in fourteen patients and osteotomy of the radius alone in six patients. The median age at the time of surgery was eighteen years (range, eleven to forty-three years). The median duration between the time of injury and the time of surgery was thirty-three months (range, five to 384 months). The minimum duration of follow-up was twenty-four months (median, twenty-nine months; range, twenty-four to forty-eight months). To evaluate the results, we compared preoperative and postoperative data from radiographs, forearm motion, grip strength, and pain.

Results.—The average radiographic deformity angle preoperatively was 21° (range, 12° to 35°) compared with the normal arm; the radiographic deformity angle was improved to 1° (range, 0° to 4°) postoperatively. The distal radioulnar joints of both sides were symmetric on postoperative radiographs regarding the relative lengths of the radius and ulna. In eighteen patients who had a restricted range of forearm motion preoperatively, the mean arc of forearm motion improved from 76° (range, 25° to 160°) preoperatively to 152° (range, 80° to 180°) postoperatively ($p < 0.01$). However, forearm supination was still restricted by $\geq 70°$ in three patients who had been younger than ten years old at the time of the initial injury and who had long-standing malunion for ninety-six months or longer. Painful recurrent dislocation of the distal ulna or radial head resolved or decreased in five patients. Average grip strength improved from 82% to 94% compared with that of the contralateral, normal side.

Conclusions.—Computer-assisted osteotomy can provide excellent radiographic and clinical outcome for the treatment of malunited diaphyseal forearm fractures. Satisfactory restoration of forearm motion can be achieved even in relatively long-standing cases in adults.

▶ Restoration of forearm rotation by corrective osteotomy of a complex, both-bone fracture malunion is a particularly challenging procedure. Success hinges on correcting the angular, rotational, and length distortions. Preoperative imaging and planning may incorporate use of 3-dimensional CT imaging, but in surgery one is faced with 2-dimensional radiographs or fluoroscopy to assess correction. This study is innovative in several areas, including development of the computer-assisted osteotomy software, but it is their incorporation of the custom-made osteotomy templates that is particularly appealing. The outcome data are favorable, considering the difficulty of the procedure, but should be considered preliminary. Their study would have been strengthened by including comparative 3-dimensional postoperative imaging.

S. D. Trigg, MD

Treatment of Unstable Distal Ulna Fractures Associated With Distal Radius Fractures in Patients 65 Years and Older
Cha S-M, Shin H-D, Kim K-C, et al (Chungnam Natl Univ School of Medicine, Daejeon, Japan)
J Hand Surg 37A:2481-2487, 2012

Purpose.—To prospectively compare the clinical and radiological outcomes of 2 treatment methods for unstable distal ulna fractures associated with distal radius fractures in patients 65 years of age and older.

Methods.—From February 2008 to March 2010, the first 29 ulnas were treated surgically (group 1) and the next 32 ulnas were treated nonoperatively (group 2). The mean final follow-up period was 34 months (range, 24–56 mo). All radiuses were fixed internally, in both groups. Clinical outcomes were compared between groups using a visual analog scale for postoperative pain; Disabilities of the Arm, Shoulder, and Hand scores; active range of motion; grip strength; and the modified system of Gartland and Werley. Radiological outcomes, including ulnar variance, were evaluated. Arthrosis was evaluated at the radiocarpal joint or distal radioulnar joint (DRUJ) according to the system of Knirk and Jupiter.

Results.—There were no significant differences between the groups in any of the clinical outcomes. No significant differences were observed for radiological outcomes including ulnar variance, distal radius, and union rate. There were no patients in either group with symptomatic arthritic changes in the radiocarpal joint or DRUJ at the final follow-up. In group 2, 1 patient had malunion (angulated, 14°) on the anteroposterior view without evidence of arthrosis in the DRUJ, and functional outcomes were good.

Conclusions.—In this population distal ulna fractures can be successfully managed nonoperatively when they occur in combination with distal radius fractures.

Type of Study/Level of Evidence.—Therapeutic II.

▶ There is a growing consensus that ulnar styloid fractures associated with distal radius fractures treated by open reduction and internal fixation (ORIF), which restores radius length and anatomic alignment, do not require internal fixation unless there is gross instability of the distal ulna. There is less agreement on the need to internally fixate combined aligned fractures of the ulnar head and shaft following satisfactory ORIF of the distal radius fracture. Further adding to the discussion are several recent studies that compare operative versus nonoperative treatment of distal radius fractures in elderly patients presenting radiographic data that did not correlate with clinical outcomes.[1]

This prospective study comparing operative vs nonoperative treatment of unstable distal ulna (excluding styloid and head) fractures in elderly patients adds valuable information to the mix of emerging information on operative treatment of distal radius fractures in this age group. My clinical experience mirrors others' experience in that internal fixation hardware about the distal ulna head and shaft is frequently troublesome postoperatively for the patient. I found the outcome data of this study valuable to my own decision process in the treatment of this population of patients.

S. D. Trigg, MD

Reference

1. Arora R, Lutz M, Deml C, Krappinger D, Huag L, Gabl M. A prospective randomized trial comparing nonoperative traetment with volar locking plate fixation for displaced and unstable distal radius fractures in patients sixty-five of age and older. *J Bone Joint Surg Am.* 2011;93:2146-2153.

The clinical and radiological outcome of pulsed electromagnetic field treatment for acute scaphoid fractures: a randomised double-blind placebo-controlled multicentre trial

Hannemann PFW, Göttgens KWA, van Wely BJ, et al (Maastricht Univ Med Centre, The Netherlands)

J Bone Joint Surg Br 94-B:1403-1408, 2012

The use of pulsed electromagnetic fields (PEMF) to stimulate bone growth has been recommended as an alternative to the surgical treatment of ununited scaphoid fractures, but has never been examined in acute fractures. We hypothesised that the use of PEMF in acute scaphoid fractures would accelerate the time to union by 30% in a randomised, double-blind, placebo-controlled, multicentre trial. A total of 53 patients in three different medical centres with a unilateral undisplaced acute scaphoid fracture were randomly assigned to receive either treatment with PEMF (n = 24) or a placebo (n = 29). The clinical and radiological outcomes were assessed at four, six, nine, 12, 24 and 52 weeks.

A log-rank analysis showed that neither time to clinical and radiological union nor the functional outcome differed significantly between the groups. The clinical assessment of union indicated that at six weeks tenderness in the anatomic snuffbox ($p = 0.03$) as well as tenderness on longitudinal compression of the scaphoid ($p = 0.008$) differed significantly in favour of the placebo group.

We conclude that stimulation of bone growth by PEMF has no additional value in the conservative treatment of acute scaphoid fractures.

▶ Prolonged healing time and the disturbingly high potential for delayed unions and nonunions of scaphoid fractures are well-known nonoperative treatment pitfalls. Much has been written about nonoperative treatment methods, but also well reported is the recognition of the significant associated socioeconomic costs in the treatment of these troublesome fractures. Use of pulsed electromagnetic field (PEMF) bone growth stimulators for scaphoid fracture nonunions is generally accepted as a treatment alternative along with operative treatment for established scaphoid fracture nonunions. Establishing a beneficial adjunct therapy to nonoperative treatment of acute scaphoid fractures that would shorten the time to union would have far-reaching economic, social, and employment benefits. This is the first prospective randomized study to investigate the effects of PEMF on acute undisplaced scaphoid fractures. Unfortunately, the results are sobering, but the information is of value to anyone who treats these injuries.

S. D. Trigg, MD

Long-Term Results of Bone-Retinaculum-Bone Autograft for Scapholunate Instability

Soong M, Merrell GA, Ortmann F IV, et al (Warren Alpert Med School of Brown Univ, Providence, RI)
J Hand Surg 38A:504-508, 2013

Purpose.—To report long-term follow-up of scapholunate interosseous ligament reconstruction with bone-retinaculum-bone autograft in patients with dynamic scapholunate instability.

Methods.—Of the 14 patients from the previously reported cohort who had bone-retinaculum-bone autograft for dynamic instability, 6 returned for clinical examination and radiographs, 3 were reached by telephone, and 2 were lost to follow-up. The remaining 3 had salvage procedures (2 total wrist arthrodeses and 1 proximal row carpectomy) between the prior report and the current study and thus reached an endpoint, at 2 to 4 years. For the 6 who returned, outcome measurements included scapholunate angle and gap, radiographic evidence of secondary arthritis, wrist extension and flexion, grip strength, and Mayo wrist score.

Results.—Follow-up averaged 11.9 years (range, 10.7—14.1 y). Clinical and radiographic outcomes deteriorated moderately from the prior report. Mayo wrist score averaged 83. There were 3 failures, resulting in 1 proximal row carpectomy and 2 total wrist arthrodeses. Findings at repeat surgery in the failed group included an intact graft without any apparent abnormalities, a partially ruptured graft (after a subsequent re-injury), and a completely resorbed graft.

Conclusions.—Bone-retinaculum-bone autograft reconstruction is a viable treatment option for dynamic scapholunate instability in which the scaphoid and lunate can be reduced. Results may deteriorate but are similar to those reported previously from other techniques. Problems with graft strength or stiffness may necessitate further surgery.

Type of Study/Level of Evidence.—Therapeutic IV.

▶ The optimum surgical treatment method for dynamic scapholunate instability is an unresolved problem. Direct repair, ligament substitution, capsulodesis, tenodesis, screw fixation, and intercarpal arthrodesis have been proposed, but data from longer-term outcome studies are inconclusive or show deterioration over the longer term. This method of direct scapholunate interosseous ligament reconstruction is intriguing on several fronts, including that the bone-retinaculum-bone graft is harvested near the repair site without further extensive dissection and offers the possibility of bone-to-bone healing with somewhat analogous tissue. Their short-term results were promising and fostered vigorous discussion at several hand surgical meetings. However, similar to other methods, their outcomes deteriorated with time. It is interesting that, at the time of subsequent salvage surgery, the graft was observed to be intact in 2 of 3 patients; therefore, the pain and arthrosis necessitating revision surgery might have been attributed to other unrecognized injury factors. Because no best treatment method for dynamic scapholunate instability is known, the careful surgeon should have several options available to him or her if direct repair cannot be accomplished, and this method is deserving of your consideration.

S. D. Trigg, MD

Early Initiation of Bisphosphonate Does Not Affect Healing and Outcomes of Volar Plate Fixation of Osteoporotic Distal Radial Fractures
Gong HS, Song CH, Lee YH, et al (Seoul Natl Univ Bundang Hosp, Seongnam, Gyeonggi-do, South Korea)
J Bone Joint Surg Am 94:1729-1736, 2012

Background.—Bisphosphonates can adversely affect fracture-healing because they inhibit osteoclastic bone resorption. It is unclear whether bisphosphonates can be initiated safely for patients who have sustained an acute distal radial fracture. The purpose of this randomized study was to determine whether the early use of bisphosphonate affects healing and outcomes of osteoporotic distal radial fractures treated with volar locking plate fixation.

Methods.—Fifty women older than fifty years of age who had undergone volar locking plate fixation of a distal radial fracture and had been diagnosed with osteoporosis were randomized to Group I (n = 24, initiation of bisphosphonate treatment at two weeks after the operation) or Group II (n = 26, initiation of bisphosphonate treatment at three months). Patients were assessed for radiographic union and other radiographic parameters (radial inclination, radial length, and volar tilt) at two, six, ten, sixteen, and twenty-four weeks, and for clinical outcomes that included Disabilities of the Arm, Shoulder and Hand (DASH) scores, wrist motion, and grip strength at twenty-four weeks. The two groups were compared with regard to the time to radiographic union, the radiographic parameters, and the clinical outcomes.

Results.—No significant differences were observed between the two groups with respect to radiographic or clinical outcomes after volar locking plate fixation. All patients obtained fracture union, and the mean times to radiographic union in Groups I and II were similar (6.7 and 6.8 weeks, respectively; $p = 0.65$). Furthermore, the time to radiographic union was not related to osteoporosis severity or fracture type.

Conclusions.—In patients with an osteoporotic distal radial fracture treated with volar locking plate fixation, the early initiation of bisphosphonate treatment did not affect fracture-healing or clinical outcomes.

Level of Evidence.—Therapeutic <u>Level I</u>. See Instructions for Authors for a complete description of levels of evidence.

▶ Biphosphonates are the most commonly used class of medications for the treatment of osteoporosis and act by inhibiting osteoclastic bone resorption. The obvious concern in the treatment of osteoporosis-related fragility fractures is that biphosphonate therapy could potentially adversely affect fracture healing biology and subsequent bone remodeling. The true effects of the medications on fracture healing remain unresolved and in need of further study. The growth in the practice of open reduction and internal fixation of distal radius fractures in adults of all age groups continues unabated, and this randomized study provides us with relevant information for anyone who operatively treats these common fractures.

S. D. Trigg, MD

Arthroscopic Repair of Ulnar-Sided Triangular Fibrocartilage Complex (Palmer Type 1B) Tears: A Comparison Between Short- and Midterm Results
Wolf MB, Haas A, Dragu A, et al (Vulpius Klinik, Bad Rappenau, Germany; Univ Hosp Heidelberg, Germany; German Cancer Res Ctr (DKFZ), Heidelberg; et al)
J Hand Surg 37A:2325-2330, 2012

Purpose.—To compare short- and midterm functional and subjective outcomes of arthroscopically repaired Palmer 1B tears.

Methods.—At 2 time points, we evaluated 49 patients with Palmer 1B tears who underwent arthroscopic repair. We examined 46 patients (23 males and 23 females) in the short-term at an average of 11 months (range, 6—23 mo) postoperatively. In a second midterm follow-up, we examined 40 patients (20 males and 20 females) an average of 4.8 years (range, 4.2—5.9 y) after repair. Between short- and midterm follow-ups, 6 patients underwent an ulnar-shortening osteotomy to alleviate persistent ulnar-sided symptoms. Objective and subjective evaluation included the determination of range of motion, grip strength, pain, and wrist scores (modified Mayo wrist score and Disabilities of Arm, Shoulder, and Hand score).

Results.—Compared with short-term repair results, midterm outcomes showed a further improvement in pain, wrist scores, grip strength, and motion. Neither static nor dynamic ulnar variance was correlated to preoperative and postoperative Disabilities of the Arm, Shoulder, and Hand scores, short-term modified Mayo wrist scores, or need for ulnar-shortening osteotomy. Five patients improved only after having received an ulnar shortening osteotomy.

Conclusions.—After repair of Palmer 1B lesions, patients continued to improve in function and comfort at least into the second year, although some needed to have the ulna shortened to achieve this result.

Type of Study/Level of Evidence.—Therapeutic IV.

▶ Palmer type 1B (posttraumatic, peripheral) tears are among the most commonly encountered types of posttraumatic triangular fibrocartilage complex (TFCC) tears. Open repairs, all-inside arthroscopic repairs, and inside-out arthroscopic repair techniques have been reported with generally favorable results, but valid comparison among these treatment methods is difficult, as selection criteria for presence of associated distal radioulnar joint instability and ulnar positive variance is not always included. Moreover, the decision to combine ulnar shortening in patients with ulnar-positive variance combined with the TFCC repair, or not, remains controversial, as level 1 outcome data are sparse. This retrospective study reviewed only type 1B lesions without distal radioulnar joint instability. Their findings that preoperative static or dynamic ulnar-positive variance did not correlate with clinical outcomes in their medium-term results is important information. However, the need to later perform ulnar-shortening osteotomy on 5 patients raises additional questions in need of future investigation.

S. D. Trigg, MD

Clinical, Radiographic, and Arthroscopic Outcomes After Ulnar Shortening Osteotomy: A Long-Term Follow-Up Study

Tatebe M, Shinohara T, Okui N, et al (Nagoya Univ School of Medicine, Showaku, Japan; Kinjo Gakuin Univ School of Human Life and Environment, Nagoya, Japan)
J Hand Surg 37A:2468-2474, 2012

Purpose.—Previous studies have investigated the long-term outcomes of ulnar shortening osteotomy (USO) in the treatment of ulnocarpal abutment syndrome (UCA), but none have used arthroscopic assessments. The purpose of this study was to investigate the long-term clinical outcomes of USO with patient-based, arthroscopic, and radiographic assessments.

Methods.—We retrospectively reviewed 30 patients with UCA after a minimum follow-up of 5 years, with arthroscopic evaluations at the time of both USO and plate removal. We confirmed the initial diagnosis of UCA by radiography and arthroscopy. Mean age at the time of index surgery was 37 years. Mean duration of follow-up was 11 years (range, 5−19 y). We obtained Disabilities of the Arm, Shoulder, and Hand and Hand20 self-assessments postoperatively for all patients. Bony spur formation was evaluated postoperatively from plain radiographs.

Results.—We detected triangular fibrocartilage complex (TFCC) disc tear in 13 wrists arthroscopically at the time of USO. Of these, 10 showed no evidence of TFCC disc tear at second-look arthroscopy. The remaining 17 cases showed no TFCC disc tear at either first- or second-look arthroscopy. Follow-up radiography revealed that bony spurs at the distal radioulnar joint had progressed in 13 wrists. Disabilities of the Shoulder, Arm, and Hand and Hand20 scores did not significantly correlate with the presence of bony spurs or TFCC disc tears. Range of motion decreased significantly with age only. Lower grip strength correlated with bony spur and lower radial inclination. Triangular fibrocartilage complex tear, male sex, and advanced age were associated with lower Disabilities of the Shoulder, Arm, and Hand and Hand20 scores.

Conclusions.—Ulnar shortening osteotomy achieved excellent long-term results in most cases. Most TFCC disc tears identified at the initial surgery had healed by long-term arthroscopic follow-up. We suggest that UCA with a TFCC disc tear is a good indication for USO.

Type of Study/Level of Evidence.—Therapeutic IV.

▶ Ulnar shortening osteotomy is a widely accepted treatment method for ulnocarpal abutment syndrome. Arthroscopy at the time of ulnar shortening is frequently performed to evaluate and address associated pathology of the triangular fibrocartilage complex (TFCC) and carpal interosseous ligaments. Unfortunately, there are few long-term studies that include arthroscopic follow-up assessment information after ulnar shortening osteotomy. Reasons for this no doubt stem from regional variations in the regular practice (or not) for removal of the ulnar shortening osteosynthesis plate at a later date, which of course provides an opportunity to reevaluate and compare TFCC pathology with a second-look arthroscopy. This retrospective study provides us with valuable radiographic and arthroscopic information on this commonly performed procedure.

S. D. Trigg, MD

Functional Results of the Darrach Procedure: A Long-Term Outcome Study
Grawe B, Heincelman C, Stern P (Univ of Cincinnati, OH)
J Hand Surg 37A:2475-2480.e2, 2012

Purpose.—To assess long-term functional outcome after ulnar head excision for distal radioulnar joint dysfunction with prior or concomitant wrist trauma. We hypothesized that long-term outcomes would reflect good functional results with satisfactory pain relief.

Methods.—A retrospective chart review identified patients who had undergone the Darrach procedure for traumatic or posttraumatic distal radioulnar joint (DRUJ) pathology. We assessed subjective outcomes using a visual analog scale questionnaire to assess pain, wrist stability, and overall satisfaction. We evaluated objective functional outcomes using the Quick Disabilities of the Shoulder, Arm, and Hand and Patient-Rated Wrist Evaluation measures. Final radiographs were compared with preoperative x-rays to investigate the effect of possible ulnar impingement syndrome (convergent instability).

Results.—A total of 98 patients with 99 wrists met our predetermined inclusion criteria. Of these, 27 patients with a total of 27 wrists were available for final follow-up, 15 of whom were available for final in-office follow-up with radiographs (6–20 y). Patients displayed an average Quick Disabilities of the Shoulder, Arm, and Hand score of 17 and a Patient-Rated Wrist Evaluation score of 14. Final average visual analog scale scores for pain (0–4), pain with activity (0–4), overall satisfaction (0–4), and wrist stability (0–10) were 0.1, 0.6, 3.7, and 1.5, respectively. Final average wrist range of motion was 85°/78° and 41°/45° for pronation-supination and flexion-extension, respectively. A total of 7 patients displayed radioulnar impingement based on dynamic radiography.

This ulnar impingement was not associated with clinical reports of pain and did not affect outcome measures in a statistically significant manner.

Conclusions.—The Darrach procedure provides reliably good long-term subjective and objective results for the treatment of a symptomatic DRUJ after a distal radius fracture. Patients can expect to have excellent forearm range of motion at long-term follow-up. Nearly one-half of patients had dynamic convergence of the DRUJ when stressed radiographically; however, the presence of radiographic dynamic convergence did not influence clinical outcomes.

▶ Posttraumatic dysfunction, pain, and degenerative arthritis about the distal radioulnar joint (DRUJ) following distal radius fracture malunions are common and perplexing problems. Distal ulna resection arthroplasty (Darrach procedure) has historically been accepted as a suitable treatment option for DRUJ dysfunction. The authors correctly point out that despite the frequency with which the Darrach procedure is performed, there is a paucity of long-term functional outcome data investigating the procedure performed exclusively for posttraumatic DRUJ dysfunction. This retrospective study has inherent limitations, but their objective outcome measurement data and conclusions are well worth your review.

S. D. Trigg, MD

Hand

Buried Kirschner wires in hand trauma: Do they reduce infection rates and is it worth the extra cost?
Koç T, Ahmed J, Aleksyeyenko S (St Thomas' Hosp, London, UK)
Eur J Plast Surg 35:803-807, 2012

There has been little research comparing rates of infectious complications between buried and percutaneous Kirschner wire (K-wire) use in hand trauma surgery. The additional cost of removing buried wires should be justified by a demonstrable reduction in the frequency and/or severity of infectious complications. We prospectively collected data on infective complications associated with K-wire use during the course of 1 year at our hand trauma unit. We observed seven (10%) infections in 70 patients where wires were left protruding and three (9%) infections in 34 patients where wires were buried. There was no statistically significant difference in the rate of infectious complications. A cost analysis was performed, taking into account infectious complications and the cost of their management. Burying K-wires resulted in an extra cost of £235.51 per patient compared to £90.80 per patient for percutaneous K-wires. Thus, the use of buried K-wires results in a £144.71 increase in cost per patient. Clinicians should consider these findings, as well as other (medical) considerations, when making the decision whether to bury K-wires.

▶ This straightforward, simple study caught my eye because it presents clinically relevant and economically important information in these challenging times in health care delivery. Although the decision to leave temporary fixation K-wires exposed or buried may be made dependent on fracture-specific factors or with regard to patient compliance and hygiene variables and acknowledging that surgery costs will vary the information presented, this study is universal and deserving of your review.

S. D. Trigg, MD

Dorsoradial Capsulodesis for Trapeziometacarpal Joint Instability

Rayan G, Do V (INTEGRIS Baptist Med Ctr, OK; Univ of Oklahoma Health Sciences Ctr, OK)
J Hand Surg 38A:382-387, 2013

We describe an alternative method for treating chronic trapeziometacarpal (TM) joint instability after acute injury or chronic repetitive use of the thumb by performing a dorsoradial capsulodesis procedure. The procedure is done by imbricating the redundant TM joint dorsoradial ligament and capsule after reducing the joint by pronating the thumb. The dorsoradial

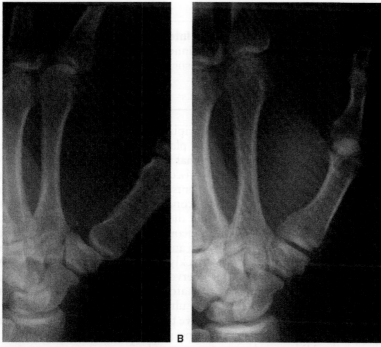

A   **B**

FIGURE 7.—A Preoperative x-ray showing TM joint subluxation. B Postoperative x-ray showing congruent TM joint after dorsoradial capsulodesis. (Reprinted from The Journal of Hand Surgery. Rayan G, Do V. Dorsoradial capsulodesis for trapeziometacarpal joint instability. *J Hand Surg.* 2013;38A:382-387, Copyright 2013, with permission from the American Society for Surgery of the Hand.)

capsulodesis is a reasonable reconstructive option for chronic TM joint instability and subluxation (Fig 7).

▶ Generally, I have not selected for review surgical technique articles that have undergone limited nonqualitative review and analysis, but this article caught my eye because it addresses an underreported clinical problem. Optimum treatment for symptomatic prearthritic hypermobility of the trapeziometacarpal joint (Eaton stage 1) in active younger women has yet to be resolved. In my own practice, I have found female dentists, dental hygienists, and surgeons with painful hypermobile trapeziometacarpal joints to be a particularly difficult group of patients for which to recommend surgical treatment, because volar oblique ligament reconstruction and arthrodesis often result in loss of motion and individually reported alterations in postoperative dexterity. These patients reported clinical information coupled with prolonged recovery time away from their practices, which has left me looking for other methods. The technique described here may have several advantages in that it burns no bridges for later arthrodesis or ligament reconstruction tendon interposition and may delay or prevent progression of trapeziometacarpal arthrosis. This will require further study. This technique as reported is straightforward and effectively restores a congruent trapeziometacarpal joint.

S. D. Trigg, MD

Nerve

Supercharged End-to-Side Anterior Interosseous to Ulnar Motor Nerve Transfer for Intrinsic Musculature Reinnervation

Barbour J, Yee A, Kahn LC, et al (Washington Univ School of Medicine, St Louis, MO)
J Hand Surg 37A:2150-2159, 2012

Functional motor recovery after peripheral nerve injury is predominantly determined by the time to motor end plate reinnervation and the absolute number of regenerated motor axons that reach target. Experimental models have shown that axonal regeneration occurs across a supercharged end-to-side (SETS) nerve coaptation. In patients with a recovering proximal ulnar nerve injury, a SETS nerve transfer conceptually is useful to protect and preserve distal motor end plates until the native axons fully regenerate. In addition, for nerve injuries in which incomplete regeneration is anticipated, a SETS nerve transfer may be useful to augment the regenerating nerve with additional axons and to more quickly reinnervate target muscle. We describe our technique for a SETS nerve transfer of the terminal anterior interosseous nerve (AIN) to the pronator quadratus muscle (PQ) end-to-side to the deep motor fascicle of the ulnar nerve in the distal forearm. In addition, we describe our postoperative therapy regimen for these transfers and an evaluation tool for monitoring progressive muscle reinnervation. Although the AIN—to—ulnar motor group SETS nerve transfer was specifically designed for ulnar nerve injuries, we believe that the SETS procedure might have broad clinical utility for second- and third-degree axonotmetic

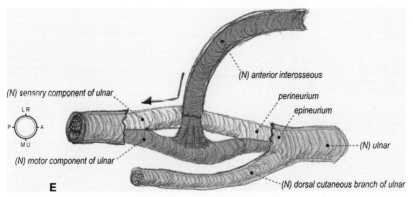

FIGURE 5.—SETS anterior interosseous—to—ulnar motor nerve transfer. E Illustration of the SETS donor anterior interosseous (*green*) to recipient motor component of the ulnar (*red*) nerve transfer. For interpretation of the references to color in this figure legend, the reader is referred to web version of this article. (Reprinted from The Journal of Hand Surgery. Barbour J, Yee A, Kahn LC, et al. Supercharged end-to-side anterior interosseous to ulnar motor nerve transfer for intrinsic musculature reinnervation. *J Hand Surg*. 2012;37A:2150-2159, Copyright 2012, with permission from the American Society for Surgery of the Hand.)

TABLE 1.—Indications for Supercharged End-to-Side Nerve Transfer for Ulnar Intrinsic Atrophy

Axonotmetic Injuries (Sunderland II, III)	Neurotmetic Injuries (Sunderland IV, V)
• Severe cubital tunnel	• Proximal to elbow with Martin Gruber anastomosis
• Failed cubital tunnel surgery	
• C8—T1 nerve root injury	
• Brachial plexus medial cord traction injury	• Injury between elbow and 10 cm proximal to wrist
• Brachial plexus neuritis (Parsonage-Turner)	
• Primary motor neuropathy (eg, Charcot-Marie-Tooth)	

nerve injuries, to augment partial recovery and/or "babysit" motor end plates until the native parent axons regenerate to target. We would consider all donor nerves currently utilized in end-to-end nerve transfers for neurotmetic injuries as candidates for this SETS technique (Fig 5E, Table 1).

▶ Gauging the level of recovery of intrinsic hand muscle function following elbow and midforearm level ulnar nerve injury repairs is difficult because of the expected delay in reinnervation of the target muscle groups along with the uncertainty of the completeness of that reinnervation. Any method of preserving motor end plate function by improving or augmenting ulnar nerve motor axons is an important advance in treatment of these challenging injuries. I found the procedure presented in this study to be particularly important and useful because the anatomy is straightforward and is potentially within the skill level of most hand surgeons.

S. D. Trigg, MD

4   Elbow

Introduction

This is the shortest section of the YEAR BOOK, as it reflects the relative limited burden of disease. For this reason I have, perhaps surprisingly given my personal interest, selected relatively few articles relating to the elbow. Nonetheless, I have tried to select a broad spectrum of topics that are relevant to those in a more general practice: trauma and overuse syndromes. While the volume is limited, the relevance, I hope, is substantive.

Bernard F. Morrey, MD

Effect of Corticosteroid Injection, Physiotherapy, or Both on Clinical Outcomes in Patients With Unilateral Lateral Epicondylalgia: A Randomized Controlled Trial

Coombes BK, Bisset L, Brooks P, et al (Univ of Queensland, St Lucia, Australia; Griffith Univ, Southport, Queensland, Australia; Univ of Melbourne, Australia)
JAMA 309:461-469, 2013

Importance.—Corticosteroid injection and physiotherapy, common treatments for lateral epicondylalgia, are frequently combined in clinical practice. However, evidence on their combined efficacy is lacking.

Objective.—To investigate the effectiveness of corticosteroid injection, multimodal physiotherapy, or both in patients with unilateral lateral epicondylalgia.

Design, Setting, and Patients.—A2 × 2 factorial, randomized, injection-blinded, placebo-controlled trial was conducted at a single university research center and 16 primary care settings in Brisbane, Australia. A total of 165 patients aged 18 years or older with unilateral lateral epicondylalgia of longer than 6 weeks' duration were enrolled between July 2008 and May 2010; 1-year follow-up was completed in May 2011.

Interventions.—Corticosteroid injection (n = 43), placebo injection (n = 41), corticosteroid injection plus physiotherapy (n = 40), or placebo injection plus physiotherapy (n = 41).

Main Outcome Measures.—The 2 primary outcomes were 1-year global rating of change scores for complete recovery or much improvement and 1-year recurrence (defined as complete recovery or much improvement at 4 or 8 weeks, but not later) analyzed on an intention-to-treat basis ($P < .01$).

Secondary outcomes included complete recovery or much improvement at 4 and 26 weeks.

Results.—Corticosteroid injection resulted in lower complete recovery or much improvement at 1 year vs placebo injection (83% vs 96%, respectively; relative risk [RR], 0.86 [99% CI, 0.75-0.99]; $P = .01$) and greater 1-year recurrence (54% vs 12%; RR, 0.23 [99% CI, 0.10-0.51]; $P < .001$). The physiotherapy and no physiotherapy groups did not differ on 1-year ratings of complete recovery or much improvement (91% vs 88%, respectively; RR, 1.04 [99% CI, 0.90-1.19]; $P = .56$) or recurrence (29% vs 38%; RR, 1.31 [99% CI, 0.73-2.35]; $P = .25$). Similar patterns were found at 26 weeks, with lower complete recovery or much improvement after corticosteroid injection vs placebo injection (55% vs 85%, respectively; RR, 0.79 [99% CI, 0.62-0.99]; $P < .001$) and no difference between the physiotherapy and no physiotherapy groups (71% vs 69%, respectively; RR, 1.22 [99% CI, 0.97-1.53]; $P = .84$). At 4 weeks, there was a significant interaction between corticosteroid injection and physiotherapy ($P = .01$), whereby patients receiving the placebo injection plus physiotherapy had greater complete recovery or much improvement vs no physiotherapy (39% vs 10%, respectively; RR, 4.00 [99% CI, 1.07-15.00]; $P = .004$). However, there was no difference between patients receiving the corticosteroid injection plus physiotherapy vs corticosteroid alone (68% vs 71%, respectively; RR, 0.95 [99% CI, 0.65-1.38]; $P = .57$).

Conclusion and Relevance.—Among patients with chronic unilateral lateral epicondylalgia, the use of corticosteroid injection vs placebo injection resulted in worse clinical outcomes after 1 year, and physiotherapy did not result in any significant differences.

Trial Registration.—anzctr.org Identifier: ACTRN12609000051246.

▶ To be honest, I read this article when it was first published, and it is in the process of changing my practice. Other than the irritation of an article by PhDs terming the condition epicondylalgia, this is an important contribution. It distresses me to see yet another study that offers data on the deleterious effect of cortisone.

The study is elegant (Fig 1 in the original article). The analysis assesses both cortisone and physical therapy. Both are mainstays to our treatment of epicondylitis. Neither, it appears, are of value (Fig 2 in the original article)! So what do we do? Look for other solutions. I believe one use of ultrasound energy in a percutaneous delivery may be the answer. Time will tell. Regardless, my use of cortisone has dropped off markedly.

B. F. Morrey, MD

Is Posterior Synovial Plica Excision Necessary for Refractory Lateral Epicondylitis of the Elbow?

Rhyou IH, Kim KW (Semyeong Christianity Hosp, Pohang, Kyeongbuk, Korea)
Clin Orthop Relat Res 471:284-290, 2013

Background.—Arthroscopic treatments for lateral epicondylitis including débridement of the extensor carpi radialis brevis (ECRB) origin (Baker technique) or resection of the radiocapitellar synovial plica reportedly improve symptoms. However the etiology of the disease and the role of the plica remain unclear.

Questions/Purposes.—We asked if posterior radiocapitellar synovial plica excision made any additional improvement in pain or function after arthroscopic ECRB release.

Methods.—We retrospectively reviewed 38 patients who had arthroscopic treatment for refractory lateral epicondylitis between November 2003 and October 2009. Twenty patients (Group A) underwent the Baker technique and 18 patients (Group B) underwent a combination of the Baker technique and posterior synovial plica excision. The minimum followup was 36 months (mean, 46 months; range, 36–72 months) for Group A and 25 months (mean, 30 months; range, 25–36 months) for Group B. Postoperatively we obtained VAS pain and DASH scores for each group.

Results.—Two years postoperatively, we found no differences in the VAS pain score or DASH: the mean VAS pain scores were 0.3 points in Group A and 0.4 points in Group B, and the DASH scores were 5.1 points and 6.1 points respectively.

Conclusions.—The addition of débridement of the posterior synovial fold did not appear to enhance either pain relief or function compared with the classic Baker technique without decortication.

▶ This is a nice study to include in the YEAR BOOK for several reasons. Tennis elbow is the most common affliction for which a patient will seek a physician's opinion. We really do not know the optimum treatment. There is a real and subtle relationship between the radiohumeral plica and tennis elbow—type symptoms. This relationship possibly justifies the arthroscopic approach as a treatment of epicondylitis. So, while the posterior plica exists and can be removed, does it improve outcomes? (See Fig 2a,b in the original article.) The answer is no. So I will continue to reserve an arthroscopic assessment and treatment for this problem only for those with documented evidence of intra-articular pathology.

B. F. Morrey, MD

Functional outcomes of surgical reconstruction for posterolateral rotatory instability of the elbow
Lin K-Y, Shen P-H, Lee C-H, et al (Natl Defense Med Ctr, Taipei, Taiwan; Taipei Med Univ Hosp, Taiwan, ROC)
Injury 43:1657-1661, 2012

Background.—The disruption or insufficiency of lateral ligament complex including lateral ulnar collateral ligament (LUCL) leads to posterolateral rotatory instability (PLRI). An accurate clinical staging is quite useful in predicting the prognosis. The purpose of our study is to review our experience with surgical reconstruction for PLRI of the elbow and to investigate the relationship between the clinical stage of elbow instability and the functional outcomes of PLRI.

Materials and Methods.—Patients with PLRI of the elbow determined by fluoroscopic stress view under anaesthesia underwent surgical reconstruction of the LUCL with autogenous tendon graft.

Results.—Thirteen of the fourteen patients (93%) were subjectively satisfied with the outcome of the surgery. The mean follow-up was 49 months (range: 24–72). The results were better in patients with stage 1 or 2 instability (group I) compared to those with stage 3 instability (group II).

Conclusions.—Reconstruction of the LUCL using an autogenous tendon graft is an effective method for patients with PLRI of elbow. Since better results were obtained in patients with stage 1 or 2 instability rather than stage 3, accurate clinical staging determined by fluoroscopic stress view under anaesthesia is important before surgery for appropriate treatment and prediction of functional outcomes.

▶ This case study is a nice example of describing an important complication of elbow trauma, that of posterior lateral rotatory instability. It is important to realize that it is due to deficiency of the lateral ulnar collateral ligament and is poorly tolerated. The authors reaffirm the means of making the diagnosis, sometimes best shown under anesthesia. Importantly, they report a success rate in excess of 90% with ligament reconstruction, which is similar to the original description as well as our subsequent experience.

B. F. Morrey, MD

Distraction Arthrolysis of Posttraumatic Elbow Stiffness With a Hinged External Fixator
Wang J, Li H, Zheng Q, et al (Med School of Zhejiang Univ, Hangzhou, China)
Orthopedics 35:e1625-e1630, 2012

The treatment of elbow stiffness remains a challenge for orthopedic surgeons. A hinged external fixator with distraction ability has recently emerged as a new option in the surgical treatment of elbow stiffness. Between January 2007 and December 2009, twenty-five posttraumatic stiff elbows (mean patient age, 29.2 years) received distraction arthrolysis

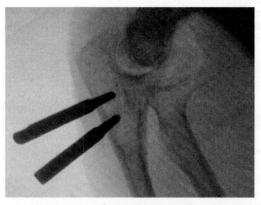

FIGURE 1.—Intraoperative image intensification showing the elbow distraction (B). (Reprinted from Wang J, Li H, Zheng Q, et al. Distraction arthrolysis of posttraumatic elbow stiffness with a hinged external fixator. *Orthopedics*. 2012;35:e1625-e1630.)

from 1 surgeon group (W.J.W., L.H., P.Z.J.) at the authors' institution. For patients with only periarticular soft tissue contracture (grade 1), close mechanical distraction was performed with the assistance of an external fixator under anesthesia; open arthrolysis was avoided as much as possible. For patients who also had heterotopic ossification (grade 2), it was removed through a limited approach before the external fixator was applied. For patients with osteoarticular surface damage or destruction (grade 3), osteoarticular integrity was restored before arthrolysis. Range of motion increased markedly, from 33.4° (range, 0°-75°) preoperatively to 105.° (range, 80°-140°) immediately postoperatively (Student's *t* test, $P < .05$).

Of the 25 patients, 23 were followed for a mean of 16 months. No serious complications occurred. Mean range of motion was 97.4° (range, 70°-130°) at final follow-up, a significant increase from preoperatively (Student's *t* test, $P < .05$). No significant loss of range of motion was found at final follow-up compared with intraoperative values (average 8.2° loss; Student's *t* test, $P > .05$). This study suggests that a hinged external distraction fixator is a less invasive option for treating posttraumatic elbow stiffness and prevents contracture recurrence after arthrolysis (Fig 1B).

▶ It is recognized that relatively few readers will be applying an external fixator as an adjunct to the management of the stiff elbow. However, elbow stiffness is the most common sequela of elbow trauma and it is important to realize the condition can be effectively treated. Use and value of an external fixator is not universally accepted.

These authors do seem to reveal it is a useful adjunct. However, it should be noted the joint is truly distracted with this technique (Fig 1B), not just "neutralized." I personally rarely leave the fixator on for more than 3 to 4 weeks and have documented increased complications with prolonged application, which apparently was not observed here. The careful additional management measures are also important in securing the final outcome.

B. F. Morrey, MD

A Prospective Randomized Controlled Trial of Dynamic Versus Static Progressive Elbow Splinting for Posttraumatic Elbow Stiffness

Lindenhovius ALC, Doornberg JN, Brouwer KM, et al (Massachusetts General Hosp, Boston)
J Bone Joint Surg Am 94:694-700, 2012

Background.—Both dynamic and static progressive (turnbuckle) splints are used to help stretch a contracted elbow capsule to regain motion after elbow trauma. There are advocates of each method, but no comparative data. This prospective randomized controlled trial tested the null hypothesis that there is no difference in improvement of motion and Disabilities of the Arm, Shoulder and Hand (DASH) scores between static progressive and dynamic splinting.

Methods.—Sixty-six patients with posttraumatic elbow stiffness were enrolled in a prospective randomized trial: thirty-five in the static progressive and thirty-one in the dynamic cohort. Elbow function was measured at enrollment and at three, six, and twelve months later. Patients completed the DASH questionnaire at enrollment and at the six and twelve-month evaluation. Three patients asked to be switched to static progressive splinting. The analysis was done according to intention-to-treat principles and with use of mean imputation for missing data.

Results.—There were no significant differences in flexion arc at any time point. Improvement in the arc of flexion (dynamic versus static) averaged 29° versus 28° at three months ($p = 0.87$), 40° versus 39° at six months ($p = 0.72$), and 47° versus 49° at twelve months after splinting was initiated ($p = 0.71$). The average DASH score (dynamic versus static) was 50 versus 45 points at enrollment ($p = 0.52$), 32 versus 25 points at six months ($p = 0.05$), and 28 versus 26 points at twelve months after enrollment ($p = 0.61$).

Conclusions.—Posttraumatic elbow stiffness can improve with exercises and dynamic or static splinting over a period of six to twelve months, and patience is warranted. There were no significant differences in improvement in motion between static progressive and dynamic splinting protocols, and the choice of splinting method can be determined by the patients and their physicians.

▶ As a level 1 prospective study, this contribution is worthy of note. To be honest, it refutes my longstanding preference for static adjustable splinting strategies. As we all know, it is very difficult to successfully complete any level 1 study, so the authors are to be commended on this effort. What is of special note is the virtual identical effectiveness at all time points (Fig 1 in the original article). Of additional note is the mean final improvement of 40°. Finally, the only reservation that remains might be whether improved brace designs might not show a difference, or, more importantly, improve the overall effectiveness.

B. F. Morrey, MD

5 Shoulder

Introduction

The growth of interest in shoulder pathology continues unabated. This, of course, is driven by the broad spectrum of pathology that presents at the shoulder: soft tissue/sport, trauma, and arthritis. In spite of the control of the rheumatoid patient, posttraumatic conditions, and primary osteoarthritis of the shoulder continue to be major clinical problems. The breakthrough design of the "reverse shoulder" dominates the arthroplasty literature, but it is not reflected in this section, because in my judgment this is not of particular relevance to the non-shoulder—focused surgeon. Rather, I have elected to depart from the balance to focus on a condition that is relevant to all orthopedic surgeons: rotator cuff. The numerous issues of open versus arthroscopic outcomes, technical considerations, and outcomes are highlighted. This focus is not characteristic, but it was thought to be the best expression of shoulder surgery evolution at this time.

Bernard F. Morrey, MD

Anterior Shoulder Dislocations in Pediatric Patients: Are Routine Prereduction Radiographs Necessary?

Reid S, Liu M, Ortega H (Children's Hosps and Clinics of Minnesota, Minneapolis/St Paul)
Pediatr Emerg Care 29:39-42, 2013

Background.—Fractures are reported to complicate anterior shoulder dislocations in up to 50% of adults. For this reason, prereduction and postreduction radiographs are recommended for the routine evaluation of shoulder dislocations in all patients. To date, few data have been reported as to the incidence of fractures or as to the value of prereduction x-rays in pediatric patients with anterior shoulder dislocations.

Objectives.—The objectives of this study were to estimate the incidence of fractures associated with anterior shoulder dislocation in pediatric patients and to examine the value of prereduction radiographs for these patients.

Methods.—This was a retrospective review of records for pediatric patients who presented to an emergency department (ED), received a diagnosis of anterior shoulder dislocation, and had at least 1 set of shoulder x-rays.

Results.—Of 119 patients who met criteria for inclusion in the study, 3 patients (3%) had a fracture identified; 6 patients (5%) had a possible fracture identified. Except for 1 patient with an avulsion fracture who was transferred without a reduction attempt or further x-rays, all patients had their dislocation reduced uneventfully in the ED.

Conclusions.—In our sample of pediatric patients with anterior shoulder dislocations due to low-energy injury mechanisms, plain radiography identified a lower incidence of fractures than those reported from adult studies. Pediatric patients with anterior shoulder dislocations clinically apparent after clinical evaluation may not benefit from prereduction radiographs. Forgoing prereduction x-rays might expedite definitive pain relief for patients, lower cost and radiation exposure, and decrease ED length of stay.

▶ Just last week at a major sports medicine clinic, the question of reducing the shoulder without a radiograph was the topic of considerable discussion. Hence, I had to include this nice study that provides some objective data to help direct our thinking. If the likelihood of reducing a fracture dislocation is about 5%, is it wrong to have a policy to reduce without the film? Extrapolated, is it acceptable to reduce a first-time dislocated shoulder on the field, which of course is a common practice? In my practice, I did reduce on the field or locker room (hockey), but then sent patient for a postreduction film. This study justifies this approach. One additional comment: The shoulder should be carefully examined for crepitus before the reduction if that is the course to be followed.

B. F. Morrey, MD

Cost-Effectiveness Analysis of Primary Arthroscopic Stabilization Versus Nonoperative Treatment for First-Time Anterior Glenohumeral Dislocations

Crall TS, Bishop JA, Guttman D, et al (Mammoth Hosp, CA; Stanford Univ, Redwood City, CA; Taos Orthopaedic Inst, NM; et al)
Arthroscopy 28:1755-1765, 2012

Purpose.—The purpose of this study was to compare the cost-effectiveness of initial observation versus surgery for first-time anterior shoulder dislocation.

Methods.—The clinical scenario of first-time anterior glenohumeral dislocation was simulated using a Markov model (where variables change over time depending on previous states). Nonoperative outcomes include success (no recurrence) and recurrence; surgical outcomes include success, recurrence, and complications of infection or stiffness. Probabilities for outcomes were determined from published literature. Costs were tabulated from Medicare Current Procedural Terminology data, as well as hospital and office billing records. We performed microsimulation and probabilistic sensitivity analysis running 6 models for 1,000 patients over a period of 15 years. The 6 models tested were male versus female patients aged 15 years versus 25 years versus 35 years.

Results.—Primary surgery was less costly and more effective for 15-year-old boys, 15-year-old girls, and 25-year-old men. For the remaining scenarios (25-year-old women and 35-year-old men and women), primary surgery was also more effective but was more costly. However, for these scenarios, primary surgery was still very cost-effective (cost per quality-adjusted life-year, <$25,000). After 1 recurrence, surgery was less costly and more effective for all scenarios.

Conclusions.—Primary arthroscopic stabilization is a clinically effective and cost-effective treatment for first-time anterior shoulder dislocations in the cohorts studied. By use of a willingness-to-pay threshold of $25,000 per quality-adjusted life-year, surgery was more cost-effective than nonoperative treatment for the majority of patients studied in the model.

Level of Evidence.—Level II, economic and decision analysis.

▶ Although the question and the conclusion is simply stated, the actual modeling and analysis of this article is very detailed. The authors are to be commended for asking the "cost-effectiveness question." As the reader would recognize, this dimension must be factored in our studies and practice in the future. As will be shown for other conditions, an initial stabilization procedure is actually a cost-effective strategy for the first-time shoulder dislocator. This is based largely on the cost of treating the recurrences, and then the high rate of subsequent stabilization procedures. Studies such as this are not easily performed, but they are extremely valuable to refine our indications for intervention.

B. F. Morrey, MD

Evolution of Nonoperatively Treated Symptomatic Isolated Full-Thickness Supraspinatus Tears

Fucentese SF, von Roll AL, Pfirrmann CWA, et al (Univ Hosp Balgrist, Zurich, Switzerland)
J Bone Joint Surg Am 94:801-808, 2012

Background.—The natural history of small, symptomatic rotator cuff tears is currently unclear. The purpose of the present study was to assess the clinical and structural outcomes for a consecutive series of patients with symptomatic, isolated full-thickness supraspinatus tears who had been offered rotator cuff repair but declined operative treatment.

Methods.—In the study period, twenty-four patients with isolated full-thickness supraspinatus tears that had been diagnosed by means of magnetic resonance arthrography were offered rotator cuff repair and elected nonoperative treatment. The twenty men and four women had an average age of fifty-two years at the time of diagnosis. At a median of forty-two months after the diagnosis, all patients were reexamined clinically according to the Constant and Murley scoring system and all shoulders underwent standard magnetic resonance imaging.

Results.—At the time of follow-up, the mean subjective shoulder score was 74% of that for a normal shoulder and the mean Constant score was

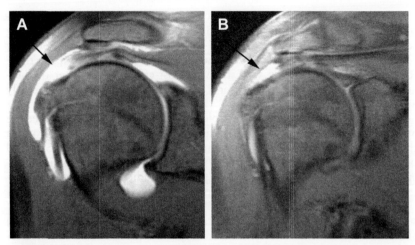

FIGURE 1.—A Coronal MRI view with arthrography, showing a full-thickness tear (*arrow*) of the supraspinatus at the time of diagnosis. **B** Coronal MRI view without arthrography, demonstrating no change in the supraspinatus tear at the time of the forty-five-month follow-up. (Reprinted from Fucentese SF, von Roll AL, Pfirrmann CWA, et al. Evolution of nonoperatively treated symptomatic isolated full-thickness supraspinatus tears. *J Bone Joint Surg Am*. 2012;94:801-808, with permission from The Journal of Bone and Joint Surgery, Incorporated.)

75 points (relative Constant score, 86%). The mean rotator cuff tear size did not change significantly over time (95% confidence interval, 0.51 to 1.12). In two shoulders, the tear was no longer detectable on magnetic resonance imaging, in nine shoulders the tear was smaller than it had been at the time of the initial diagnosis, in nine patients the tear had not changed, and in six patients the tear had increased in size. There was a slight but significant progression of fatty muscle infiltration of the supraspinatus, but no patient had fatty infiltration beyond stage 2 at the time of the latest follow-up (95% confidence interval, 0% to 14%).

Conclusions.—In a consecutive series of patients who had been offered repair of an isolated, symptomatic supraspinatus tear, the refusal of operative treatment resulted in surprisingly high clinical patient satisfaction and no increase of the average size of the rotator cuff tear 3.5 years after the recommendation of operative repair. This study confirms that the size of small rotator cuff tears does not invariably increase over a limited period of time. Distinguishing tears that will increase in size from those that will not needs further study (Fig 1).

▶ This is an interesting and important study from an experienced investigative team. With the ever-increasing emphasis on technique and predictable outcomes, it is refreshing to see a study such as this. The quality of the study allows one to believe the conclusion. In spite of accepted dogmas, small tears do not necessarily progress (Fig 1 A,B). The key is to try to determine how one determines which of these will and will not progress. Regardless, without question, they do not all progress to more substantial tears over time. Hence, observation is appropriate care in some individuals.

B. F. Morrey, MD

Biologically Enhanced Healing of the Rotator Cuff
Gordon NM, Maxson S, Hoffman JK (Coordinated Health, Bethlehem, PA; Osiris Therapeutics, Inc, Columbia, MD)
Orthopedics 35:498-504, 2012

Failure of rotator cuff repair is a well-documented problem. Successful repair is impeded by muscle atrophy, fat infiltration, devascularization, and scar tissue formation throughout the fibrocartilagenous transition zone. This case study exemplifies a technique to biologically augment rotator cuff healing. Clinically, pain and function improved. Postoperative magnetic resonance imaging evaluation confirmed construct integrity. Biological enhancement of the healing process and physiologically based alterations in rehabilitation protocols can successfully treat complicated rotator cuff tears. Prospective studies with larger sample sizes and continued follow-up are necessary to assess the definitive efficacy of this treatment modality.

▶ As a rule, I do not review case reports, as these are more "gee whiz" than offering any insights that are of substantive value. The rationale of including this report, of just 1 patient, is to introduce this approach that is being actively investigated around the globe. The use of biological enhancement to assist in the healing of rotator cuff tears is now widespread. The science to support the concept is strong. The clinical data to prove the proper formula or procedure have been described is lacking. The use of platelet-rich plasma, so widespread in the United States, is largely dues to its safety and conceptual attractiveness, not its proven efficacy. However, the thrust will continue, and I feel we will develop reliable processes and procedures in the not too distant future. And they will be scientifically justified.

B. F. Morrey, MD

Biomechanical Evaluation of Transosseous Rotator Cuff Repair: Do Anchors Really Matter?
Salata MJ, Sherman SL, Lin EC, et al (Univ Hosps Case Med Ctr, Cleveland, OH; Missouri Orthopaedic Inst, Columbia; Northwestern Univ, Chicago, IL; et al)
Am J Sports Med 41:283-290, 2013

Background.—Suture anchor fixation has become the preferred method for arthroscopic repairs of rotator cuff tears. Recently, newer arthroscopic repair techniques including transosseous-equivalent repairs with anchors or arthroscopic transosseous suture passage have been developed.

Purpose.—To compare the initial biomechanical performance including ultimate load to failure and localized cyclic elongation between transosseous-equivalent repair with anchors (TOE), traditional transosseous repair with a curved bone tunnel (TO), and an arthroscopic transosseous repair technique utilizing a simple (AT) or X-box suture configuration (ATX).

Study Design.—Controlled laboratory study.

Methods.—Twenty-eight human cadaveric shoulders were dissected to create an isolated supraspinatus tear and randomized into 1 of 4 repair groups (TOE, TO, AT, ATX). Tensile testing was conducted to simulate the anatomic position of the supraspinatus with the arm in 60° of abduction and involved an initial preload, cyclic loading, and pull to failure. Localized elongation during testing was measured using optical tracking. Data were statistically assessed using analysis of variance with a Tukey post hoc test for multiple comparisons.

Results.—The TOE repair demonstrated a significantly higher mean ± SD failure load (558.4 ± 122.9 N) compared with the TO (325.3 ± 79.9 N), AT (291.7 ± 57.9 N), and ATX (388.5 ± 92.6 N) repairs ($P < .05$). There was also a significantly larger amount of first-cycle excursion in the AT group (8.19 ± 1.85 mm) compared with the TOE group (5.10 ± 0.89 mm). There was no significant difference between repair groups in stiffness during maximum load to failure or in normalized cyclic elongation. Failure modes were as follows: TOE, tendon (n = 4) and bone

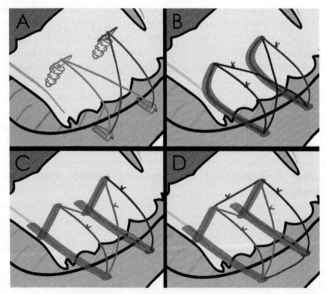

FIGURE 2.—Suture configurations: (A) transosseous equivalent (TOE), (B) transosseous (TO), (C) ArthroTunneler (AT), and (D) ArthroTunneler X-box (ATX). (Reprinted from Salata MJ, Sherman SL, Lin EC, et al. Biomechanical evaluation of transosseous rotator cuff repair: do anchors really matter? *Am J Sports Med.* 2013;41:283-290, with permission from The Author(s).)

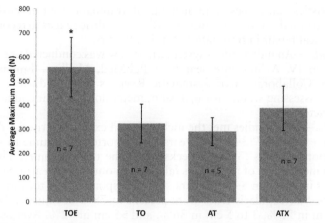

FIGURE 6.—Maximum load to failure with standard deviation. *The transosseous-equivalent (TOE) group exhibited a statistically greater maximum load than the transosseous (TO), ArthroTunneler (AT), and ArthroTunneler X-box (ATX) groups. (Reprinted from Salata MJ, Sherman SL, Lin EC, et al. Biomechanical evaluation of transosseous rotator cuff repair: do anchors really matter? *Am J Sports Med.* 2013;41:283-290, with permission from The Author(s).)

(n = 3); TO, suture (n = 6) and bone (n = 1); AT, tendon (n = 2) and bone (n = 3) and suture (n = 1); ATX, tendon (n = 7).

Conclusion.—This study demonstrates that anchorless repair techniques using transosseous sutures result in significantly lower failure loads than a repair model utilizing anchors in a TOE construct.

Clinical Relevance.—Suture anchor repair appears to offer superior biomechanical properties to transosseous repairs regardless of tunnel or suture configuration (Figs 2 and 6).

▶ The question of which cuff repair technique to use is important and has been extensively studied. I was attracted to this specific study as it assessed 3 different suture strategies compared with a single suture anchor design (Fig 2). The authors are experienced surgeons and investigators. The conclusions clearly showed the superiority of the suture anchors (Fig 6). Given this was a cadaver experiment, the osteoporosis associated with the specimens can sometimes give inaccurate information. Nonetheless, even in this setting, the anchor was superior.

B. F. Morrey, MD

An Evidenced-Based Examination of the Epidemiology and Outcomes of Traumatic Rotator Cuff Tears

Mall NA, Lee AS, Chahal J, et al (Rush Univ Med Ctr, Chicago, IL; et al)
Arthroscopy 29:366-376, 2013

Purpose.—The purpose of this study was to systematically review the literature to better define the epidemiology, mechanism of injury, tear characteristics, outcomes, and healing of traumatic rotator cuff tears. A secondary goal was to determine if sufficient evidence exists to recommend early surgical repair in traumatic rotator cuff tears.

Methods.—An independent systematic review was conducted of evidence Levels I to IV. A literature search of PubMed, Medline, Embase, and Cochrane Collaboration of Systematic Reviews was conducted, with 3 reviewers assessing studies for inclusion, methodology of individual study, and extracted data.

Results.—Nine studies met the inclusion and exclusion criteria. Average patient age was 54.7 (34 to 61) years, and reported mean time to surgical intervention, 66 days (3 to 48 weeks) from the time of injury. The most common mechanism of injury was fall onto an outstretched arm. Supraspinatus was involved in 84% of tears, and infraspinatus was torn in 39% of shoulders. Subscapularis tears were present in 78% of injuries. Tear size was <3 cm in 22%, 3 to 5 cm in 36%, and >5 cm in 42%. Average active forward elevation improved from 81° to 150° postoperatively. The weighted mean postoperative UCLA score was 30, and the Constant score was 77.

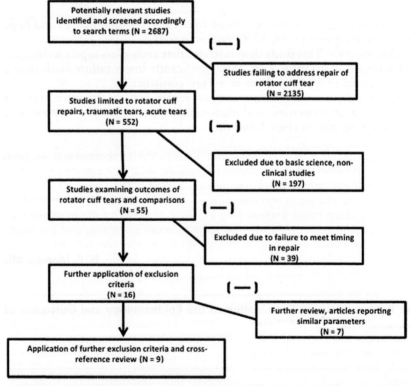

FIGURE 1.—Search strategy results. (Reprinted from Mall NA, Lee AS, Chahal J, et al. An evidenced-based examination of the epidemiology and outcomes of traumatic rotator cuff tears. *Arthroscopy.* 2013;29:366-376, with permission from Elsevier.)

Conclusions.—Traumatic rotator cuff tears are more likely to occur in relatively young (age 54.7), largely male patients who suffer a fall or trauma to an abducted, externally rotated arm. These tears are typically large and involve the subscapularis, and repair results in acceptable results. However, insufficient data prevent a firm recommendation for early surgical repair.

Level of Evidence.—Level IV, systematic review Levels III and IV studies (Fig 1).

▶ My disclosure is I am recognizably biased toward analytical assessments of the literature, especially when the topic is so clinically relevant. In fact, I have discussed this approach with the senior author, Dr Romeo, on occasion. I, and I am sure many others, have wondered whether we should treat the acute, traumatic cuff tear differently than the chronic lesion. Sadly, this study does not answer the question, but it does offer valuable demographic information. The lesions occur in younger, 57-year-old men, and the tears tend to be larger. The study protocol is worth noting (Fig 1). Of interest to me is the relative lack of acceptable studies, not an uncommon observation. Take-home message—we need to do better with our literature and improve the level of evidence.

B. F. Morrey, MD

Diagnostic Performance and Reliability of Ultrasonography for Fatty Degeneration of the Rotator Cuff Muscles

Wall LB, Teefey SA, Middleton WD, et al (Washington Univ School of Medicine, St Louis, MO)
J Bone Joint Surg Am 94:e83.1-e83.9, 2012

Background.—Diagnostic evaluation of rotator cuff muscle quality is important to determine indications for potential operative repair. Ultrasonography has developed into an accepted and useful tool for evaluating rotator cuff tendon tears; however, its use for evaluating rotator muscle quality has not been well established. The purpose of this study was to investigate the diagnostic performance and observer reliability of ultrasonography in grading fatty degeneration of the posterior and superior rotator cuff muscles.

Methods.—The supraspinatus, infraspinatus, and teres minor muscles were prospectively evaluated with magnetic resonance imaging (MRI) and ultrasonography in eighty patients with shoulder pain. The degree of fatty degeneration on MRI was graded by four independent raters on the basis of themodified Goutallier grading system. Ultrasonographic evaluation of fatty degeneration was performed by one of three radiologists with use of a three-point scale. The two scoring systems were compared to determine the diagnostic performance of ultrasonography. The interobserver and intraobserver reliability of MRI grading by the four raters were determined. The interobserver reliability of ultrasonography among the three radiologists was determined in a separate group of thirty study subjects. The weighted Cohen kappa, percentage agreement, sensitivity, and specificity were calculated.

Results.—The accuracy of ultrasonography for the detection of fatty degeneration, as assessed on the basis of the percentage agreement with MRI, was 92.5% for the supraspinatus and infraspinatus muscles and 87.5% for the teres minor. The sensitivity was 84.6% for the supraspinatus, 95.6% for the infraspinatus, and 87.5% for the teres minor. The specificity was 96.3% for the supraspinatus, 91.2% for the infraspinatus, and 87.5% for the teres minor. The agreement between MRI and ultrasonography was substantial for the supraspinatus and infraspinatus (kappa = 0.78 and 0.71, respectively) and moderate for the teres minor (kappa = 0.47). The interobserver reliability for MRI was substantial for the supraspinatus and infraspinatus (kappa = 0.76 and 0.77, respectively) and moderate for the teres minor (kappa = 0.59). For ultrasonography, the interobserver reliability was substantial for all three muscles (kappa = 0.71 for the supraspinatus, 0.65 for the infraspinatus, and 0.72 for the teres minor).

Conclusions.—The diagnostic performance of ultrasonography in identifying and grading fatty degeneration of the rotator cuff muscles was comparable with that of MRI. Ultrasonography can be used as the primary diagnostic imaging modality for fatty changes in rotator cuff muscles.

▶ For shoulder surgeons this is really an important study. Gerber has shown that the presence of fatty degeneration portends the outcome of intervention for rotator cuff tears. Hence, this study is quite relevant, as it compares 2 diagnostic modalities for fatty degeneration of the cuff tendons/muscle. The fact that the less-expensive and more readily available ultrasound modality (Fig 2 in the original article) is as reliable and sensitive as is the magnetic resonance imaging (Fig 1 in the original article) is revealing, and relevant. We must consider this option going forward.

B. F. Morrey, MD

Does Open Repair of Anterosuperior Rotator Cuff Tear Prevent Muscular Atrophy and Fatty Infiltration?

Di Schino M, Augereau B, Nich C (European Hosp of Paris, France)
Clin Orthop Relat Res 470:2776-2784, 2012

Background.—Repair of cuff tears involving rotator interval reportedly improves function. However, it is unclear whether successful repair prevents shoulder degenerative changes.

Questions/Purposes.—Therefore, we (1) documented the minimal 4-year function of patients who underwent open surgical repair for rotator interval tears; (2) evaluated repaired tendon healing with postoperative MRI; and (3) sought to determine the influence of tendon healing on muscular and glenohumeral joint changes.

Methods.—We retrospectively analyzed 22 patients (23 shoulders) treated by open transosseous reinsertion of supraspinatus and subscapularis tendons. The mean age of the patients was 53 years (range, 37—64 years). The tear was traumatic in four cases. Repair healing and muscular changes were assessed using MRI. The minimum followup was 46 months (mean, 75 months; range, 46—103 months).

Results.—We observed an improvement in the absolute Constant-Murley score from 63 points preoperatively to 76 points postoperatively. With the last followup MRI, the supraspinatus tendon repair had failed in two of the 23 shoulders, whereas the subscapularis tendon repair had healed in all cases. Once healing of the repaired tendon occurred, supraspinatus muscle atrophy never worsened. However, on MRI fatty infiltration of the rotator cuff muscles increased despite successful tendon repair. Glenohumeral arthritis remained stable. Postoperative abduction and internal rotation strengths were better when the standardized supraspinatus muscle area was greater than 0.5 at the final evaluation.

Conclusion.—Durable functional improvement and limited degenerative articular and muscular changes can be expected in most patients 4 to 10 years after open repair of anterosuperior cuff tears provided that healing of the cuff is obtained.

Level of Evidence.—Level IV, therapeutic study. See Guidelines for Authors for a complete description of levels of evidence.

▶ As we become more technically competent in performance of rotator cuff repair, some biologic issues will continue to frustrate our efforts to obtain long-term restoration of function. Although this study covers relatively few patients, the surveillance period is more than 4 years. More importantly is the specific question being asked—does a successful repair prevent progressive muscle/tendon degeneration-fatty infiltration? In a word, no. This insight is important when trying to understand the long-term efficacy of various intervention or treatment strategies.

B. F. Morrey, MD

Analysis of Rotator Cuff Repair Trends in a Large Private Insurance Population

Zhang AL, Montgomery SR, Ngo SS, et al (David Geffen School of Medicine at UCLA)
Arthroscopy 29:623-629, 2013

Purpose.—The purpose of this study was to identify current trends in open and arthroscopic surgical treatment of rotator cuff tears across sex, age, and region in the United States.

Methods.—Using the PearlDiver Patient Record Database (PearlDiver, Fort Wayne, IN), a publicly available national database of insurance records, patients who underwent rotator cuff repair from 2004 through 2009 were identified. The number of open (CPT codes 23410, 23412, 23420) and arthroscopic (CPT code 29827) rotator cuff repairs were quantified in isolation and in combination with acromioplasty (CPT codes 23415, 29826). The type of procedure, date, sex, and region of the country

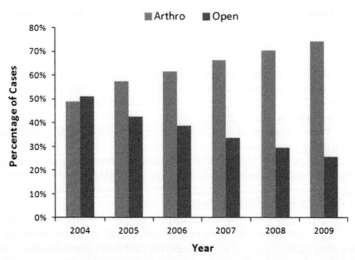

FIGURE 1.—Percentage of arthroscopic versus open rotator cuff repair by year. In 2004, 49% of rotator cuff repairs were performed arthroscopically, whereas 51% were open repairs. There was a steady increase in the proportion of arthroscopic repairs; in 2009, 74% were performed arthroscopically and only 26% were open repairs. Cochran-Armitage trend testing revealed these trends to be statistically significant, with a P value less than .0001. (Reprinted from Arthroscopy: The Journal of Arthroscopic and Related Surgery. Zhang AL, Montgomery SR, Ngo SS, et al. Analysis of rotator cuff repair trends in a large private insurance population. *Arthroscopy*. 2013;29:623-629, Copyright 2013, with permission from the Arthroscopy Association of North America.)

was identified for each patient. Trend tests (χ^2 and Cochran-Armitage) were used to determine statistical significance.

Results.—There were 151,866 rotator cuff repair procedures identified in the database from 2004 through 2009, which represented an incidence of 13.6 for every 1,000 patients assigned an orthopaedic International Classification of Diseases, Ninth Revision (ICD-9) or Current Procedural Terminology (CPT) code. Male patients accounted for 60% of the repairs and female patients for 40%. There were 98,174 arthroscopic cuff repairs (65%) and 53,692 open repairs (35%). The annual percentage of arthroscopic cases increased from 48.8% in 2004 to 74.3% in 2009, whereas the percentage of open cases decreased from 51.2% in 2004 to 25.7% in 2009 ($P < .0001$). Acromioplasty was also performed in 47.3% of cases, and the rate showed only a slight increase (from 46.6% to 47.8%) between 2004 and 2009 ($P < .01$). All regions of the United States showed similar surgical trends and trends for sex and age distributions.

Conclusions.—Our analysis shows that the majority of rotator cuff repairs in the United States are now performed arthroscopically (>74%) and there has been a recent steady decline in performance of open rotator cuff repair. Concomitant acromioplasty is performed approximately half the time, and this trend is increasing slightly. These findings were consistent across age, sex, and region in the United States.

Level of Evidence.—IV, cross-sectional study (Fig 1).

▶ Rotator cuff repair is the most frequently performed shoulder procedure. The issue is very important from a shear volume perspective and hence has been the subject of a guideline issued in 2010 by the American Academy of Orthopaedic Surgeons (AAOS). Currently an "Appropriate Use Criteria" statement is being formulated by the AAOS. It is a major practice shift to see the procedure has gone from a 50% to 50% ration of scope to open procedure in 2004 to a 75% to 25% ratio of scope to open procedure in 2009 (Fig 1). This trend will not reverse. Another particularly noteworthy observation is that 50% had an associated acromioplasty. Of even greater interest is the lack of wide variation in use and practice patterns geographically.

B. F. Morrey, MD

Clinical Outcome in All-Arthroscopic Versus Mini-Open Rotator Cuff Repair in Small to Medium-Sized Tears: A Randomized Controlled Trial in 100 Patients With 1-Year Follow-up
van der Zwaal P, Thomassen BJW, Nieuwenhuijse MJ, et al (Med Ctr Haaglanden, The Hague, The Netherlands; Leiden Univ Med Ctr, The Netherlands; et al)
Arthroscopy 29:266-273, 2013

Purpose.—The purpose of this study was to compare clinical outcomes in the first postoperative year of patients with full-thickness small to medium-sized tears undergoing all-arthroscopic (AA) versus mini-open (MO) rotator cuff repair.

Methods.—One hundred patients were randomized to either AA or MO rotator cuff repair at the time of surgery on an intention-to-treat basis. Patients were evaluated before and 6, 12, 26, and 52 weeks after surgery using the Disabilities of the Arm, Shoulder, and Hand (DASH) score as a primary outcome score and the Constant—Murley score, visual analog scale (VAS)—pain/impairment score, and measurement of active forward flexion/external rotation as secondary outcome measures. Ultrasound evaluation was used to assess structural integrity of the repair 1 year postoperatively.

Results.—Forty-seven patients were analyzed in the AA group and 48 in the MO group. Five patients were lost to follow-up. Mean age was 57.2 (SD 8.0) years in the AA group and 57.8 (SD 7.9) years in the MO group. Primary and secondary outcome measures significantly improved in both groups postoperatively. Overall mean primary and secondary postoperative outcome scores did not statistically significantly differ between the treatment groups (DASH between-group mean difference: -3.4; 95% confidence interval [CI], -10.2 to 3.4; $P = .317$). However, at the 6-week follow-up, DASH score, VAS—pain and —impairment, and active forward flexion were significantly more improved in the AA group than in the MO group. A retear was seen in 8 patients (17%) in the AA group and 6 patients

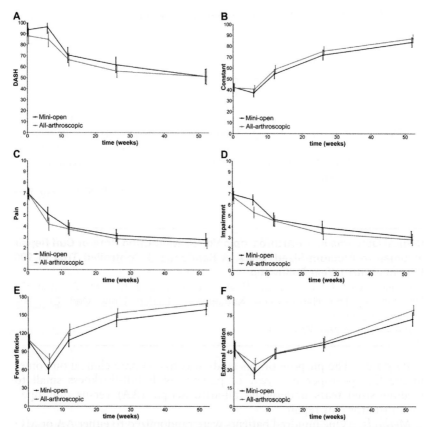

FIGURE 2.—Mean outcome scores (± SD) of patients undergoing the all-arthroscopic (black line) and mini-open (gray line) procedures over time (weeks). (A) DASH score. (B) Constant score (B). (C) Visual analog scale—pain. (D) Visual analog scale—impairment. (E) Active forward flexion in degrees. (F) Active external rotation in degrees. (Reprinted from Arthroscopy: The Journal of Arthroscopic and Related Surgery. van der Zwaal P, Thomassen BJW, Nieuwenhuijse MJ, et al. Clinical outcome in all-arthroscopic versus mini-open rotator cuff repair in small to medium-sized tears: a randomized controlled trial in 100 patients with 1-year follow-up. *Arthroscopy.* 2013;29:266-273, Copyright 2013, with permission from the Arthroscopy Association of North America.)

(13%) in the MO group. Five patients in the AA group (11%) and 6 patients (13%) in the MO group developed adhesive capsulitis.

Conclusions.—Functional outcome, pain, range of motion, and complications do not significantly differ between patients treated with all-arthroscopic repair and those treated with mini-open repair in the first year after surgery. Patients do attain the benefits of treatment somewhat sooner (6 weeks) with the arthroscopic procedure.

Level of Evidence.—Level II, randomized controlled trial without postoperative blinding (Fig 2).

▶ The ability to successfully perform prospective randomized studies in our specialty is quite difficult. It is appropriate, therefore, to highlight a well-done

prospective study that addresses a controversial question. The bulk of the literature does tend to show no difference between the 2 techniques studied here. This
study would seem to be definitive with 100 patients followed for a year. If there is
an advantage it is in the earlier recovery in the all arthroscopic patients (Fig 2). So
what should be the determining factor, or the next logical study? Cost! To study
this, accurate surgical costs must be fully allocated, and the analysis must of
course include the additional rehabilitative resources required to achieve comparable results. I'll keep my eye out for that study.

B. F. Morrey, MD

A Comparison of Outcomes After Arthroscopic Repair of Partial Versus Small or Medium-Sized Full-Thickness Rotator Cuff Tears

Peters KS, McCallum S, Briggs L, et al (Univ of New South Wales, Sydney, Australia)
J Bone Joint Surg Am 94:1078-1085, 2012

Background.—Little is known about the outcomes after repair of partial-
thickness rotator cuff tears. The aim of this study was to assess the outcome
after repair of partial-thickness rotator cuff tears compared with full-
thickness tears. Our hypothesis was that repair of partial-thickness tears
leads to more shoulder stiffness but fewer retears compared with repair of
full-thickness tears.

Methods.—A group of 105 consecutive patients who had a full-thickness
tear measuring <3 cm^2 was compared with a group of sixty-four patients
who had a partial-thickness tear. All tears were repaired with use of a knotless single-row arthroscopic repair. The American Shoulder and Elbow
Surgeons (ASES) score and standardized patient and examiner-determined
outcomes were obtained preoperatively and at six, twelve, and twenty-
four weeks and at two years after surgery. Rotator cuff integrity was determined by ultrasound examination at six months and two years after surgery.

Results.—Examiner-determined postoperative stiffness at six weeks was
common in both groups (50% of those with a partial-thickness tear and
47% of those with a full-thickness tear) but was decreased compared
with preoperative findings in both groups to 21% and 19%, respectively,
at three months and to 15% and 14% at six months. The ultrasound-
determined retear rate was small (5% in the partial-thickness group and
10% in the full-thickness group) at six months, but increased to 10% and
20%, respectively, at twenty-four months. The ASES score, patient-
determined overall shoulder function, and all pain scores were superior to
preoperative scores at six months ($p < 0.001$) and at twenty-four months
($p < 0.001$) in both groups.

Conclusions.—Arthroscopic repair of partial-thickness and small and
medium-sized full-thickness rotator cuff tears was associated with excellent
medium-term clinical outcomes with low retear rates. The data did not
support our hypothesis: the differences in retear rate and postoperative

shoulder stiffness rate found between the two groups did not reach significance.

▶ This is a nice prospective study of a relevant clinical question: Do partial tears do better than small full-thickness tears when repaired arthroscopically? The authors conclude that there is no statistical difference. However, one reason for selecting this article is to underscore a growing concern that I have with our literature. The obsession with statistical analysis sometimes distorts clinical truth. While there is no statistical difference, the retear rates are twice as common in the full-thickness than in the partial-thickness tears (Fig 2 in the original article). For this clinician, complication rates that differ by 100% are significant to me and my patient.

All of that said, this is a very nice, clean, and relevant study that does disprove one assumption—the partial tear will have greater postoperative stiffness. This was not found to be the case.

B. F. Morrey, MD

Arthroscopic Single-Row Versus Double-Row Rotator Cuff Repair: A Meta-analysis of the Randomized Clinical Trials
Sheibani-Rad S, Giveans MR, Arnoczky SP, et al (McLaren Regional Med Ctr/ Michigan State Univ, Flint; Minnesota Sports Medicine and Twin Cities Orthopedics, Minneapolis; Michigan State Univ, East Lansing; et al)
Arthroscopy 29:343-348, 2013

Purpose.—The purpose of this meta-analysis was to critically assess whether there are differences in clinical outcomes between single-row and double-row rotator cuff repair in prospective randomized Level I studies.

Methods.—Using Medline, Scopus, Scirus, CINAHL (Cumulative Index to Nursing and Allied Health Literature), and the Cochrane Library, as well as a hand search, we searched for randomized prospective trials comparing single-row and double-row rotator cuff repair. The functional outcome scores included the American Shoulder and Elbow Surgeons shoulder scale, the Constant shoulder score, and the University of California, Los Angeles shoulder rating scale. A test of heterogeneity was performed to determine whether there was a difference across the included studies.

Results.—Five studies met our inclusion criteria. A test of heterogeneity showed no difference across these studies. The functional American Shoulder and Elbow Surgeons; Constant; and University of California, Los Angeles outcomes scores showed no difference between single- and double-row rotator cuff repair.

Conclusions.—We found no significant differences in clinical outcomes between single-row and double-row rotator cuff repair in a meta-analysis of Level I studies.

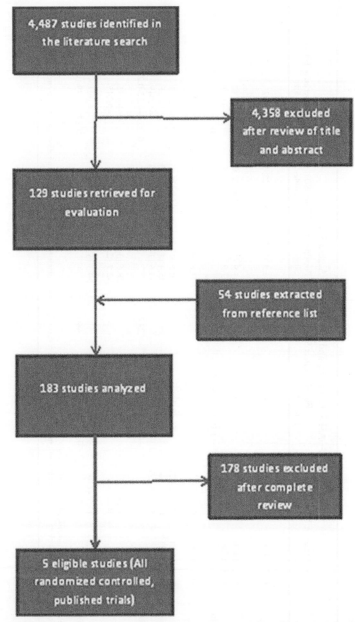

FIGURE 1.—Flowchart showing studies retrieved for systematic review and meta-analysis of randomized clinical trials on single-row versus double-row arthroscopic rotator cuff repair. (Reprinted from Arthroscopy: The Journal of Arthroscopic and Related Surgery. Sheibani-Rad S, Giveans MR, Arnoczky SP, et al. Arthroscopic single-row versus double-row rotator cuff repair: a meta-analysis of the randomized clinical trials. *Arthroscopy*. 2013;29:343-348, Copyright 2013, with permission from the Arthroscopy Association of North America.)

TABLE 2.—ASES, Constant, and UCLA Scores Across Studies

Study	Preoperative Mean (SD)		Preoperative Effect Size		Postoperative Mean (SD)		Postoperative Effect Size	
	Single	Double	Effect Size	P Value	Single	Double	Effect Size	P Value
ASES score								
Burks et al.[13]	41.0 (21.5)	37.6 (19.3)	0.166		85.9 (14.0)	85.5 (20.0)	0.023	
Franceschi et al.[17]								
Grasso et al.[14]								
Koh et al.[16]	38.8 (14.0)	38.1 (11.1)	0.055		85.9 (15.2)	83.4 (20.9)	0.137	
Lapner et al.[15]	47.8 (17.6)	54 (19)	-0.338		87.9 (16.9)	89.3 (17.5)	-0.081	
Weighted effect size			-0.10 (-0.34-0.18)	.357			0.01 (-0.27-0.29)	.484
Constant score								
Burks et al.[13]	44.1 (18.8)	45.6 (20.3)	-0.077		77.8 (9.0)	74.4 (18.4)	0.235	
Franceschi et al.[17]								
Grasso et al.[14]	73.2 (19.0)	77.5 (14.7)	-0.235		100.5 (17.8)	104.9 (21.8)	-0.221	
Koh et al.[16]	61.4 (18.1)	63.5 (17.6)	-0.118		85.4 (13.8)	82.5 (21.9)	0.158	
Lapner et al.[15]	55.1 (15)	58.2 (19.2)	-0.179		85.6 (14)	86.3 (14.2)	-0.049	
Weighted effect size			-0.17 (-0.41-0.08)	.247			0.01 (-0.25-0.24)	.490
UCLA score								
Burks et al.[13]	12.1 (3.9)	13.6 (4.6)	-0.352		28.6 (3.6)	29.5 (5.6)	-0.191	
Franceschi et al.[17]	11.6 (2.1)	10.2 (2.6)	0.592		32.9 (2.4)	33.4 (1.6)	-0.245	
Grasso et al.[14]								
Koh et al.[16]	18.0 (4.8)	17.7 (4.0)	0.068		29.3 (5.2)	29.8 (6.7)	-0.083	
Weighted effect size			0.13 (-0.19-0.55)	.660			-0.17 (-0.49-0.15)	.301

Editor's Note: Please refer to original journal article for full references.
NOTE. Weighted effect sizes are reported with 95% confidence intervals in parentheses. Positive effect sizes reflect greater single-row scores, whereas negative effect sizes show greater double-row scores.

Level of Evidence.—Level I, meta-analysis of Level I randomized controlled studies (Fig 1, Table 2).

▶ Although not receiving the same attention as does the anterior cruciate ligament to the sports surgeon, the issues of single- or double-row suture for full-thickness cuff tears does occupy a considerable portion of the shoulder literature. Of note is that of the almost 4500 articles on the general topic, only 5 were of sufficient focus and rigor to be included in the study (Fig 1). So beware, the conclusions are based on only 5 studies. However, there is no suggestion of a hint of difference between the 2 techniques (Table 2). Enough said. So, because suture anchors are expensive, it would seem clear that the single-row technique would be the treatment of choice.

B. F. Morrey, MD

A Multicenter Randomized Controlled Trial Comparing Single-Row with Double-Row Fixation in Arthroscopic Rotator Cuff Repair
Lapner PLC, Sabri E, Rakhra K, et al (Univ of Ottawa, Ontario, Canada; Pan Am Clinic, Winnipeg, Manitoba, Canada; Univ of Manitoba, Winnipeg, Canada)
J Bone Joint Surg Am 94:1249-1257, 2012

Background.—Controversy exists regarding the optimal technique for arthroscopic rotator cuff repair. The purpose of this multicenter, randomized, double-blind controlled study was to compare the functional outcomes and healing rates after use of single-row and double-row suture techniques for repair of the rotator cuff.

Methods.—Ninety patients undergoing arthroscopic rotator cuff repair were randomized to receive either a single-row or a double-row repair. The primary objective was to compare the Western Ontario Rotator Cuff Index (WORC) score at twentyfour months. Secondary objectives included comparison of the Constant and American Shoulder and Elbow Surgeons (ASES) scores and strength between groups. Anatomical outcomes were assessed with magnetic resonance imaging (MRI) or ultrasonography to determine the postoperative healing rates.

Results.—Baseline demographic data including age ($p = 0.29$), sex ($p = 0.68$), affected side ($p = 0.39$), and rotator cuff tear size ($p = 0.28$) did not differ between groups. The WORC score did not differ significantly between groups at any time point ($p = 0.48$ at baseline, $p = 0.089$ at three months, $p = 0.52$ at six months, $p = 0.83$ at twelve months, and $p = 0.60$ at twenty-four months). The WORC score at each postoperative time point was significantly better than the baseline value. The Constant score, ASES score, and strength did not differ significantly between groups at any time point. Logistic regression analysis demonstrated that a smaller initial tear size and double-row fixation were associated with higher healing rates.

Conclusions.—No significant differences in functional or quality-of-life outcomes were identified between single-row and double-row fixation techniques. A smaller initial tear size and a double-row fixation technique

TABLE 3.—Demographics and Final Treatment Outcomes According to Healing Status

	Intact* (N = 55)	Retear* (N = 21)	P Value[†]
Age (yr)	56.8 ± 7.2	58.6 ± 10.4	0.479
Initial tear size (mm)			
Coronal	20.4 ± 9.4 (20)	28.4 ± 10 (30)	0.0018[‡]
Sagittal	17.9 ± 6.9 (17)	22.8 ± 9.1 (20)	0.016[‡]
ASES score[§]	87.7 ± 16.84 (94)	81.3 ± 19.6 (90)	0.180
Constant score	83.0 ± 16.5 (87)	74.3 ± 15.3 (80)	0.044[‡]
WORC score[#]	83.9 ± 20.4 (93)	77.3 ± 20.3 (86)	0.22
Strength (kg)	7.2 ± 3.2 (7.4)	4.9 ± 1.8 (4.5)	0.0013[‡]

*The values are given as the mean and standard deviation, with the median in parentheses.
[†]Calculated with use of a t test.
[‡]Significant.
[§]ASES = American Shoulder and Elbow Surgeons.
[#]WORC = Western Ontario Rotator Cuff Index.

were associated with higher healing rates as assessed with ultrasonography or MRI.

Level of Evidence.—Therapeutic Level I. See Instructions for Authors for a complete description of levels of evidence (Table 3).

▶ This is a simple yet elegant prospective study of a clinically relevant question. The controversy that surrounds the utility of single- or double-row fixation strategies for rotator cuff tears is a dominant one in shoulder circles. This study is adequately powered and executed to seem to resolve this issue; there is no advantage in the tear size treated using a double-row fixation strategy (Table 3). What is known is that suture anchors are expensive and the double-row surgery often takes longer to accomplish. Hence the more expensive procedure is not more beneficial—that is, is not cost-effective. Although this may not be the central message or the author's intent, going forward this is the kind of information that we will need to make the appropriate patient care decisions.

B. F. Morrey, MD

Good function after shoulder arthroplasty
Fevang B-TS, Lygre SHL, Bertelsen G, et al (Haukeland Univ Hosp, Bergen, Norway; et al)
Acta Orthop 83:467-473, 2012

Background and Purpose.—Different results after shoulder arthroplasty have been found for different diagnostic groups. We evaluated function, pain, and quality of life after shoulder arthroplasty in 4 diagnostic groups.

Patients and Methods.—Patients with shoulder arthroplasties registered in the Norwegian Arthroplasty Register from 1994 through 2008 were posted a questionnaire in 2010. 1,107 patients with rheumatoid arthritis (RA), osteoarthritis (OA), acute fracture (AF), or fracture sequela (FS) returned completed forms (65% response rate). The primary outcome

TABLE 5.—Preoperative OSS, Current OSS, and Change in OSS, Divided into Pain and Function Scores, for Patients With the Four Major Diagnoses

Diagnosis[a]	Mean (SD) Preoperatively	Mean (SD) Currently	Mean Change[b]	Adjusted Difference[c]	P-value
OSS pain					
Rheumatoid arthritis	3.6 (2.2)	9.8 (4.5)	6.7	Ref.	
Fracture sequelae	4.6 (4.1)	8.4 (4.3)	4.4	−2.4	<0.001
Acute fracture	13 (5.2)	9.6 (4.1)	−3.7	−	−
Osteoarthritis	3.6 (2.3)	9.5 (4.7)	6.4	−0.3	0.5
OSS function					
Rheumatoid arthritis	12 (6)	20 (8)	9.2	Ref.	
Fracture sequelae	13 (9)	19 (9)	7.0	−2.2	0.02
Acute fracture	27 (10)	20 (9)	−7.0	−	−
Osteoarthritis	14 (7)	23 (8)	9.5	0.4	0.7

[a]The patients who were operated due to acute fractures were excluded from the regression analysis.
[b]For RA, FS, and OA, the mean changes were adjusted for sex, age, and revision status while unadjusted mean change is given for acute fractures since they were not included in the analyses.
[c]The difference in change compared to the reference group, with corresponding p-values, calculated using linear regression analysis with adjustment for age, sex, and prosthesis type.

measure was the Oxford shoulder score (OSS), which assesses symptoms and function experienced by the patient on a scale from 0 to 48. A secondary outcome measure was the EQ-5D, which assesses life quality. The patients completed a questionnaire concerning symptoms 1 month before surgery, and another concerning the month before they received the questionnaire.

Results.—Patients with RA and OA had the best results with a mean improvement in OSS of 16 units, as opposed to 11 for FS patients. Both shoulder pain and function had improved substantially. The change in OSS for patients with AF was negative (−11), but similar end results were obtained for AF patients as for RA and OA patients. Quality of life had improved in patients with RA, OA, and FS.

Interpretation.—Good results in terms of pain relief and improved level of function were obtained after shoulder arthroplasty for patients with RA, OA, and—to a lesser degree—FS. A shoulder arthropathy had a major effect on quality of life, and treatment with shoulder replacement substantially improved it (Table 5).

▶ Although this is a questionnaire study, the question is interesting and the analysis carefully done. Knowing the expected outcome as a function of age and underlying diagnosis are of course important parameters of which to be aware for any surgical intervention. For joint replacement, these questions have been addressed in the past. Hence, the findings here are not really new, but do depict an international experience with a large database. We have documented similar differences at the elbow. That posttraumatic arthritis does less well regarding pain and function (Table 5), and almost certainly relates to the soft-tissue alteration associated with the injury, its prior surgical treatment, or both.

B. F. Morrey, MD

6 Spine

Introduction

With the continued explosion in online medical and surgical content available to the orthopedic practitioner, I believe the value for readers of the Spine section of the 2013 YEAR BOOK OF ORTHOPEDICS continues to be high, and I am grateful to be a part of this service. This year's selections represent the best of over 900 articles reviewed. While the depth and breadth of the selections will satisfy those wanting a synthesis of the relevant literature of the day in the Spine space, the emphasis continues to be on evidence-based clinical, quality, and outcomes studies. Readers will have the opportunity to get up to date on the latest investigations involving motion-sparing technologies in the cervical and lumbar spine. The use of robotics in spine surgery and issues with complications of minimal access surgery have been selected. Several articles related to medicolegal issues from epidural abscess and hematoma and wrong level spine surgery are available, as well as prehospital interventions for spinal injuries in the sports arena. Pediatric spine selections detail patient outcome variability across children's hospitals in the United States and the validation of a smart phone app for scoliosis measurements. Topics such as vertebroplasty, obesity, preoperative embolization on blood loss in oncologic surgeries, and retrograde ejaculation are reviewed. It was a pleasure reviewing last year's available literature, and I hope these selections provide insight, opinion, and enthusiasm for all that was worth reading in spine last year and look forward to having this YEAR BOOK as a useful reference for the future!

Paul M. Huddleston, MD

Meta-Analysis of Vertebral Augmentation Compared With Conservative Treatment for Osteoporotic Spinal Fractures

Anderson PA, Froyshteter AB, Tontz WL Jr (Univ of Wisconsin, Madison; Coastal Orthopedics, Bradenton, FL)
J Bone Miner Res 28:372-382, 2013

Cement augmentation is a controversial treatment for painful vertebral compression fractures (VCF). Our research questions for the meta-analysis were: Is there a clinical and statistical difference in pain relief, functional improvement, and quality of life between conservative care and cement augmentation for VCF and, if so, are they maintained at longer time points? We conducted a search of MEDLINE from January 1980 to July 2011 using PubMed, Cochrane Database of Systematic Reviews and Controlled Trials, CINAHL, and EMBASE. Searches were performed from Medical Subject Headings. Terms "vertebroplasty" and "compression fracture" were used. The outcome variables of pain, functional measures, health-related quality of life (HRQOL), and new fracture risk were analyzed. A random effects model was chosen. Continuous variables were calculated using the standardized mean difference comparing improvement from baseline of the experimental group with the control group. New vertebral fracture risk was calculated using log odds ratio. Six studies met the criteria. The pain visual analog scale (VAS) mean difference was 0.73 (confidence interval [CI] 0.35, 1.10) for early (<12 weeks) and 0.58 (CI 0.19, 0.97) for late time points (6 to 12 months), favoring vertebroplasty ($p < 0.001$). The functional outcomes at early and late time points were statistically significant with 1.08 (CI 0.33, 1.82) and 1.16 (CI 0.14, 2.18), respectively. The HRQOL showed superior results of vertebroplasty compared with conservative care at early and late time points of 0.39 (CI 0.16, 0.62) and 0.33 (CI 0.16, 0.51), respectively. Secondary fractures were not statistically different between the groups, 0.065 (CI −0.57, 0.70). This meta-analysis showed greater pain relief, functional recovery, and health-related quality of life with cement augmentation compared with controls. Cement augmentation results were significant in the early (<12 weeks) and the late time points (6 to 12 months). This meta-analysis provides strong evidence in favor of cement augmentation in the treatment of symptomatic VCF fractures.

▶ The recent medical evidence and professional enthusiasm for the procedures of vertebroplasty and kyphoplasty have waned over the recent years following the publication of 2 negative articles showing no definitive value.[1,2] Since 2009, the American Academy of Orthopedic Surgeons has issued a position paper strongly opposing the use of "vertebroplasty for patients who present with an osteoporotic spinal compression fracture on imaging with correlating clinical signs and symptoms and who are neurologically intact."[3] I believe that with this report from the department of orthopedic surgery, University of Wisconsin, that the debate has not yet been settled. The authors correctly point out that although the 2 predominant negative studies from Kallmes et al[2] and Buchbinder et al[1] were well done, methodologically sound investigations, they were both underpowered and suffered from study subject crossover. I suspect there is an optimal time and patient for these procedures and that it will be early in the disease process and in those with little deformity. I would recommend not yet giving up on this treatment option for your patients.

P. Huddleston, MD

References

1. Buchbinder R, Osborne RH, Ebeling PR, et al. A randomized trial of vertebroplasty for painful osteoporotic vertebral fractures. *N Engl J Med.* 2009;361: 557-568.
2. Kallmes DF, Comstock BA, Heagerty PJ, et al. A randomized trial of vertebroplasty for osteoporotic spinal fractures. *N Engl J Med.* 2009;361:569-579.
3. American Academy of Orthopaedic Surgeons. The Treatment of Symptomatic Osteoporotic Spinal Compression Fractures: Guideline and Evidence Report. http://www.aaos.org/research/guidelines/SCFguideline.pdf. Accessed February 1, 2013.

Variability in Spinal Surgery Outcomes Among Children's Hospitals in the United States
Erickson MA, Morrato EH, Campagna EJ, et al (Children's Hosp Colorado, Aurora)
J Pediatr Orthop 33:80-90, 2013

Background.—We performed a retrospective cohort study of 7637 spinal fusion surgical cases from 2004 to 2006 at 38 children's hospitals participating in the Pediatric Health Information System database to evaluate the variability of in-hospital outcomes by patient factors and between facilities in children who underwent spinal surgery.

Methods.—Outcomes were stratified by whether children did or did not have neurological impairment. Multilevel multivariate logistic regression models were used to determine patient and hospital factors associated with in-hospital infections, surgical complications, and length of stay (LOS) ≥ 10 days.

Results.—Neurologically impaired (NI) children (N = 2117 out of 7637) represented 28% of the cases. The interhospital interquartile range of LOS for NI children was 6 to 8 days (median 7 d) and for non-neurologically impaired (NNI) children was 5 to 6 days (median 5 d). Children with NI had roughly 6 times higher rates of in-hospital infection and 3 times higher complication rates: major interhospital variation was seen for both of these outcomes. Hospital rates of infection ranged from 0% to 27% (median 10%) for NI and from 0% to 14% (median 2%) for NNI children. Complication rates ranged from 0% to 89% (median 33%) for NI and from 3% to 68% (median 9%) for NNI children. The following factors were associated with a LOS ≥ 10 days: in-hospital infection ($P < 0.0001$), surgical complication ($P < 0.0001$), and anterior/posterior versus posterior-only surgery ($P < 0.0001$). Hospital case volume was not associated with infection, surgical complication, or LOS ≥ 10 days.

Conclusions.—Substantial variation exists in reported outcomes for children undergoing spinal surgery in children's hospitals within the United

States. Further study is needed to characterize hospital-level factors related to surgical outcome to direct future quality improvement.

▶ The results from this study by authors from the Children's Hospital Colorado and the University of Colorado demonstrate a high variation in patient outcomes among 38 different children's hospitals across the United States for spine surgery. Although some practitioners and public policymakers might suggest that this is justification to stop spine surgery at some of the lower-performing hospitals and funnel the remainder to the higher-performing hospitals, with the expectation of better outcomes consummate with higher volumes, I think the issue is more basic. The issue is really that there is no real "system" for care of the children who have these complex surgeries. A true "system" would allow the best-known care to be known and accepted by all the caregivers with special attention to the truly vulnerable neurologically impaired patients. I hope that studies such as this one will serve as a clarion for better communication among hospitals and a concerted effort to move past ritual and routine to disseminate best practice. Shared surgical site infection prevention bundles and multidisciplinary care pathways would be great opportunities for the large systems of children's hospitals to rally around.

P. Huddleston, MD

Segmental mobility, disc height and patient-reported outcomes after surgery for degenerative disc disease: a prospective randomised trial comparing disc replacement and multidisciplinary rehabilitation
Johnsen LG, Brinckmann P, Hellum C, et al (Norwegian Univ of Science and Technology (NTNU), Trondheim, Norway)
Bone Joint J 95-B:81-89, 2013

This prospective multicentre study was undertaken to determine segmental movement, disc height and sagittal alignment after total disc replacement (TDR) in the lumbosacral spine and to assess the correlation of biomechanical properties to clinical outcomes.

A total of 173 patients with degenerative disc disease and low back pain for more than one year were randomised to receive either TDR or multidisciplinary rehabilitation (MDR). Segmental movement in the sagittal plane and disc height were measured using distortion compensated roentgen analysis (DCRA) comparing radiographs in active flexion and extension. Correlation analysis between the range of movement or disc height and patient-reported outcomes was performed in both groups. After two years, no significant change in movement in the sagittal plane was found in segments with TDR or between the two treatment groups. It remained the same or increased slightly in untreated segments in the TDR group and in this group there was a significant increase in disc height in the operated segments. There was no correlation between segmental movement or disc height and patient-reported outcomes in either group.

In this study, insertion of an intervertebral disc prosthesis TDR did not increase movement in the sagittal plane and segmental movement did not correlate with patient-reported outcomes. This suggests that in the lumbar spine the movement preserving properties of TDR are not major determinants of clinical outcomes.

▶ This article from the Norwegian authors details a prospective, randomized study of lumbar total disc arthroplasty (TDA) and results that may seem surprising to spine surgeons—that TDA does not increase range of motion (ROM) compared with nonoperative management. I don't perform total knee arthroplasty anymore but do remember counseling patients that one of the predictors of postoperative ROM was preoperative ROM. It should seem no surprise then when applying this experience to the spine that stiff, arthritic motion segments don't seem to move much after replacement. It is easy to see and measure the change in height of the disc space after placing the ProDisc 2 lumbar TDA. One of the challenges I have experienced in these operations is judging what size to accept when trialing the prosthesis. The irresolvable tradeoff becomes the limitation of ROM when trying to restore normal anatomic height, especially at the lumbosacral junction. Because the surgeon has to perform a much greater release than when performing an arthrodesis, there is a tendency to imbalance the motion segment, leaving a "fish mouth" deformity. The prosthesis cannot then be placed posterior enough and fails to approximate the center of rotation of the motion segment or is placed through the posterior end plate leading to subsidence and a fixed extension position. Even if the surgeon balances the disc space well, there is no way to release the posterior elements from the anterior approach again biasing toward extending the motion segment. Attempting to achieve a more normal disc height will only overstuff the disc joint, leading to a tight joint with decreased ROM.

A second very interesting observation is that motion gained or retained did not approach normal values in either randomized group, and ROM did not correlate with patient-reported outcome. Both of these challenge the basic argument justifying the placement of the devices in the first place.[1] As the old medical saying goes, "Nothing ruins great surgical results like long-term follow-up!"

P. Huddleston, MD

Reference

1. Zigler J, Delamarter R, Spivak JM, et al. Results of the prospective, randomized, multicenter Food and Drug Administration investigational device exemption study of the ProDisc-L total disc replacement versus circumferential fusion for the treatment of 1-level degenerative disc disease. *Spine (Phila Pa 1976)*. 2007;32: 1155-1162.

Cervical Intervertebral Disc Replacement
Cason GW, Herkowitz HN (William Beaumont Hosp, Royal Oak, MI)
J Bone Joint Surg Am 95:279-285, 2013

Symptomatic adjacent-level disease after cervical fusion has led to the development and testing of several discreplacement prostheses.

Randomized controlled trials of cervical disc replacement (CDR) compared with anterior cervical discectomy and fusion (ACDF) have demonstrated at least equivalent clinical results for CDR with similar or lower complication rates.

Biomechanical, kinematic, and radiographic studies of CDR reveal that the surgical level and adjacent vertebral level motion and center of rotation more closely mimic the native state.

Lower intradiscal pressures adjacent to CDR may help decrease the incidence of adjacent spinal-level disease, but long-term follow-up is necessary to evaluate this theory.

▶ This is a detailed and comprehensive review of the state of knowledge concerning the use of cervical disc replacement (CDR) technology. The authors remind us of the recurring theme that CDR has repeatedly been shown to be equivalent to anterior cervical discectomy and fusion (ACDF) when measuring short and intermediate outcomes. The devices benefit from many positive arguments based on morbidity, cost reductions from earlier return to work, and biomechanical arguments for a more accurate replication of a natural state. Unfortunately, follow-up to date has not demonstrated a difference over ACDF.

Although it is tempting to assume the development of adjacent disc joint pathology is predominantly based on restoring a mostly normal motion, this assumes little or no contribution from genetics or natural history. Rationalizing the eventual wear of adjacent levels as the normal progression of chronic disease allows the clinician to adjust the expectations and patient education to be open to the possibility of further symptoms in the future. If symptomatic wear of adjacent levels is an inevitability, then more consideration of the cost, safety, and global value of both interventions to large populations of patients must be ascertained to properly assign treatment options.

P. Huddleston, MD

Preoperative Embolization Significantly Decreases Intraoperative Blood Loss During Palliative Surgery for Spinal Metastasis
Kato S, Murakami H, Minami T, et al (Kanazawa Univ School of Medicine, Japan)
Orthopedics 35:e1389-e1395, 2012

Several studies have evaluated the efficacy of preoperative embolization in devascularizing tumors. However, no study has measured intraoperative blood loss in a single palliative surgery compared with a control group without preoperative embolization. The purpose of this retrospective study was to evaluate the efficacy of preoperative embolization on intraoperative blood loss in palliative decompression and instrumented surgery using a posterior approach for spinal metastasis.

Between 2000 and 2010, forty-six patients underwent palliative decompression and instrumented surgery using a posterior approach for spinal metastasis in the thoracic and lumbar spine. Preoperative embolization was performed in 23 patients (embolization group), and surgery was performed within 3 days after embolization. The embolic materials used were polyvinyl alcohol particles, gelatin sponge, and metallic coils. Twenty-three patients did not undergo embolization (no embolization group). Pain and neurologic symptoms in all 46 patients were relieved postoperatively. Average intraoperative blood loss was 520 mL (range, 140-1380 mL) in the embolization group and 1128 mL (range, 100-3260 mL) in the no embolization group ($P < .05$). In the embolization group, intraoperative blood loss was not correlated with the degree of tumor vascularization, completeness of embolization, or time between embolization and surgery.

Intraoperative blood loss after preoperative embolization was less than half that after no preoperative embolization.

▶ Although I have used preoperative embolization for highly vascular tumors such as paraganglioma and renal cell for many years, it has not been a standard in my spine practice to preoperatively embolize metastatic spine tumors in general. I was surprised to see that the results from the department of orthopedic surgery in Kanazawa, Japan, showed a reduction of 50% on average blood loss when using the technique. Although pure operative tumor embolization is not a new technique, and I would generally consider it a safe procedure, it is not without risk. It is becoming more clear that much of the risk of length of stay and postoperative infection can be minimized by reducing blood transfusions. It may well be that the authors' results can be repeated in another care setting, but the dramatic decrease in preoperative bleeding seen in this randomized study should at least merit consideration by surgeons performing any volume of spine surgeries for metastatic disease in the near future.

P. Huddleston, MD

Intervertebral Disc Height Changes After Weight Reduction in Morbidly Obese Patients and Its Effect on Quality of Life and Radicular and Low Back Pain
Lidar Z, Behrbalk E, Regev GJ, et al (Tel Aviv Sourasky Med Ctr, Israel; et al)
Spine 37:1947-1952, 2012

Study Design.—Prospective study in a morbidly obese population after bariatric surgery.

Objective.—To document the effect of significant weight reduction on intervertebral disc space height, axial back pain, radicular leg pain, and quality of life.

Summary of Background Data.—Low back pain is a common complaint in obese patients, and weight loss is found to improve low back pain and quality of life. The mechanism by which obesity causes low back pain is not fully understood.

On acute axial loading and offloading, intervertebral disc changes its height; there are no data on intervertebral disc height changes after significant weight reduction.

Methods.—Thirty morbidly obese adults who underwent bariatric surgery for weight reduction were enrolled in the study. Disc space height was measured before and 1 year after surgery. Visual analogue scale was used to evaluate axial and radicular pain. The 36-Item Short Form Health Survey and Moorehead-Ardelt questionnaires were used to evaluate changes in quality of life.

Results.—Body weight decreased at 1 year after surgery from an average of 119.6 ± 20.7 kg to 82.9 ± 14.0 kg corresponding to an average reduction in body mass index of 42.8 ± 4.8 kg/m^2 to 29.7 ± 3.4 kg/m^2 ($P < 0.001$).

The L4—L5 disc space height increased from 6 ± 1.3 mm, presurgery to 8 ± 1.5 mm 1 year postsurgery ($P < 0.001$).

Both axial and radicular back pain decreased markedly after surgery ($P < 0.001$). Patients' Moorehead-Ardelt score significantly improved after surgery ($P < 0.001$). Although the 36-Item Short Form Health Survey score did not show any statistically significant improvement after surgery, the physical component of the questionnaire showed a positive trend for improvement.

No correlation was noted between the amount of weight reduction and the increment in disc space height or back pain improvement.

Conclusion.—Bariatric surgery, resulting in significant weight reduction, was associated with a significant decrease in low back and radicular pain as well as a marked increase in the L4—L5 intervertebral disc height.

Reduction in body weight after bariatric surgery in morbidly obese patients is associated with a significant radiographical increase in the L4—L5 disc space height as well as a significant clinical improvement in axial back and radicular leg pain.

▶ Physicians have known for years that being overweight and deconditioned could predispose or aggravate preexisting back pain, but these researchers from Israel have quantified it in this clever study in patients undergoing bariatric surgery. With an average weight loss of about 39 kg 1 year postoperatively, their series of morbidly obese patients gained an average of 2 mm in disc height and axial and radicular pain decreased markedly. I am just surprised the discs did not bounce back even more. A more interesting long-term outcome would be to follow the patients longer to see if the effects, both radiographic and clinical, are durable. I wonder if the small vessel disease that is present in patients with diabetes mellitus will doom them to disc degeneration and painful radicular leg discomfort secondary to peripheral neuropathy. What are the potential effects of long-term malnutrition that is common postoperatively? Nevertheless, the results can provide all those caring for obese, deconditioned patients with low back pain more information for better patient counseling and education.

P. Huddleston, MD

Sports prehospital-immediate care and spinal injury: not a car crash in sight
Hanson JR, Carlin B (Dr Mackinnon Memorial Hosp, Isle of Skye, Scotland; Univ College Dublin, Ireland)
Br J Sports Med 46:1097-1101, 2012

The prehospital management of serious injury is a key skill required of pitch-side medical staff. Previously, specific training in sports prehospital-immediate care was lacking or not of a comparable standard to other aspects of emergency care. Many principles have been drawn from general prehospital care or in-hospital training courses. This article discusses sports prehospital-immediate care as a niche of general prehospital care, using spinal injury management as an illustration of the major differences. It highlights the need to develop the sport-specific prehospital evidence base, rather than relying exclusively on considerations relevant to prolonged immobilisation of multiply injured casualties from motor vehicle accidents, falls from height or burns.

▶ It has been several years since I have been the sideline physician at any of the local high school or college games, but I still remember the fun and excitement of the "big game" and the fact that fortunately not too many of the athletes were ever seriously injured. The lion's share of most of the problems were bumps and bruises, sprains, and strains that ice and early physical therapy could more than handle. Although our care and knowledge of sports-related head trauma has grown logarithmically since then, I believe that most of the families, coaches, and athletes saw me as a "sport medicine doctor," as in ankle, shoulder, knee specialist. I have come to think that many in the field of sports medicine see themselves in the same light: highly trained arthroscopists ever ready to repair and rehabilitate whatever bone or joint that happens to be limiting your athletic prowess, unless it's your spine, of course. But as I remember prior to my spine fellowship days, a spine or spinal cord injury in a game or practice was actually the injury I feared having to care for the most. This wonderful article is a fantastic review of the current knowledge and techniques of prehospital immediate care for the spine-injured athlete and should prove beneficial to all health care providers standing on the sidelines or in the stands. While mastering all the common care tactics for the usual bumps and bruises, providers owe it to themselves, the coaches, the public, and most of all the players to be thoroughly comfortable assessing and managing the potentially spine-injured athlete. There will be plenty of time to fix the anterior cruciate ligament or to rehabilitate the shoulder, but you may have only one brief moment to protect and safely transport the spine-injured player to avoid a catastrophic injury and ensure the best possible outcome.

P. Huddleston, MD

Errors of level in spinal surgery: An evidence-based systematic review
Longo UG, Loppini M, Romeo G, et al (Centre for Sport and Exercise Medicine, London, UK)
J Bone Joint Surg Br 94-B:1546-1550, 2012

Wrong-level surgery is a unique pitfall in spinal surgery and is part of the wider field of wrong-site surgery. Wrong-site surgery affects both patients and surgeons and has received much media attention. We performed this systematic review to determine the incidence and prevalence of wrong-level procedures in spinal surgery and to identify effective prevention strategies. We retrieved 12 studies reporting the incidence or prevalence of wrong-site surgery and that provided information about prevention strategies. Of these, ten studies were performed on patients undergoing lumbar spine surgery and two on patients undergoing lumbar, thoracic or cervical spine procedures. A higher frequency of wrong-level surgery in lumbar procedures than in cervical procedures was found. Only one study assessed preventative strategies for wrong-site surgery, demonstrating that current site-verification protocols did not prevent about one-third of the cases. The current literature does not provide a definitive estimate of the occurrence of wrong-site spinal surgery, and there is no published evidence to support the effectiveness of site-verification protocols. Further prevention strategies need to be developed to reduce the risk of wrong-site surgery.

▶ This is possibly the most important article of the year for the spine section of the YEAR BOOK, and I commend the authors for their intellectual courage and honesty in addressing such an important and taboo subject as wrong-level surgery. I agree that the incidence of wrong-level surgery in spine is grossly underreported. This can occur for many reasons. Surgeons practicing in hospitals or surgery centers may not be participating, either covertly or overtly, in an official program or checklist to prevent such events. I can imagine a scenario where the pathology of arthritis may be present at multiple levels of the spine and the intent may be to decompress only a specific degenerative level, but during the case, there arises confusion as to the correct level and a decompression is performed erroneously. The surgeon may recognize the error during the case and correct the situation by performing another decompression at the adjacent spinal level, which may be only 1.5 cm away. It would seem like such a small "detour" that many likely do not report the event or even acknowledge any real morbidity. I have heard rationalizations suggesting that "those levels were worn out anyway" to "I did not have to enlarge the incision" or "the patient would not have known anyway" when talking with other surgeons about their thoughts on the matter. I agree with the authors' findings that although the published risk may be in the 3% to 5% range, the actual risk may be up to 15%. Surgeons should make use of all the tools available (such as the American Academy of Orthopedic Surgeons'[1] and the North American Spine Society's[2] checklists) to prevent this potentially serious mistake. Most important would be having a surgical pause at the beginning of the case and a second, hard stop marking the spine with a metal marker and verifying the correct level prior to any destructive work on the spine.

P. Huddleston, MD

References

1. American Academy of Orthopedic Surgeons. Advisory Statement: Wrong Site Surgery. http://www.aaos.org/about/papers/advistmt/1015.asp. Accessed July 23, 2012.
2. North American Spine Society. Prevention of Wrong Site Surgery: Sign. Mark and X-Ray (SMaX). http://www.spine.org/Pages/PracticePolicy/ClinicalCare/SMAX/Default.aspx. Accessed July 23, 2012.

Thirty-day readmissions after elective spine surgery for degenerative conditions among US Medicare beneficiaries
Wang MC, Shivakoti M, Sparapani RA, et al (Med College of Wisconsin, Milwaukee; et al)
Spine J 12:902-911, 2012

Background Context.—Readmissions within 30 days of hospital discharge are undesirable and costly. Little is known about reasons for and predictors of readmissions after elective spine surgery to help plan preventative strategies.

Purpose.—To examine readmissions within 30 days of hospital discharge, reasons for readmission, and predictors of readmission among patients undergoing elective cervical and lumbar spine surgery for degenerative conditions.

Study Design.—Retrospective cohort study.

Patient Sample.—Patient sample includes 343,068 Medicare beneficiaries who underwent cervical and lumbar spine surgery for degenerative conditions from 2003 to 2007.

Outcome Measures.—Readmissions within 30 days of discharge, excluding readmissions for rehabilitation.

Methods.—Patients were identified in Medicare claims data using validated algorithms. Reasons for readmission were classified into clinically meaningful categories using a standardized coding system (Clinical Classification Software).

Results.—Thirty-day readmissions were 7.9% after cervical surgery and 7.3% after lumbar surgery. There was no dominant reason for readmissions. The most common reasons for readmissions were complications of surgery (26%–33%) and musculoskeletal conditions in the same area of the operation (15%). Significant predictors of readmission for both operations included older age, greater comorbidity, dual eligibility for Medicare/Medicaid, and greater number of fused levels. For cervical spine readmissions, additional risk factors were male sex, a diagnosis of myelopathy, and a posterior or combined anterior/posterior surgical approach; for lumbar spine readmissions, additional risk factors were black race, Middle Atlantic geographic region, fusion surgery, and an anterior surgical approach. Our model explained more than 60% of the variability in readmissions.

Conclusions.—Among Medicare beneficiaries, 30-day readmissions after elective spine surgery for degenerative conditions represent a target for improvement. Both patient factors and operative techniques are associated with readmissions. Interventions to minimize readmissions should be specific to surgical site and focus on high-risk subgroups where clinical trials of interventions may be of greatest benefit.

▶ I enjoy reading reports from the large Medicare databases, despite their inherent limitation of having a large dataset. National trends can often be more apparent when viewed across large geographic areas, and as the baby boomer population ages, Medicare-specific data will become more relevant to general spine practices. This article from the researchers at the University of Wisconsin details many surprising points. Foremost would be the acknowledgment of the importance of the 30-day readmission rate. It seems that I often spend a lot of time, effort, and organization on managing service-related issues such as length of stay and surgical site infection rate and obsessing over implant costs and cost per case, but I cannot remember recently considering a 30-day readmission rate as part of the value equation.[1] The readmission rates stated by these authors are surprisingly high; 7% for both cervical and lumbar spine postoperative Medicare patients with risk factors being male, black, and from the mid-Atlantic geographic region. Practitioners should temper these results from what they know is relevant to their practice in anticipation of the coming "tidal wave" of baby boomers in need of spinal stenosis care!

P. Huddleston, MD

Reference

1. Porter E. What Is Value in Health Care? *N Engl J Med.* 2010;363:2477-2481.

What Is the Prevalence of MRSA Colonization in Elective Spine Cases?

Chen AF, Chivukula S, Jacobs LJ, et al (Univ of Pittsburgh Med Ctr, PA)
Clin Orthop Relat Res 470:2684-2689, 2012

Background.—The incidence of methicillin-resistant Staphylococcus aureus (MRSA) infection is increasing. However, the prevalence of MRSA colonization among patients undergoing spine surgery is unclear.

Questions/Purposes.—We therefore (1) determined the prevalence of MRSA colonization in a population of patients scheduled for elective spine surgery; and (2) evaluated whether MRSA screening and treatment reduce the rate of early wound complications.

Methods.—We retrospectively reviewed prospectively collected data from 1002 patients undergoing elective spine surgery in 2010. There were 719 primary and 283 revision surgeries. Instrumentation was used in 72.0% cases and autologous iliac crest bone graft was taken in 65.1%. Twelve patients were lost to followup; of the remaining 990 patients, 503 were screened for MRSA and 487 were not. MRSA-colonized patients were treated with mupirocin and chlorhexidine. An early wound complication was defined as wound drainage or the presence of an abscess. Patients were followed for a minimum of 3 months (average, 7 months; range, 3–545 days).

Results.—Of the patients undergoing elective spine surgery and screened for MRSA, 14 of 503 (2.8%) were colonized with MRSA. The rates of early wound complications were similar for patients who were screened and pretreated for MRSA (17 of 503 [3.4%]) compared with those who were not (17 of 487 [3.5%]).

Conclusions.—The colonization rate for MRSA in our elective spine surgery population was comparable to that in the arthroplasty literature.

Level of Evidence.—Level III, retrospective comparative study. See the Guidelines for Authors for a complete description of levels of evidence.

▶ The investigators from the University of Pittsburgh have made a great contribution with their article describing methicillin-resistant *Staphylococcus aureus* (MRSA) colonization rates in elective spine cases. In what can only be described as a growing public health disaster, the emergence, spread, and increased resistance of MRSA in hospitals and the community will be an enormous drain of resources and a source of morbidity and mortality in the future for spine surgery patients. Although the colonization of patients and staff can be the cause of lost productivity and delays in treatment resulting in expensive decolonization procedures, it is the infection with this organism that is the real tragedy. Treating an MRSA deep wound infection can be an ordeal for patients and surgeons alike, but with the increasing use of instrumentation in spinal surgeries, an implant-associated spinal infection is catastrophic. The formation of biofilm on retained spinal implants often necessitates their removal, often after multiple surgeries and a prolonged antibiotic course. Hence, here is the real value in this article—it details the baseline prevalence of 2.8% in an elective population. I am surprised that the subsequent infection rate was not lower in the decolonized patient population, and the authors reported a surgical site infection rate of about 3.5%, which seems excessively high, but it may be that weaknesses in the study design are to blame. The more interesting question may be if the authors' recommendation of twice a day for 5 days intranasal mupirocin and 2 chlorhexidine baths prior to surgery don't improve the deep wound infection rate compared with baseline, what can we do differently? I see promise in better topical soaps as barriers to infection as well as improved patient education to increase compliance with their suggested preoperative surgical skin preparations. I believe the best practices will avoid irresponsible use of antibiotics to prevent the further development of antibiotic resistance.

P. Huddleston, MD

Medicolegal Cases for Spinal Epidural Hematoma and Spinal Epidural Abscess

French KL, Daniels EW, Ahn UM, et al (SUNY Upstate Med Univ, Syracuse, NY; Univ Hosps Case Med Ctr, Cleveland, OH)
Orthopedics 36:48-53, 2013

Spinal epidural hematoma and spinal epidural abscess are rare surgical emergencies resulting in significant neurologic deficits. Making the diagnosis for spinal epidural hematoma and spinal epidural abscess can be challenging; however, a delay in recognition and treatment can be devastating. The objective of this retrospective analysis study was to identify risk factors for an adverse outcome for the provider.

The LexisNexis Academic legal search database was used to identify a total of 19 cases of spinal epidural hematoma and spinal epidural abscess filed against medical providers. Outcome data on trial verdicts, age, sex, initial site of injury, time to consultation, time to appropriate imaging studies, time to surgery, and whether a rectal examination was performed or not were recorded. The results demonstrated a significant association between time to surgery more than 48 hours and an unfavorable verdict for the provider. The degree of permanent neurologic impairment did not appear to affect the verdicts. Fifty-eight percent of the cases did not present with an initial deficit, including loss of bowel or bladder control.

All medical professionals must maintain a high level of suspicion and act quickly. Physicians who are able to identify early clinical features, appropriately image, and treat within a 48 hour time frame have demonstrated a more favorable medicolegal outcome compared with their counterparts in filed lawsuits for spinal epidural hematoma and spinal epidural abscess cases (Table 1).

▶ Talking about spine surgery without talking about medico-legal issues may seem like talking about the duck without the water. Although the vast majority of practitioners may feel competent about the care they provide, there will always be poor outcomes. And in Western society that means there will always be lawsuits.

TABLE 1.—Comparison of Cases Won by the Plantiff Versus the Defendant

Variable	Plaintiff (n = 4)	Defendant (n = 15)
Sex distribution, %	Male, 75; female, 25	Male, 80; female, 20
Postoperation, %	No, 50; yes, 50	No, 47; yes, 53
Mean time to surgery, d	33.5	18.9
Mean time to imaging, d	33.75	4
Mean time to consultation, d	32.7	2.8
Surgical specialty consulted, %	Ortho, 0; NS, 50	Ortho, 33; NS, 33
Other consultation, %[a]	50	33

Abbreviations: Ortho, orthopedic surgeon; NS, neurosurgeon.
[a]Infectious disease, urology, pain management, and anesthesia.

This novel article reviews the LexisNexis Academic legal search database for malpractice cases concerning epidural abscess and epidural hematoma. These 2 entities, although different in etiology, have a similar pathophysiology, with both causing increasing pain, neurologic dysfunction, and the threat of permanent deficit from space-occupying lesions within the spinal canal. Clinically, both entities can be considered emergencies, and the authors describe the case details and outcomes of 19 cases that went to trial, approximately 50% of which occurred postoperatively (Table 1). Fifty-eight percent presented to the emergency department and 32% to the outpatient clinic. In none of the cases reviewed was a rectal examination documented, in spite of the often severe lower extremity complaints. The most significant threshold for return of function or return of judgment in favor of the plaintiff was time to surgery more than 48 hours after onset of symptoms. Plaintiffs were 100% successful in their litigations with a verdict of failure to diagnose and treat after this time. It is most illuminating to appreciate the difference in what the patients and providers value and how presence or absence of transient or permanent neurologic deficit, or lack of thorough physical examination, was important in predicting the verdicts. All providers caring for postoperative spine surgery patients or patients with risk factors for epidural hematoma or abscess should be aware of the presentation and shape their evaluation and treatment in a measured but rapid manner to preserve patient function and minimize malpractice risk.

P. Huddleston, MD

Comparison of Superior-Level Facet Joint Violations During Open and Percutaneous Pedicle Screw Placement

Babu R, Park JG, Mehta AI, et al (Duke Univ School of Medicine, Durham, NC)
Neurosurgery 71:962-969, 2012

Background.—Superior-level facet joint violation by pedicle screws may result in increased stress to the level above the instrumentation and may contribute to adjacent segment disease. Previous studies have evaluated facet joint violations in open or percutaneous screw cases, but there are no reports describing a direct institutional comparison.

Objective.—To compare the incidence of superior-level facet violation for open vs percutaneous pedicle screws and to evaluate patient and surgical factors that affect this outcome.

Methods.—We reviewed 279 consecutive patients who underwent an index instrumented lumbar fusion from 2007 to 2011 for degenerative spine disease with stenosis with or without spondylolisthesis. We used a computed tomography grading system that represents progressively increasing grades of facet joint violation. Patient and surgical factors were evaluated to determine their impact on facet violation.

Results.—Our cohort consisted of 126 open and 153 percutaneous cases. Percutaneous procedures had a higher overall violation grade ($P = .02$) and a greater incidence of high-grade violations ($P = .006$) compared with open procedures. Bivariate analysis showed significantly greater violations in

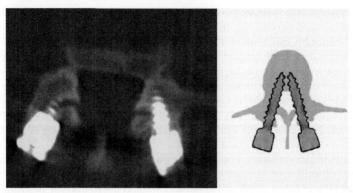

FIGURE 3.—Grade 3 violation: screw lies within the articular facet surface (*bilateral*). (Reprinted from Babu R, Park JG, Mehta AI, et al. Comparison of superior-level facet joint violations during open and percutaneous pedicle screw placement. *Neurosurgery.* 2012;71:962-970, with permission from the Congress of Neurological Surgeons.)

percutaneous cases for age < 65 years, obesity, pedicle screws at L4, and 1- and 2-level surgeries. Multivariate analysis showed the percutaneous approach and depth of the spine to be independent risk factors for high-grade violations.

Conclusion.—This study demonstrates greater facet violations for percutaneously placed pedicle screws compared with open screws (Fig 3).

▶ These researchers from Duke University Medical Center have reported a multi-surgeon, large, single-center series of spinal fusions revealing an increased incidence of high-grade facet joint violations at the cranial end of instrumented constructs when compared with an open technique. Although the study was retrospective in nature, it was interesting to note the 8-fold higher incidence in subsequent adjacent segment disease in 3-year follow-up within the group having high-grade facet violations (Fig 3). Although it is tempting to blame the high-grade facet violations on high body mass index or the increased lordosis present at the L4 spinal level, it is likely both methods of implant placement would benefit from a standardized classification of facet violation and its universal application intraoperatively. It remains to be seen whether newer technologies such as navigated implant placement using 3-dimensional imaging from the O-arm can minimize this iatrogenic event.

P. Huddleston, MD

Validation of a Scoliometer Smartphone App to Assess Scoliosis
Franko OI, Bray C, Newton PO (Univ of California, San Diego; Rady Children's Hosp and Health Ctr, San Diego, CA)
J Pediatr Orthop 32:e72-e75, 2012

Background.—Surgeons and software developers recognize that apps can improve patient care by replicating the function of existing medical devices. However, the incorporation of new tools requires that the clinical data being recorded is accurate and valid. This study attempts to validate a new iPhone app to measure scoliotic rotation. The objective of this study was to validate the scoliogauge iPhone application by comparing the results to simultaneous readings from a standard Scoliometer.

Methods.—Four orthopaedic medical providers (attending surgeon, fellow, resident, and nurse practitioner) each read a standard scoliometer at 60 randomly selected angular measurements between −30 and 30 degrees, whereas a blinded observer simultaneously recorded the angular measurement derived from the scoligauge app. The correlation between the 2 measurements were calculated using a Pearson correlation coefficient with a *P*-value set to <0.05 for significance.

Results.—The Pearson correlation values ranged from 0.9994 to 0.9996 for all providers and all *P*-values <0.001. There was no increase in time associated with using the app compared with the standard device.

Conclusions.—The scoligauge app is a convenient novel tool that replicates the function of a standard clinical scoliometer but with a potentially decreased financial cost and greater convenience for providers.

Clinical Relevance.—Validation of this new device demonstrates the potential to increase the distribution of cost-effective scoliosis screening tools to a broad population of medical providers (Fig 1).

▶ With the explosion of applications for the seemingly ubiquitous smart phones, I suppose it was only a matter of time before someone adapted the accelerometer built into the current generation iPhone as a scoliometer (Fig 1). I find the current phones indispensable in managing my clinic appointments and interfacing with patients' medical records, including viewing laboratory test results and advanced imaging. The scoliometer smart phone tested out almost perfect in a blind

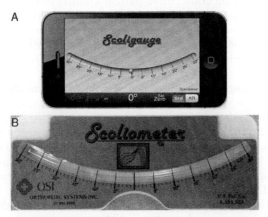

FIGURE 1.—Images of the scoligauge iPhone app (A) and scoliometer (B) used for the validation study. During actual testing, the iPhone was turned to face the reverse direction so that the 2 investigators could read the results simultaneously and blinded. (Reprinted from Franko OI, Bray C, Newton PO. Validation of a scoliometer smartphone app to assess scoliosis. *J Pediatr Orthop.* 2012;32:e72-e75, with permission from Lippincott Williams & Wilkins.)

comparison with a standard scoliometer and with very little training. The authors appear to have addressed the issue of a plastic adapter to interface with the patient's back (yet to be mass produced), and the app is currently available on the Apple App Store. Although I am not advocating for the medical use of a non-Food and Drug Administration—approved product (iPhone), I think this idea has promise and believe we will see more of this app in the future. Now if it could only help the surgeon with selecting a scoliosis brace!

P. Huddleston, MD

Retrograde ejaculation after anterior lumbar interbody fusion with and without bone morphogenetic protein-2 augmentation: A 10-year cohort controlled study
Comer GC, Smith MW, Hurwitz EL, et al (Stanford Univ School of Medicine, Redwood City, CA; Univ of Hawaii, Honolulu; et al)
Spine J 12:881-890, 2012

Background Context.—Retrograde ejaculation (RE) is a complication of anterior lumbar interbody fusion (ALIF) techniques. Most commonly, this results from mechanical or inflammatory injury to the superior hypogastric plexus near the aortic bifurcation. Bone morphogenetic protein-2 (BMP-2) has been used in spinal fusions and has been associated with inflammatory and neuroinflammatory adverse reactions, which may contribute to RE development after anterior lumbar surgery.

Purpose.—While controlling for anterior approach technique, we compared the incidence of RE with and without rhBMP-2 exposure, in large, matched cohorts of patients after ALIF.

Study Design.—Retrospective analysis of 10 years of prospectively gathered outcomes data on consecutive-patient cohorts having the same anterior exposure technique for ALIF with and without rhBMP-2 use.

Patient Sample.—All male patients without baseline sexual incapacity and having ALIF for lumbar spondylosis or spondylolisthesis of the lowest one or two lumbar levels with and without rhBMP-2, from 2002 through 2011.

Outcome Measures.—Diagnosis of RE as a new finding after ALIF compared against BMP-2 exposure, comorbid conditions, and other urological complications after ALIF surgery.

Methods.—From the comprehensive surgical database at a high volume, university practice, male subjects having ALIF at one (L5/S1) or two levels (L4/5, L5/S1) from 2002 to 2011 were identified. Baseline comorbid factors, postoperative urinary catheter/retention events, and RE events were recorded and comparative incidence compared.

Results.—There were four consecutive-patient cohorts identified: one before rhBMP-2 use was adopted (n = 174), two cohorts in which BMP-2 use was routine (n = 88 and n = 151), and one final cohort after BMP-2 use was discontinued from routine use (n = 59). The cohorts with and without BMP-2 exposure were closely comparable for age, approach, levels of surgery, comorbid factors affecting RE. Of 239 patients with ALIF and exposure to BMP-2, RE was diagnosed in 15 subjects (6.3%), compared with an RE diagnosis rate of two of 233 control patients without BMP-2 exposure (0.9%; $p = .0012$). Urinary retention after bladder catheter removal was also more frequently observed in patients exposed to BMP-2 (9.7%) compared with control patients (4.6%; $p = .043$). Of the baseline comorbid factors, medical or surgical treatment for prostatic hypertrophy disease was associated with an increased risk of RE in the BMP-2 patients ($p = .034$).

Conclusions.—This study confirms previous reports of a higher rate of RE in ALIF procedures using rhBMP-2 and an open anterior approach to the spine. This effect may be associated with an increased risk of postoperative urinary retention after BMP-2 exposure. The magnitude of the RE effect may be increased with concomitant prostatic disease treatments.

▶ This article from Stanford University School of Medicine highlights the continued reporting of increased complication rates postoperatively when using bone morphogenic protein-2 (BMP-2). There has been much reported recently about the potential minimizing of reported complication rates in the initial US Food and Drug Administration studies that were performed prior to the public release of the drug and the possible effect that industry conflicts and money may have played.[1] This study finds rates of retrograde ejaculation after anterior lumbar interbody fusion that were similar to the initial reported rates, but also confirms that the use of BMP-2 was associated with a significantly higher rate. The authors speculate that this pathology may be induced by the same irritating phenomena that is seen with posterior spine procedures after placement of the drug near the nerve roots. Regardless of the mechanism, it is unfortunately not too surprising to see once again that great initial reported results fade with time and that complications may be minimized in the initial excitement surrounding users' experience with a new drug, technique, or implant. Anytime someone says "but this time it is different" I have come to believe that it really is not, regardless of whether they are speaking of interbody cages, minimally invasive surgery techniques, or new bone graft extenders. I think even in spine care, if something seems too good to be true, then it probably is!

P. Huddleston, MD

Reference

1. Carragee EJ, Hurwitz EL, Weiner BK. A critical review of recombinant human bone morphogenetic protein-2 trials in spinal surgery: emerging safety concerns and lessons learned. *Spine J.* 2011;11:471-491.

Do Lumbar Motion Preserving Devices Reduce the Risk of Adjacent Segment Pathology Compared With Fusion Surgery? A Systematic Review

Wang JC, Arnold PM, Hermsmeyer JT, et al (UCLA Comprehensive Spine Ctr, Santa Monica; Univ of Kansas Med Ctr, Kansas City; Spectrum Research, Inc, Tacoma, WA)

Spine 37:S133-S143, 2012

Study Design.—A systematic review of the literature.

Objective.—To compare total disc replacement (TDR) with fusion, other motion-sparing devices with fusion, and motion-sparing devices with other motion-sparing devices to determine which devices may be associated with a lower risk of radiographical or clinical adjacent segment pathology (ASP).

Summary of Background Data.—Adjacent segment pathology, also termed adjacent segment disease (ASD) or adjacent segment degeneration, is a controversial phenomenon that can occur after a spinal fusion; it is thought to be either related to the altered mechanics or loss of motion from the fusion or to be part of the natural history of progressive arthritis. Motion preservation devices theoretically may decrease or prevent ASP from occurring.

Methods.—A systematic search was conducted in PubMed and the Cochrane Library for literature published between January 1990 and February 2012. For all key questions, we identified all cohort studies and randomized controlled trials, making the comparison of interest independent of the outcomes measured. We searched each full-text article to determine whether it reported any type of structural or degenerative condition specifically occurring at an adjacent segment. We included articles reporting adult lumbar patients who had degenerative disc disease, disc herniation, radiculopathy, kyphosis, scoliosis, and spondylolisthesis, and who were treated with TDR, other motion-sparing procedures, or fusion. The overall strength of the evidence for each key question was rated using the Grades of Recommendation Assessment, Development and Evaluation (GRADE) criteria.

Results.—There is moderate evidence to suggest that patients who undergo fusion may be nearly 6 times more likely to be treated for ASP than those who undergo TDR. From 2 randomized trials, the pooled risk of clinical ASP treated surgically was 1.2% and 7.0% in the TDR and fusion groups, respectively ($P = 0.009$). The increased risk of clinical ASP treated surgically associated with fusion is 5.8%. For every 17 operations, one might expect a new clinical ASP event requiring surgery when treated with fusion in those otherwise not harmed by TDR. There was insufficient literature to answer the other key questions, resulting in low to insufficient evidence that other motion-sparing operations are superior to fusion in preventing clinical ASP.

Conclusion.—There does seem to be a low rate of ASP after lumbar spinal fusion. The evidence suggests that the risk of clinical ASP following fusion is higher when compared with TDR, but there is limited evidence that fusion may increase the risk of developing clinical ASP compared with other motion-sparing procedures.

Consensus Statement.—1. Evidence demonstrates that the risk of clinical ASP requiring surgery is likely greater after fusion but the risk is still quite rare. The increased risk compared to TDR could be as small as less than 1% or as great as 10%.

Strength of Statement: Weak.

2. There is insufficient evidence to make a definitive statement regarding fusion *versus* other motion-sparing devices with respect to the risk of ASP.

▶ This article serves as a nice pairing with the article by Zigler et al[1] and is a meta-analysis of 22 years of literature concerning lumbar fusion and lumbar disc replacement. I like the terminology used by the authors of adjacent segment pathology (ASP) to indicate symptomatic disease and adjacent segment disease (ASD) to indicate asymptomatic imaging changes. Another strength of the article includes the use of statements of evidence to rank the references by Grades of Recommendation Assessment, Development and Evaluation (GRADE) criteria. Literature reviews that fail to follow the GRADE criteria can be flawed, as they may bias their conclusion toward lower-evidence studies or reports. The authors' conclusion follows my thoughts on the Zigler et al study, that there may be a higher risk of ASD with lumbar fusion, but with current follow-up it has yet to be shown that total disc replacement (TDR) is superior in preventing ASP. What remains to be seen is whether the hope of a reduced risk of ASP will overcome the potential of a generation of failed or worn-out TDR to become unreplaceable or revisable to fusion.

P. Huddleston, MD

Reference

1. Zigler JE, Glenn J, Delamarter RB. Five-year adjacent-level degenerative changes in patients with single-level disease treated using lumbar total disc replacement with ProDisc-L versus circumferential fusion. *J Neurosurg Spine.* 2012;17:504-511.

The Influence of Obesity on the Outcome of Treatment of Lumbar Disc Herniation: Analysis of the Spine Patient Outcomes Research Trial (SPORT)
Rihn JA, Kurd M, Hilibrand AS, et al (Thomas Jefferson Univ Hosp, Philadelphia, PA; et al)
J Bone Joint Surg Am 95:1-8, 2013

Background.—Questions remain as to the effect that obesity has on patients managed for symptomatic lumbar disc herniation. The purpose of this study was to determine if obesity affects outcomes following the treatment of symptomatic lumbar disc herniation.

Methods.—An as-treated analysis was performed on patients enrolled in the Spine Patient Outcomes Research Trial for the treatment of lumbar disc herniation. A comparison was made between patients with a body mass index of <30 kg/m^2 (nonobese) (n = 854) and those with a body mass index of ≥30 kg/m^2 (obese) (n = 336). Baseline patient demographic and clinical characteristics were documented. Primary and secondary outcomes were measured at baseline and at regular follow-up time intervals up to four years. The difference in improvement from baseline between operative and nonoperative treatment was determined at each follow-up period for both groups.

Results.—At the time of the four-year follow-up evaluation, improvements over baseline in primary outcome measures were significantly less for obese patients as compared with nonobese patients in both the operative treatment group (Short Form-36 physical function, 37.3 compared with 47.7 points [$p < 0.001$], Short Form-36 bodily pain, 44.2 compared with 50.0 points [$p = 0.005$], and Oswestry Disability Index, −33.7 compared with −40.1 points [$p < 0.001$]) and the nonoperative treatment group (Short Form-36 physical function, 23.1 compared with 32.0 points [$p < 0.001$] and Oswestry Disability Index, −21.4 compared with −26.1 points [$p < 0.001$]). The one exception was that the change from baseline in terms of the Short Form-36 bodily pain score was statistically similar for obese and nonobese patients in the nonoperative treatment group (30.9 compared with 33.4 points [$p = 0.39$]). At the time of the four-year follow-up evaluation, when compared with nonobese patients who had been managed operatively, obese patients who had been managed operatively had significantly less improvement in the Sciatica Bothersomeness Index and the Low Back Pain Bothersomeness Index, but had no significant difference in patient satisfaction or self-rated improvement. In the present study, 77.5% of obese patients and 86.9% of nonobese patients who had been managed operatively were working a full or part-time job. No significant differences were observed in the secondary outcome measures between obese and nonobese patients who had been managed nonoperatively. The benefit of surgery over nonoperative treatment was not affected by body mass index.

Conclusions.—Obese patients realized less clinical benefit from both operative and nonoperative treatment of lumbar disc herniation. Surgery provided similar benefit over nonoperative treatment in obese and nonobese patients.

▶ In this spinoff analysis of the Spine Patient Outcomes Research Trial (SPORT) for the treatment of lumbar disc herniation, the researchers suggest that the outcomes of obese patients were worse at 2 years poststudy than for nonobese patients, regardless of whether they had surgery or were treated nonoperatively. I cannot say I am surprised, because this also reflects the outcomes in my practice. Because of increased body habitus, these patients can be difficult to position in the operating room and take longer to finish because their distorted anatomy can make identifying the correct surgical levels difficult and visualization of the anatomy challenging, because standard surgical instruments are too short. The increased prevalence of diabetes and its many comorbidities can challenge wound healing and increase infection rates, making postoperative glucose management challenging. I was surprised to see that obese patients preferred surgical treatment to nonoperative management when compared with nonobese patients' preferences. Is this because they perceive surgical treatment as a quick fix for their health issues when most of the other options for their obese state and its comorbidities are nonoperative and part of a lifelong chronic disease management strategy? The authors cannot say, but their data are enlightening enough to be incorporated into every physician's medical counseling to those suffering from a herniated lumbar disc and sciatica. My main critique of the article would be that it is common in my practice to see obese patients with a body mass index (BMI) higher than 40. It would be interesting to see the study repeated with this subgroup analyzed as a separate group. This may be more useful to those patients and practitioners living in states where the average BMI is much higher than in the northeastern states.

P. Huddleston, MD

A Prospective Multicenter Registry on the Accuracy of Pedicle Screw Placement in the Thoracic, Lumbar, and Sacral Levels With the Use of the O-arm Imaging System and StealthStation Navigation
Van de Kelft E, Costa F, Van der Planken D, et al (AZ Nikolaas, Sint Niklaas, Belgium; Istituto Clinico Humanitas, Rozzano, Milan, Italy; Clinique Saint Joseph, Liége, Belgium)
Spine 37:E1580-E1587, 2012

Study Design.—An international, multicenter, prospective, postmarketing clinical registry to record the accuracy of pedicle screw placement, using the O-arm Complete Multidimensional Surgical Imaging System with StealthStation Navigation.

Objective.—To evaluate the accuracy of pedicle screw placement in common neurosurgical practice and assess the patient's radiation exposure.

Summary of Background Data.—Several imaging techniques have been used to increase accurate pedicle screw placement. The O-arm 3-dimensional (3D) imaging (Medtronic Navigation, Louisville, CO), an intraoperative computed tomographic (CT) scan, combined with an existing navigation system was reported to further increase accuracy of screw placement, especially because an intraoperative 3D scan provides information for screw adjustment before wound closure.

Methods.—Patients already planned for instrumented spinal surgery were operated while using the O-arm as imaging device and the StealthStation Navigation (Medtronic Navigation, Louisville, CO) as navigation tool. At the end of all pedicle screw insertions, the placement was classified according to a validated method. The accuracy of pedicle screw placement based on the intraoperative 3D scan and the surgeon's perception of correct screw placement were assessed as well as the radiation doses the patient received during the entire procedure.

Results.—During a 16-month period, a total of 1922 screws in 353 patients were evaluated. In 97.5%, the screws were correctly placed. Only

2.5% of the screws were considered as misplaced, and 1.8% of the screws were revised during the same procedure. When the surgeon perceived the screws to be correctly placed, the CT scan verified his assessment in 98.5% of the cases. The mean radiation dose was comparable with half the dose of a 64 multislice CT scan.

Conclusion.—The use of the O-arm in combination with a navigation system increases the accuracy of pedicle screw placement. The accuracy of the surgeon's perception and the need to limit the radiation dose for the patient justify an additional CT scan only after careful assessment of the potential additional value (Fig 4).

▶ The advent of the O-arm imaging device once again proves spine surgery to be at the forefront of technology, safety, and a messy conversation about the appropriate balance between innovation and sustainability. The 3-dimensional nature

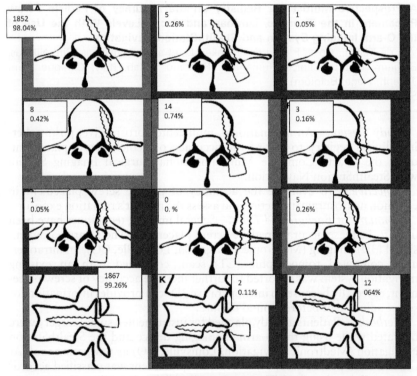

FIGURE 4.—Types of screw placement according to the grading system. Placement in red boxes is classified as unacceptable. Placement in the green boxes is classified as acceptable. The figure indicates the number of screws and the percentage that have that type of placement. For interpretation of the references to color in this figure legend, the reader is referred to web version of this article. (Reprinted from Van de Kelft E, Costa F, Van der Planken D, et al. A prospective multicenter registry on the accuracy of pedicle screw placement in the thoracic, lumbar, and sacral levels with the use of the O-arm imaging system and StealthStation navigation. *Spine.* 2012;37:E1580-E1587, with permission from Lippincott Williams & Wilkins.)

of spine instrumentation procedures is not in itself novel. Unlike many other orthopedic procedures, much of the anatomy is hidden and must be "seen" by experience and what the sailors of yore would call "dead reckoning." Additionally, the consequences of implant misplacement can result in death, paralysis, or permanent morbidity, which cannot be remedied by a poly-exchange or higher offset stem. The O-arm, also referred to as an in operating room CT scan, can be coupled with a computerized navigation module to assist the surgeon with placement of spinal implants in the most complicated spinal anatomy but at the cost of increased radiation exposure to the patient and potentially the staff.

This prospective study, which was performed by separate surgeons in Italy and Belgium, demonstrated a high degree of accuracy of placement for pedicle instrumentation using a standardized, computer-navigation—assisted technique. The authors additionally performed a postimplant placement repeat CT to verify the accuracy of the initial attempt. This allowed the testing of a second hypothesis, that if the surgeon felt good about the initial guided placement based on his or her past surgical experience, then the effort was seen to be accurate and only 1.5% of screws were "misplaced" (Fig 4) and 1% needed to be revised. When the surgeon's "gut instinct" judged the initial pedicle hole to be misguided, 12% of implants were misplaced and 10% needed to be revised.

This study raises many questions. If current spine surgeons' guesstimates about implant placement are highly accurate, will this experience fade over time and generations if future surgeons are trained on computer navigation? Five percent of the time the O-arm experienced a breakdown or malfunction during the surgical cases. What will future surgeons have to fall back on for guidance? Additionally, up to 3 different CT scans were performed in patients who had implants revised: the first for planning, the second to check the implants, and a third to check any implants that had revised. I am not sure of the value of this much time in the operating room and radiation exposure to any particular patient or large populations of surgical patients. I agree with the authors that the tool can be highly accurate, but prospective studies should be performed with free-hand technique or fluoroscopic guidance as controls.

P. Huddleston, MD

Five-year adjacent-level degenerative changes in patients with single-level disease treated using lumbar total disc replacement with ProDisc-L versus circumferential fusion
Zigler JE, Glenn J, Delamarter RB (Texas Back Inst, Plano; Core Orthopaedic Med Ctr, Encinitas, CA; Cedars-Sinai Spine Ctr, Los Angeles, CA)
J Neurosurg Spine 17:504-511, 2012

Object.—The authors report the 5-year results for radiographically demonstrated adjacent-level degenerative changes from a prospective multicenter study in which patients were randomized to either total disc replacement (TDR) or circumferential fusion for single-level lumbar degenerative disc disease (DDD).

Methods.—Two hundred thirty-six patients with single-level lumbar DDD were enrolled and randomly assigned to 2 treatment groups: 161 patients in the TDR group were treated using the ProDisc-L (Synthes Spine, Inc.), and 75 patients were treated with circumferential fusion. Radiographic follow-up data 5 years after treatment were available for 123 TDR patients and 43 fusion patients. To characterize adjacent-level degeneration (ALD), radiologists at an independent facility read the radiographic films. Adjacent-level degeneration was characterized by a composite score including disc height loss, endplate sclerosis, osteophytes, and spondylolisthesis. At 5 years, changes in ALD (ΔALDs) compared with the preoperative assessment were reported.

Results.—Changes in ALD at 5 years were observed in 9.2% of TDR patients and 28.6% of fusion patients ($p = 0.004$). Among the patients without adjacent-level disease preoperatively, new findings of ALD at 5 years posttreatment were apparent in only 6.7% of TDR patients and 23.8% of fusion patients ($p = 0.008$). Adjacent-level surgery leading to secondary surgery was reported for 1.9% of TDR patients and 4.0% of fusion patients ($p = 0.6819$). The TDR patients had a mean preoperative index-level range of motion ([ROM] of 7.3°) that decreased slightly (to 6.0°) at 5 years after treatment ($p = 0.0198$). Neither treatment group had significant changes in either ROM or translation at the superior adjacent level at 5 years posttreatment compared with baseline.

Conclusions.—At 5 years after the index surgery, ProDisc-L maintained ROM and was associated with a significantly lower rate of ΔALDs than in the patients treated with circumferential fusion. In fact, the fusion patients were greater than 3 times more likely to experience ΔALDs than were the TDR patients. Clinical trial registration no.: NCT00295009.

▶ The most important point in this 5-year follow-up of a randomized trial of Synthes' ProDisc-L versus lumbar fusion can be summed up by saying "treat patients, not x-rays!" The authors describe a 3 times more likely chance for fusion patients to develop radiographic signs of adjacent segment disease when compared with fusion patients, but with no differences in range of motion (ROM) or translation at the superior adjacent level at 5 years and no significant difference in surgery for adjacent-level degeneration (ALD) (see Figs 1-3 in the original article). When I hear patients and referring physicians ask about the option of total disc replacement (TDR), it is usually based on either the desire for the new technology or the perception that it will prevent symptomatic ALD. Although it may be that even longer follow-up will show a change in results, based on this study and its reported results I do not believe we can say that the TDR has prevented more surgeries or increased physiologic ROM. The truly cynical might say we have "discovered" the world's most expensive interbody fusion implant!

P. Huddleston, MD

7   Total Hip Arthroplasty

Introduction

Since hip joint replacement surgery is so reliable, a veritable dearth of the literature relates to case series documenting high success rates, even with increasingly long follow-up. This literature has been included in previous years, but less so this year. The reason is that we have intentionally focused more on evidence-based studies, information that is gained from large population-based National Registries as well as meta-analysis or analytical reviews of controversial or problematic topics. The hope is that this year's selections will not only provide insight into the current status and direction of hip joint replacement but will also provide a better understanding of what we have learned through the years. Hopefully, this will also serve as a glimpse of what is to come in our practice in the years ahead.

Bernard F. Morrey, MD

Detection of Total Hip Prostheses at Airport Security Checkpoints: How Has Heightened Security Affected Patients?

Johnson AJ, Naziri Q, Hooper HA, et al (Sinai Hosp of Baltimore, MD)
J Bone Joint Surg Am 94:e44.1-e44.4, 2012

Background.—The sensitivity of airport security screening measures has increased substantially during the past decade, but few reports have examined how this affects patients who have undergone hip arthroplasty. The purpose of this study was to determine the experiences of patients who had hip prostheses and who passed through airport security screenings.

Methods.—A consecutive series of 250 patients who presented to the office of a high-volume surgeon were asked whether they had had a hip prosthesis for at least one year and, if so, whether they had flown on a commercial airline within the past year. Patients who responded affirmatively to both questions were asked to complete a written survey that included questions about which joint(s) had been replaced, the number of encounters with airport security, the frequency and location of metal detector activation, any additional screening procedures that were utilized, whether security officials requested documentation regarding the prosthesis, the degree of inconvenience, and other relevant information.

Results.—Of the 143 patients with hip replacements who traveled by air, 120 (84%) reported triggering the alarm and required wanding with a hand-held detector. Twenty-five of these patients reported subsequently having to undergo further inspection, including additional wanding, being patted down, and in two cases having to undress in a private room to show the incision. Ninety-nine (69%) of the 143 patients reported that the prosthetic joint caused an inconvenience while traveling.

Conclusions.—This study provides interesting and critical information that allows physicians to understand the real-world implications of implanted orthopaedic devices for patients who are traveling where there has been heightened security since September 11, 2001. Patients should be counseled that they should expect delays and be prepared for such inconveniences, but that these are often only momentary. This information could relieve some anxiety and concerns that patients may have prior to traveling.

▶ After reading this I was prompted to say, "duh." But on second thought, maybe my colleagues would be interested in the specific, objective findings. About 85% will set off the surveillance equipment, and of these, 70% of patients consider themselves inconvenienced when traveling. Because it is a common question for total hip patients, we can now give them the specific expectations.

B. F. Morrey, MD

Does Impact Sport Activity Influence Total Hip Arthroplasty Durability?

Ollivier M, Frey S, Parratte S, et al (Aix-Marseille Univ, Marseille, France)

Clin Orthop Relat Res 470:3060-3066, 2012

Background.—Return to sport is a key patient demand after hip arthroplasty and some patients are even involved in high-impact sports. Although polyethylene wear is related to the number of cycles and the importance of the load, it is unclear whether high-impact sport per se influences THA durability.

Questions/Purposes.—Therefore, we compared (1) function between the patients involved in high-impact sports and the patients with lower activities as measured by the Harris hip score (HHS) and the Hip Osteoarthritis Outcome Score (HOOS); (2) linear wear rates; and (3) survivorships considering revision for mechanical failure with radiographic signs of aseptic loosening as the end point.

Methods.—We retrospectively identified 70 patients who engaged in high-impact sports and 140 with low activity levels from among 843 THAs from a prospectively collected database performed between September 1, 1995, and December 31, 2000. Patients were evaluated at a minimum followup of 10 years (mean, 11 years; range, 10–15 years) by two independent observers. We obtained a HHS and HOOS at each followup.

Results.—The mean HOOS was higher in the high-impact group for three of the five subscales of the HOOS. Mean linear wear was higher in

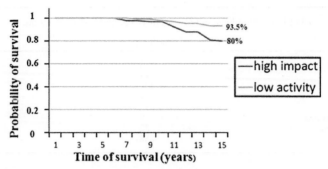

FIGURE 2.—Results of the Kaplan-Meier analysis showing a worse survivorship in the high-activity group at 15 years followup. (With kind permission from Springer Science+Business Media: Ollivier M, Frey S, Parratte S, et al. Does impact sport activity influence total hip arthroplasty durability? *Clin Orthop Relat Res.* 2012;470:3060-3066, with permission from The Association of Bone and Joint Surgeons®.)

the high-impact group than in the low-activities group. We also found a higher number of revisions in the high-activity group.

Conclusions.—Our observations confirm concern about the risk of THA mechanical failures related to high-impact sport, and patient and surgeons alike should be aware of these risks of mechanical failures.

Level of Evidence.—Level III, therapeutic study. See the Guidelines for Authors for a complete description of levels of evidence (Fig 2).

▶ As the population with replacement creeps ever younger and the expectation of normalcy increases relentlessly, formal studies such as this one take on increased relevance. As might be expected, impact activities decrease the longevity of the implant (Fig 2). I have long advised my patients they can glide on their replacement, but they can't bang on it. QED.

B. F. Morrey, MD

Higher risk of reoperation for bipolar and uncemented hemiarthroplasty
Leonardsson O, Kärrholm J, Åkesson K, et al (Lund Univ, Malmö, Sweden; Swedish Hip Arthroplasty Register, Göteborg, Sweden)
Acta Orthop 83:459-466, 2012

Background and Purpose.—Hemiarthroplasty as treatment for femoral neck fractures has increased markedly in Sweden during the last decade. In this prospective observational study, we wanted to identify risk factors for reoperation in modular hemiarthroplasties and to evaluate mortality in this patient group.

Patients and Methods.—We assessed 23,509 procedures from the Swedish Hip Arthroplasty Register using the most common surgical approaches with modular uni- or bipolar hemiarthroplasties related to fractures in the period 2005—2010. Completeness of registration (individual

TABLE 5.—Numbers and Causes of Reoperations and Revisions

	Reoperation	Revision
Dislocation	393	373
Infection	275	174
Fracture	131	93
Acetabular erosion	41	41
Pain	17	16
Aseptic loosening	9	9
Other reasons	22	9
Total	888	715

procedures) was 89–96%. The median age was 85 years and the median follow-up time was 18 months.

Results.—3.8% underwent reoperation (any further hip surgery), most often because of implant dislocation or infection. The risk of reoperation (Cox regression) was higher for uncemented stems (hazard ratio (HR) = 1.5), mainly because of periprosthetic femoral fractures. Bipolar implants had a higher risk of reoperation irrespective of cause (HR = 1.3), because of dislocation (1.4), because of infection (1.3), and because of periprosthetic fracture (1.7). The risk of reoperation due to acetabular erosion was lower (0.30) than for unipolar implants, but reoperation for this complication was rare (1.7 per thousand). Procedures resulting from failed internal fixation had a more than doubled risk; the risk was also higher for males and for younger patients. The surgical approach had no influence on the risk of reoperation generally, but the anterolateral transgluteal approach was associated with a lower risk of reoperation due to dislocation (HR = 0.7). At 1 year, the mortality was 24%. Men had a higher risk of death than women (1.8).

Interpretation.—We recommend cemented hemiarthroplasties and the anterolateral transgluteal approach. We also suggest that unipolar implants should be used, at least for the oldest and frailest patients (Table 5).

▶ This is another example of the value of national registries. This simple question of whether type of implant or fixation made a difference in the management of a hip fracture in an elderly patient was rather clearly answered. The uncemented stem has a higher frequency of fracture, and the bipolar has a higher rate of dislocation. The uncemented bipolar is more expensive, by the way. The leading complications of dislocation, infection, and fracture account for 90% of all complications (Table 5). The take-home message: Cement the stem of a monopolar implant in the elderly patient.

B. F. Morrey, MD

Cost savings of using a cemented total hip replacement: an analysis of the National Joint Registry data
Griffiths EJ, Stevenson D, Porteous MJ (West Suffolk NHS Trust, Bury St Edmunds, UK)
J Bone Joint Surg Br 94-B:1032-1035, 2012

The debate whether to use cemented or uncemented components in primary total hip replacement (THR) has not yet been considered with reference to the cost implications to the National Health Service.

We obtained the number of cemented and uncemented components implanted in 2009 from the National Joint Registry for England and Wales. The cost of each component was established. The initial financial saving if all were cemented was then calculated. Subsequently the five-year rates of revision for each type of component were reviewed and the predicted number of revisions at five years for the actual components used was compared with the predicted number of revisions for a cemented THR. This was then multiplied by the mean cost of revision surgery to provide an indication of the savings over the first five years if all primary THRs were cemented.

The saving at primary THR was calculated to be £10 million with an additional saving during the first five years of between £5 million and £8.5 million. The use of cemented components in routine primary THR in the NHS as a whole can be justified on a financial level but we recognise individual patient factors must be considered when deciding which components to use.

▶ These two articles are reviewed together because they obviously are addressing the same high-level, cost-effective surgery. However, the methodology is dramatically different. In the study of the femoral neck fracture, the follow-up is short, so the analysis is primarily based on purchase price and utilization. The finding that the cementless implant was less expensive is mainly due to the extreme cost of the cement, greater than $1000 per case. How sad. All this reflects is supply and demand and the philosophy of the materials management group and effective cost negotiations. The study from the United Kingdom, on the other hand, assessed a large number of patients with significant follow-up. They thus took into consideration the initial cost, as well as that of subsequent procedures. In this setting, the cemented implanted patients outperformed the cementless group by 10 million pounds initially, with an additional saving of 5 to 8 million over the next 5 years based on clinical performance. Admittedly, there are many variables. However, we have experience in our country with this same analysis and found that at the Mayo Clinic, a similar savings was realized with the cemented implants. This study was performed 10 years ago. The work was rejected for publication.

B. F. Morrey, MD

Comparison of Ten-Year Survivorship of Hip Prostheses with Use of Conventional Polyethylene, Metal-on-Metal, or Ceramic-on-Ceramic Bearings
Milošev I, Kovač S, Trebše R, et al (Valdoltra Orthopaedic Hosp, Ankaran, Slovenia)
J Bone Joint Surg Am 94:1756-1763, 2012

Background.—To improve the long-term performance of hip prostheses, alternative bearings with metal-on-metal (MoM) and ceramic-on-ceramic (CoC) couples have been introduced. Although currently the results from the use of these bearings are in the midterm stage, there have been few comparative studies of these different bearings.

Methods.—From 2000 to 2002, 487 total hip replacements were performed with use of a BICON-PLUS acetabular cup and an SL-PLUS femoral stem (Plus Orthopedics, Rotkreuz, Switzerland, now Smith & Nephew Orthopaedics). The patients were divided into three groups according to the type of bearing that was used: an MoM group (sixty-nine prostheses), a metal-on-polyethylene (MoP) group (200 prostheses), and a CoC group (218 prostheses). Patient demographic data and data with regard to revision operations were evaluated from the hospital computer database. The mean follow-up period was 8.5 years (range, 6.9 to 10.5 years). Patient activity was assessed with use of the University of California at Los Angeles activity scale.

Results.—The mean patient age was sixty years at the time of the index arthroplasty in the MoM and CoC groups, and seventy-one years in the MoP group. Based on a scale of ten, the mean postoperative activity level was six in the CoC group, five in the MoM group, and four in the MoP group. Survival at ten years with regard to revision for any reason was 0.984, 0.956, and 0.879 for the MoP, CoC, and MoM groups, respectively. When revision for any reason was considered as the end point, survival of the MoM bearings was significantly worse than that of the MoP bearings ($p = 0.005$). Survival at ten years with regard to revision for aseptic loosening was 0.995, 0.990, and 0.894 for the MoP, CoC, and MoM groups, respectively. When revision for aseptic loosening was considered as the end point, survival of the MoM group was significantly worse than that of either the MoP group ($p = 0.001$) or the CoC group ($p = 0.003$).

Conclusions.—When comparing two groups of patients of similar mean age and mean activity level undergoing total hip arthroplasty with the use of alternative bearings, CoC bearings had better survival than did MoM bearings at the ten-year follow-up; the difference was significant when revision for aseptic loosening was defined as a failure. However, neither the CoC nor the MoM alternative bearings provided improved midterm results when compared with the results of the conventional MoP bearings. For older, less active patients, traditional metal-on-polyethylene bearings are the appropriate choice.

Level of Evidence.—Therapeutic <u>Level III</u>. See Instructions for Authors for a complete description of levels of evidence.

▶ Realizing the implant being studied was not one typically used in the United States almost made me pass on this article. But after I read it, I could not help but include it; not only does this tend to confirm my personal preference and practice, the data are sound and convincing. Few studies have compared the long-term outcome of the 3 articulations discussed here. Unfortunately, the sample size is too small to stratify by age. Regardless, the analysis does consider age and activity to some extent (Table 3 in the original article). Most importantly, it reveals the poorer performance of metal on metal bearing as well as the superior performance of the metal on polyethylene articulation (Fig 4 in the original article). Recognizing the variation in design and manufacturer are important variables; this study does cause one to pause.

B. F. Morrey, MD

Clinical and radiological results of the collarless polished tapered stem at 15 years follow-up
Burston BJ, Barnett AJ, Amirfeyz R, et al (Avon Orthopaedic Centre, Bristol, UK)
J Bone Joint Surg Br 94-B:889-894, 2012

We prospectively followed 191 consecutive collarless polished tapered (CPT) femoral stems, implanted in 175 patients who had a mean age at operation of 64.5 years (21 to 85). At a mean follow-up of 15.9 years (14 to 17.5), 86 patients (95 hips) were still alive. The fate of all original stems is known. The 16-year survivorship with re-operation for any reason was 80.7% (95% confidence interval 72 to 89.4). There was no loss to follow-up, with clinical data available on all 95 hips and radiological assessment performed on 90 hips (95%). At latest follow-up, the mean Harris hip score was 78 (28 to 100) and the mean Oxford hip score was 36 (15 to 48). Stems subsided within the cement mantle, with a mean subsidence of 2.1 mm (0.4 to 19.2). Among the original cohort, only one stem (0.5%) has been revised due to aseptic loosening. In total seven stems were revised for any cause, of which four revisions were required for infection following revision of the acetabular component. A total of 21 patients (11%) required some sort of revision procedure; all except three of these resulted from failure of the acetabular component. Cemented acetabular components had a significantly lower revision burden (three hips, 2.7%) than Harris Galante uncemented components (17 hips, 21.8%) ($p < 0.001$).

The CPT stem continues to provide excellent radiological and clinical outcomes at 15 years following implantation. Its results are consistent with other polished tapered stem designs.

▶ By accepting this article, I feel like I'm swimming upstream. I know for most surgeons the bus has left the station on the use of cemented hip replacement. Yet, the data do not support this decision. Notice the mean age of this cohort is

65 years, and the revision rate of the femoral stem for loosening is less than 10% at 15 years (Fig 3 in the original article). The reason for failure is mostly on the acetabular side of the joint. The message is that with a polished, tapered stem, a cemented femoral component is a reliable option for those 65 years and older. But, these data will probably not change our practice. Too bad.

B. F. Morrey, MD

Constrained Cups Appear Incapable of Meeting the Demands of Revision THA

Noble PC, Durrani SK, Usrey MM, et al (Baylor College of Medicine, Houston, TX; The Inst of Orthopedic Res and Education, Houston, TX; et al)
Clin Orthop Relat Res 470:1907-1916, 2012

Background.—Failure rates of constrained cups for treating recurrent dislocation in revision THA range from 40% to 100%. Although constrained liners are intended to stabilize the hip by mechanically preventing dislocation, the resulting loss of range of motion may lead to impingement and, ultimately, implant failure.

Questions/Purposes.—We therefore documented the mechanisms of failure of constrained acetabular cups in revision THA and determined the type and severity of damage (wear, fracture, and impingement) that occurs in situ.

Methods.—We retrieved 57 constrained components of four different designs at revision THA and examined for the presence of rim impingement, oxidation, cracks within the liner, backside wear, pitting, scratching, abrasion, burnishing, and the presence of embedded particles. Articular wear was calculated from the volume of the concave articular bearing surface, which was measured using the fluid displacement method.

Results.—Failure of the locking ring was responsible for 51% of failures, whereas 28% of revisions were the result of acetabular cup loosening, 6% backside wear, and 22% infection. Impingement damage of the rim of the polyethylene liner was seen in all retrievals with moderate or severe damage in 54%. The average volumetric wear rate of the articular surface was 95 mm^3/year.

Conclusions.—Failure of the locking liner ring and loosening of the acetabular cup are the primary causes of mechanical failure with constrained liners; polyethylene is an inadequate material for restricting motion of the hip to prevent instability. The durability of these devices is unlikely to improve unless the mechanical demands are modified through increased range of motion leading to less frequent rim impingement.

▶ Because dislocation remains the most frequent early major complication of hip replacement, the orthopedic community has turned to larger heads and more constrained articulations. This group of seasoned investigators has provided a clear demonstration of a central truth—constraining the articulation comes at a cost. The high failure rate occurs from failure of the constraining mechanism in about half of the failures studied. Cup loosening accounted for another 25%, and sepsis accounts for most of the remainder of the failures. The message is NEVER use a constrained articulation in a setting where it is not needed: rarely in primary procedures; only if elevated rims, larger heads, and assuring abductor function is not adequate in the revision hip. Note the conclusion of the study. Failure basically occurs because the constrained implant decreases motion, and polyethylene is an inferior material to resist impingement over a long period.

B. F. Morrey, MD

Acetabular Components in Total Hip Arthroplasty: Is There Evidence That Cementless Fixation Is Better?
Toossi N, Adeli B, Timperley AJ, et al (Thomas Jefferson Univ, Philadelphia, PA; Royal Devon & Exeter Hosp, UK; et al)
J Bone Joint Surg Am 95:168-174, 2013

Background.—The use of cementless acetabular components in total hip arthroplasty has gained popularity over the past decade. Most total hip arthroplasties being performed in North America currently use cementless acetabular components. The objective of this systematic review and meta-analysis was to compare the survivorship and revision rate of cemented and cementless acetabular components utilized in total hip arthroplasty.

Methods.—A primary literature search in PubMed identified 3488 articles, of which 3407 did not meet the inclusion criteria and were excluded. Only English-language articles on either the survivorship or revision rate of primary total hip arthroplasty at a minimum of ten years of follow-up were included. The present study analyzed forty-five articles reporting the long-term outcome of cementless acetabular components, twenty-nine reporting the outcome of cemented acetabular components, and seven comparing cemented and cementless acetabular components. Meta-analysis (with a random-effects model) was performed on the data from the seven comparative studies, and study-level logistic regression analysis (with a quasibinomial model) was performed on the pooled data on the eighty-one included articles to determine a consensus. The studies were weighted according to the number of total hip arthroplasties performed.

Results.—The meta-analysis did not reveal any effect of the type of acetabular component fixation on either survivorship or revision rate. The regression analysis revealed the estimated odds ratio for survivorship of a cemented acetabular component to be 1.60 (95% confidence interval, 1.32 to 2.40; $p = 0.002$) when adjustments for factors including age, sex, and mean duration of follow-up were made.

Conclusions.—The preference for cementless acetabular components on the basis of improved survivorship is not supported by the published evidence. Although concerns regarding aseptic loosening of cemented acetabular components may have led North American surgeons toward the nearly exclusive use of cementless acetabular components, the available literature suggests that the fixation of cemented acetabular components is more reliable than that of cementless components beyond the first postoperative decade.

▶ Dr Parvizi has a knack for studying topics that are of importance to the orthopedic community—or at least are important to me. I, of course, did not know the outcome of this study until I read it, but I was determined to accept it because of the method and validity of the observations (Fig 1 in the original article). It is sad that of almost 3500 articles, only 81 satisfied the study criteria. Yet, these data were sufficient to document a better survival rate in the cemented cup compared with the modular uncemented cup (Fig 2 in the original article). To put it another way, there were fewer revisions in the cemented compared with the cementless modular cup design (Fig 3 in the original article). These findings pleased me, as I continue to cement the cup in patients older than 70. The data, but not the orthopedic community, support this practice.

B. F. Morrey, MD

Cemented, cementless, and hybrid prostheses for total hip replacement: cost effectiveness analysis
Pennington M, Grieve R, Sekhon JS, et al (London School of Hygiene and Tropical Medicine, UK; Univ of California, Berkeley; et al)
BMJ 346:f1026, 2013

Objective.—To compare the cost effectiveness of the three most commonly chosen types of prosthesis for total hip replacement.

Design.—Lifetime cost effectiveness model with parameters estimated from individual patient data obtained from three large national databases.

Setting.—English National Health Service.

Participants.—Adults aged 55 to 84 undergoing primary total hip replacement for osteoarthritis.

Interventions.—Total hip replacement using either cemented, cementless, or hybrid prostheses.

Main Outcome Measures.—Cost (£), quality of life (EQ-5D-3L, where 0 represents death and 1 perfect health), quality adjusted life years (QALYs), incremental cost effectiveness ratios, and the probability that each prosthesis type is the most cost effective at alternative thresholds of willingness to pay for a QALY gain.

Results.—Lifetime costs were generally lowest with cemented prostheses, and postoperative quality of life and lifetime QALYs were highest with hybrid prostheses. For example, in women aged 70 mean costs were £6900 ($11 000; €8200) for cemented prostheses, £7800 for cementless prostheses, and £7500 for hybrid prostheses; mean postoperative EQ-5D scores were 0.78, 0.80, and 0.81, and the corresponding lifetime QALYs were 9.0, 9.2, and 9.3 years. The incremental cost per QALY for hybrid compared with cemented prostheses was £2500. If the threshold willingness to pay for a QALY gain exceeded £10 000, the probability that hybrid prostheses were most cost effective was about 70%. Hybrid prostheses have the highest probability of being the most cost effective in all subgroups, except in women aged 80, where cemented prostheses were most cost effective.

Conclusions.—Cemented prostheses were the least costly type for total hip replacement, but for most patient groups hybrid prostheses were the most cost effective. Cementless prostheses did not provide sufficient improvement in health outcomes to justify their additional costs.

▶ As we near completion of our reviews for this volume, I had to include this study. The topic is one I investigated about 15 years ago and concluded that cemented hips were more cost-effective than uncemented ones. The journals rejected it, although I had a statistician develop the study design and participate in the writing of the manuscript. Now 15 years later, this much more elegant study from the United Kingdom reaffirms what we found. Overall, cemented implants are the most cost-effective option. What I was not expecting was that the hybrid had a better quality outcome, was not too much more expensive, and has a 70% chance of being the most cost-effective option.

Will this make a difference in utilization patterns? Absolutely not, at least in the near term. But when we lose further control in our choices, this type of study will be used to explain why implant usage will be dictated to us. Preference is at risk, as well it should be.

B. F. Morrey, MD

Association Between Low Admission Norton Scale Scores and Postoperative Complications After Elective THA in Elderly Patients

Asleh K, Sever R, Hilu S, et al (Tel-Aviv Univ, Israel; Sourasky Med Ctr, Tel-Aviv, Israel)
Orthopedics 35:e1302-e1306, 2012

The Norton scoring system is used by nurses to evaluate pressure ulcer risk. The authors have previously shown that low admission Norton scale scores (ANSS) are associated with postoperative complications other than pressure ulcers following hip fracture and spine fracture surgery in elderly patients. The purpose of this retrospective, cross-sectional study study was to determine whether low ANSS are associated with postoperative complications other than pressure ulcers following elective total hip arthroplasty (THA) in elderly patients. The medical charts of consecutive elderly (older than 65 years) patients admitted between February 2008 and November 2010 were studied for acute renal failure, cardiovascular events, confusion, pneumonia, pressure ulcers, urinary infection, urinary retention, venous thromboembolism, wound infection, and other complications. The final cohort included 166 patients (108 [65.1%] women; aged 75.2 ± 6.4 years). Overall, 24 (14.5%) patients had low (16 or less) ANSS. Patients with low ANSS had significantly more postoperative complications other than pressure ulcers compared with patients with high ANSS (0.5 ± 0.7 vs 0.2 ± 0.4, respectively; $P = .018$). Binary regression analysis showed that low ANSS were independently associated with

TABLE 2.—Characteristics of Patients With Low and High ANSS

Characteristic	High (n = 142)	Low (n = 24)	OR (95% CI)	P
Demographic				
Age, y, mean±SD	74.7±6.2	77.9±6.9	NA	.038
Female sex	91 (64.1)	17 (70.8)	1.36 (0.53-3.50)	.646
Comorbidity				
Hypertension	82 (57.7)	16 (66.7)	1.46 (0.59-3.64)	.504
Hyperlipidemia	52 (36.6)	6 (25.0)	0.57 (0.21-1.54)	.356
Diabetes mellitus	28 (19.7)	6 (25.0)	1.36 (.49-3.73)	.587
Ischemic heart disease	19 (13.4)	4 (16.7)	29 (.39-4.20)	.749
Osteoporosis	14 (9.9)	4 (16.7)	1.82 (.54-6.11)	.300
Hypothyroidism	14 (9.9)	3 (12.5)	1.30 (.34-4.93)	.716
Atrial fibrillation	13 (9.1)	3 (12.5)	1.41 (.37-5.40)	.706
Stroke	7 (4.9)	3 (12.5)	2.76 (.66-11.50)	.160
Depression	4 (2.8)	1 (4.2)	1.50 (.16-14.02)	.547
Chronic lung disease	4 (2.8)	1 (4.2)	1.50 (.16-14.02)	.547
Parkinson's disease	2 (1.4)	1 (4.2)	3.04 (.27-34.94)	.376
Postoperative complication				
Wound infection	8 (5.6)	4 (16.7)	3.35 (.92-12.15)	.075
Urinary infection	8 (5.6)	2 (8.3)	1.52 (.30-7.64)	.639
Urinary retention	3 (2.1)	1 (4.2)	2.01 (.20-20.20)	.468
Acute renal failure	0 (0.0)	3 (12.5)	NA	.003
Pressure ulcer	1 (0.7)	2 (8.3)	12.81 (1.11-147.37)	.055
Pneumonia	2 (1.4)	0 (0.0)	NA	.999
Cholecystitis	1 (0.7)	1 (4.2)	6.13 (.37-101.48)	.269
Other[a,b]	4 (2.8)	1 (4.2)	1.50 (.16-14.02)	.547

Abbreviations: ANSS, admission Norton scale scores; CI, confidence interval; NA, not applicable; OR, odds ratio.
[a]Acute gastroenteritis (n = 1), confusion (n = 1), Creutzfeldt-Jakob disease (n = 1), heart failure exacerbation (n = 1), and pseudogout arthritis (n = 1).
[b]Patients may have had more than 1 comorbidity, postoperative complication, or both.

all postoperative complications other than pressure ulcers (P = .039). In addition to predicting pressure ulcer risk, the Norton scoring system may be used for predicting other postoperative complications in elderly patients following elective THA (Table 2).

▶ This is an interesting article because it shows the correlation between complication after hip replacement and a standardized score to assess risk of pressure ulcers. A moment's thought would support the concept that the same factors that contribute to pressure ulcers also pertain to other medical problems as well (Table 2). Of particular interest is that the correlation is so strong, and the assessment is easily done. It would seem to be worth considering the introduction of the Norton assessment for all patients undergoing major orthopedic procedures.

B. F. Morrey, MD

Heterotopic ossification following total hip replacement for acetabular fractures

Chémaly O, Hebert-Davies J, Rouleau DM, et al (Univ of Montreal, Québec, Canada)

Bone Joint J 95-B:95-100, 2013

Early total hip replacement (THR) for acetabular fractures offers accelerated rehabilitation, but a high risk of heterotopic ossification (HO) has been reported. The purpose of this study was to evaluate the incidence of HO, its associated risk factors and functional impact. A total of 40 patients with acetabular fractures treated with a THR weres retrospectively reviewed. The incidence and severity of HO were evaluated using the modified Brooker classification, and the functional outcome assessed. The overall incidence of HO was 38% (n = 15), with nine severe grade III cases. Patients who underwent surgery early after injury had a fourfold increased chance of developing HO. The mean blood loss and operating time were more than twice that of those whose surgery was delayed ($p = 0.002$ and $p < 0.001$, respectively). In those undergoing early THR, the incidence of grade III HO was eight times higher than in those in whom THR was delayed ($p = 0.01$). Only three of the seven patients with severe HO showed good or excellent Harris hip scores compared with eight of nine with class 0, I or II HO ($p = 0.049$). Associated musculoskeletal injuries, high-energy trauma and head injuries were associated with the development of grade III HO.

The incidence of HO was significantly higher in patients with a displaced acetabular fracture undergoing THR early compared with those

TABLE 2.—Surgical Data, Incidence of Heterotopic Ossification and Other Complications Following Total Hip Replacement (THR)

	Early THR	Late THR	Total	p-value
Mean operating time (mins) (range)	171 (105 to 315)	76 (39 to 140)		<0.001*
Mean blood loss (cc) (range)	992 (300 to 2000)	416 (200 to 1500)		0.002*
Heterotopic ossification (n, %)	n = 19	n = 20		
Grade 0 (none)	7 (37)	17 (85)	24 (61.5)	
Grade I	2 (10.5)	2 (10)	4 (10)	
Grade II	2 (10.5)	0 (0)	2 (5)	
Grade III	8 (42)	1 (5)	9 (23)	
Grade IV	0	0	0	
Grades 0 to II	11 (58)	19 (95)	30 (77)	
Grades III and IV	8 (42)	1 (5)	9 (23)	0.01†
Complications (n, %)				
Thrombotic event	3	1		
Dislocation	1	0		
Infection	0	0		
Death	1	2		

*Student's *t*-test.
†chi-squared test.

undergoing THR later and this had an adverse effect on the functional outcome (Table 2).

▶ Although, fortunately, fractured acetabuli are not too frequent, they have a well-deserved reputation for subsequent arthritis requiring hip replacement. Although this is a retrospective cohort study, the findings are clear and important to our management of such fractures. The impressive difference in those undergoing replacement less than 2 months after injury compared with those who have the surgery longer than one year after the fracture is shown in Table 2. Note the difference in blood loss and other complications as well as in the development of ectopic bone. This study does not address when the temporal associated risk subsides, so it seems prudent to wait a year if possible before the definitive reconstruction.

B. F. Morrey, MD

Highly Crosslinked Polyethylene Does Not Reduce Aseptic Loosening in Cemented THA 10-year Findings of a Randomized Study
Johanson P-E, Digas G, Herberts P, et al (Univ of Gothenburg, Sweden; Xanthi Hosp, Greece; et al)
Clin Orthop Relat Res 470:3083-3093, 2012

Background.—Polyethylene (PE) wear particles are believed to cause aseptic loosening and thereby impair function in hip arthroplasty. Highly crosslinked polyethylene (XLPE) has low short- and medium-term wear rates. However, the longterm wear characteristics are unknown and it is unclear whether reduced wear particle burden improves function and survival of cemented hip arthroplasty.

Questions/Purposes.—We asked whether XLPE wear rates remain low up to 10 years and whether this leads to improved implant fixation, periprosthetic bone quality, and clinical function compared to conventional PE.

Methods.—We randomized 60 patients (61 hips) to receive either PE or XLPE cemented cups combined with a cemented stem. At 10 years postoperatively, 51 patients (52 hips) were evaluated for polyethylene wear and component migration estimation by radiostereometry, for radiolucent lines, bone densitometry, and Harris hip and pain scores. Revisions were recorded.

Results.—XLPE cups had a lower mean three-dimensional wear rate between 2 and 10 years compared to conventional PE hips: 0.005 mm/year versus 0.056 mm/year. We found no differences in cup migration, bone mineral density, radiolucencies, functional scores, and revision rate. There was a trend toward improved stem fixation in the XLPE group. The overall stem failure rate was comparably high, without influencing wear rate in XLPE hips.

Conclusions.—XLPE displayed a low wear rate up to 10 years when used in cemented THA, but we found no clear benefits in any other parameters. Further research is needed to determine whether cemented THA designs with XLPE are less prone to stem loosening.

Level of Evidence.—Level I, therapeutic study. See the Instructions for Authors for a complete description of levels of evidence.

▶ We benefit, yet again, from registry data. With large numbers, the authors ask a relevant question. Does the emerging documented enhancement in the wear characteristics of x-linked polyethylene translate into enhanced cemented implant survival, free of loosening? No. The improvement in wear is again demonstrated (see Fig 2 in the original article). However, this difference in survival free of revision for loosening did not change (see Fig 3 in the original article). What does this mean? I suspect, as previously conjectured, the value of highly x-linked polyethylene is more in the modular design than in the cemented cup design.

B. F. Morrey, MD

Comparison of Complications in Single-Incision Minimally Invasive THA and Conventional THA

Li N, Deng Y, Chen L (Zhongnan Hosp of Wuhan Univ, Wuhan, People's Republic of China)
Orthopedics 35:e1152-e1158, 2012

The purpose of this meta-analysis was to investigate whether single-incision minimally invasive total hip arthroplasty (THA) is superior to conventional incision THA by comparing postoperative complication rates, Harris Hip Scores, and Western Ontario and McMaster Universities Arthritis Index (WOMAC) scores. Randomized, controlled trials comparing single-incision minimally invasive THA and conventional THA were reviewed. The methodological quality of each randomized, controlled trial was assessed using the Physiotherapy Evidence Database (PEDro) scale (Centre for Evidence-based Physiotherapy, The George Institute for Global Health, New South Wales, Australia). The Grading of Recommendations Assessment, Development and Evaluation (GRADE) approach was used to determine the quality of the evidence. Fourteen studies involving 1254 patients (1329 hips) were included in the meta-analysis, comprising 659 single-incision minimally invasive THAs (mean patient age, 63.9 years) and 670 conventional incision THAs (mean patient age, 65.0 years). A funnel plot of postoperative complication rates showed that a slight publication bias existed in the study.

According to the meta-analysis, no significant statistical difference was observed in complication rates in no more than 3 postoperative years (odds ratio = 1.06; 95% confidence interval, 0.69 to 1.63; $P = .79$), in Harris Hip Scores in no more than 2 postoperative years (weighted mean difference = 0.71; 95% confidence interval, -3.09 to 4.51; $P = .71$), and in WOMAC scores at 6 weeks postoperatively (weighted mean difference = -0.55; 95% confidence interval, -3.54 to 2.44; $P = .72$) between single-incision minimally invasive THA and conventional THA. Therefore, single-incision minimally invasive THA is not superior to conventional THA in early postoperative recovery, hip function, and complication rate.

▶ We hear less about minimally invasive surgery (MIS) these days, as most have decided either for or against. Now that some time has passed, it is interesting to see the topic revisited with a meta-analysis from China. Of a literature base of more than 200 articles on the subject, only 14 (~7%) were of adequate quality to be considered. The first question we always ask is the complication rate. In this assessment, there was no real difference as exhibited in Forest graft (Fig 3 in the original article). The second essential question is whether one provides superior outcomes. The answer is no, at least based on the relatively poor standard of the Harris Hip Score (Fig 4 in the original article). So, this confirms what is well known and accepted. Dealer's choice. But my informed bias: I do not accept the considerable learning curve and my observed complication rate associated with MIS to justify teaching it, or doing it.

B. F. Morrey, MD

High complication rate in the early experience of minimally invasive total hip arthroplasty by the direct anterior approach

Spaans AJ, van den Hout JAAM, Bolder SBT (Amphia Hosp, Breda, the Netherlands)
Acta Orthop 83:342-346, 2012

Background and Purpose.—There is growing interest in minimally invasive surgery techniques in total hip arthroplasty (THA). In this study, we investigated the learning curve and the early complications of the direct anterior approach in hip replacement.

Methods.—In the period January through December 2010, THA was performed in 46 patients for primary osteoarthritis, using the direct anterior approach. These cases were compared to a matched cohort of 46 patients who were operated on with a conventional posterolateral approach. All patients were followed for at least 1 year.

Results.—Operating time was almost twice as long and mean blood loss was almost twice as much in the group with anterior approach. No learning effect was observed in this group regarding operating time or blood loss. Radiographic evaluation showed adequate placement of the implants in both groups. The early complication rate was higher in the anterior approach group. Mean time of hospital stay and functional outcome

TABLE 2.—Operative Outcome. Numbers are Mean (SD)

	DAA Group	PLA Group	*p*-Value
Blood loss, mL	704 (426)	364 (174)	<0.001
Operation time, min	84 (28)	46 (9)	<0.001
Hospital stay, days	4.8 (2.0)	4.7 (2.1)	0.8

TABLE 4.—Complications		
	DAA Group	PLA Group
Intraoperative complications with conversion to the posterolateral approach		
Insufficient visibility	1	
Insertion of a cemented prothesis	1	
Acetabular fissure	1	1
Trochanteric fracture	1	
Postoperative complications		
Periprosthetic fracture		1
Dislocation	1	1
Revision		
cup migration/luxation	2	
femoral stem collapse	1	
M. quadriceps weakness	1	
Other complications		
Ischemic cerebrovascular accident	1	
Pneumonia	1	
Ogilvie syndrome		1

(with Harris hip score and Oxford hip score) were similar in both groups at the 1-year follow-up.

Interpretation.—The direct anterior approach is a difficult technique, but adequate hip placement was achieved radiographically. Early results showed no improvement in functional outcome compared to the posterolateral approach, but there was a higher early complication rate. We did not observe any learning effect after 46 patients (Tables 2 and 4).

▶ The authors offer an interesting assessment, not just of the outcome and complication of 2 cohorts, but also of addressing the so-called learning curve. I must disclose I am not a fan of limited invasive techniques unless there is a true and measurable value in assuming the burden of the learning curve. Although these surgeons' experience may not be able to be extrapolated to others, the findings are sobering. As expected, the direct anterior approach took more time, but the increased blood loss surprised me (Table 2). I was not the least bit surprised by the lack of measurable improved function of 1 over the other; this is a universal finding. Although we must cut a little slack for the learning curve, it seems a complication rate that is 3 times in excess of the standard is a little high (Table 4). But for me the hook is that the operative times, blood loss, and complications have not been reduced after 46 procedures. This seems like an excessive learning sample. I guess this is why I don't use this approach.

B. F. Morrey, MD

Comparative Long-Term Survivorship of Uncemented Acetabular Components in Revision Total Hip Arthroplasty

Kremers HM, Howard JL, Loechler Y, et al (Mayo Clinic, Rochester, MN)
J Bone Joint Surg Am 94:e82.1-e82.8, 2012

Background.—It is unknown whether the long-term survival of uncemented acetabular components in revision total hip arthroplasty varies according to component type. The purpose of this study was to compare the survivorship of historical and current uncemented acetabular components following revision total hip arthroplasty.

Methods.—The study population included 3236 patients who underwent 3448 revision total hip arthroplasty procedures with an uncemented acetabular component at a large United States medical center between January 1, 1984, and December 31, 2004. Patients were actively followed up at regular intervals to ascertain details of subsequent revision surgical procedures, including cup (metal shell plus liner) and liner revisions. The overall survival and the cause-specific survival of ten different acetabular components were compared with use of Cox proportional-hazards regression models, adjusting for age and sex.

Results.—A total of 605 repeat revisions, including 386 cup revisions, were performed. The corresponding overall survival rate at fifteen years was 69% (95% confidence interval [CI], 67% to 72%). Compared with titanium wire mesh designs, cup revision for aseptic loosening was significantly more common with beaded designs (hazard ratio [HR], 2.01; 95% CI, 1.44 to 2.80) but less common with trabecular metal designs (HR, 0.25; 95% CI, 0.06 to 1.04). There were no liner revisions for wear and/ or osteolysis during a median of 5.2 years of follow-up of 534 total hip arthroplasties with cross-linked polyethylene liners, resulting in a

TABLE 1.—Baseline Characteristics of the 3448 Revision Total Hip Arthroplasty Procedures Using Uncemented Acetabular Components

Acetabular Shell/ Polyethylene Type*	Time Period	No. of Revision Total Hip Arthroplasty Procedures	Age at Revision Surgery† (yr)	No. (%) of Women
HG-I/conventional	1984−1992	251	57 ± 14	114 (45%)
HG-II/conventional	1988−1997	637	64 ± 13	338 (53%)
PCA/conventional	1984−1988	64	52 ± 15	29 (45%)
Omnifit PSL/conventional	1990−2004	895	66 ± 13	454 (51%)
Spherical/conventional	1987−1990	101	62 ± 14	60 (59%)
Trilogy/conventional	1993−2004	591	66 ± 14	297 (50%)
Trilogy/cross-linked	1999−2004	184	59 ± 14	89 (48%)
Pinnacle/cross-linked	2000−2004	83	63 ± 12	44 (53%)
TM Revision Shell/ conventional	2000−2004	292	71 ± 13	181 (62%)
TM Revision Shell/ cross-linked	1999−2004	350	63 ± 13	198 (57%)
Total		3448	64 ± 14	1804 (52%)

*HG = Harris-Galante, PCA = Porous-Coated Anatomic, PSL = Peripheral Self Locking, and TM = Trabecular Metal.
†Values are given as the mean and the standard deviation.

significantly lower risk of wear-related revision with cross-linked polyethylene compared with conventional liners. Femoral head size and use of an elevated liner were not associated with the risk of repeat revision.

Conclusions.—In the setting of revision total hip arthroplasty, cup survival was worse with beaded acetabular designs compared with titanium wire mesh or highly porous designs. Cross-linked polyethylene liners were associated with a reduced risk of wear-related liner revision (Table 1).

▶ Now that joint replacement is the standard procedure of the orthopedic surgeon today, information on the second-level salvage of failure is very worthwhile. This study offers a large cohort of almost 3500 revisions with study of 605 repeat revisions. The important messages are that the 15-year survival rate of the second revision is 70%: not too bad. Of special interest is the demonstration of a difference in survival according to implant design. Over the period of study, numerous designs were used (Table 1). The outcomes varied considerably as a function of these designs (Fig 1 in the original article). The beaded cup surface treatment fared the worst. This surprised me.

B. F. Morrey, MD

Increased one-year risk of symptomatic venous thromboembolism following total hip replacement: a nationwide cohort study
Pedersen AB, Johnsen SP, Sørensen HT (Aarhus Univ Hosp, Denmark)
J Bone Joint Surg Br 94-B:1598-1603, 2012

We examined the one-year risk of symptomatic venous thromboembolism (VTE) following primary total hip replacement (THR) among Danish patients and a comparison cohort from the general population. From the Danish Hip Arthroplasty Registry we identified all primary THRs performed in Denmark between 1995 and 2010 (n = 85 965). In all, 97% of patients undergoing THR received low-molecular-weight heparin products during hospitalisation. Through the Danish Civil Registration System we sampled a comparison cohort who had not undergone THR from the general population (n = 257 895). Among the patients undergoing THR, the risk of symptomatic VTE was 0.79% between 0 and 90 days after surgery and 0.29% between 91 and 365 days after surgery. In the comparison cohort the corresponding risks were 0.05% and 0.12%, respectively. The adjusted relative risks of symptomatic VTE among patients undergoing THR were 15.84 (95% confidence interval (CI) 13.12 to 19.12) during the first 90 days after surgery and 2.41 (95% CI 2.04 to 2.85) during 91 to 365 days after surgery, compared with the comparison cohort. The relative risk of VTE was elevated irrespective of the gender, age and level of comorbidity at the time of THR.

We concluded that THR was associated with an increased risk of symptomatic VTE up to one year after surgery compared with the general population, although the absolute risk is small.

▶ This article addresses what is probably the most written about subject in joint replacement: deep venous thrombosis (DVT). The value of the article is that it compares the risk of hip replacement to the general population, not one treatment over the other. Remember, the general population does experience DVT and pulmonary embolism (PE), albeit at a very low incidence rate. So the key is not so much the incidence of these problems, but rather does joint replacement with current avoidance strategies still place the patient at risk? The answer is yes (see Fig 1 in the original article). However, the risk is extremely low, especially for PE (as shown in Fig 1C in the original article). I liken it to the lottery. You can increase your chances of winning the lottery 5-fold by buying 5 tickets instead of 1 ticket. Does it really matter? Of course it matters, but it appears we are, fortunately, significantly reducing the risk of this dreaded complication.

B. F. Morrey, MD

Do Retained Pediatric Implants Impact Later Total Hip Arthroplasty?
Woodcock J, Larson AN, Mabry TM, et al (Mayo Clinic, Rochester, MN)
J Pediatr Orthop 33:339-344, 2013

Background.—It is debated whether all pediatric implants in the proximal femur should be removed in childhood. Hardware removal requires an additional surgical procedure and may put the child at risk for postoperative fracture. However, the impact of retained pediatric implants on future surgeries such as total hip arthroplasty (THA) is not well-understood. We undertook this case-control study to evaluate the effect of retained pediatric implants on surgical complexity and complications at the time of THA. This may offer insight as to whether pediatric proximal femoral implants should be removed in childhood.

Methods.—Case-control study. Between 1990 and 2007, 15,601 primary THAs were performed at a tertiary referral center. Of those, 31 hips had pediatric hardware that had been implanted at a mean of 31 years before the time of THA. Perioperative course and complications were compared with an age-matched, sex-matched, and BMI-matched cohort of 31 patients with no retained implants. Mean follow-up after arthroplasty was 7 years.

Results.—Operative time was significantly longer in the retained implant group compared with the control group (230 vs. 159 min; $P < 0.0001$), as was the hospital stay (5.2 vs. 3.8 d; $P = 0.02$). Four of the 14 patients with retained plates required a strut allograft at the time of primary THA. Revision femoral stems and bone grafting were more frequently required in the retained implant cohort. Estimated blood loss was also higher in the retained implant cohort (886 vs. 583 mL; $P = 0.031$). Seven patients in the retained hardware group had a major complication, including

TABLE 2.—Perioperative Results and Complications

	Control [N = 31 Hips (Range)]	Retained Hardware [N = 31 Hips (Range)]	P
Operative time (min)	159 (73-235)	230 (84-434)	<0.0001
Blood loss (mL)	583 (100-1200)	886 (250-3000)	0.031
Hospital stay (d)	3.8 (3-7)	5.2 (3-11)	0.02
Revision stem at the time of primary THA	1	13	0.0005
Bone graft (any)	0	15	<0.0001
Allograft strut	0	4	—
Intraoperative complications	0	7	0.017
Fracture	0	5	—
Nerve palsy	0	1	—
Excessive bleeding	0	1	—
Revision for aseptic loosening	2	4	0.69
Minor complications	3	1	0.61
Superficial infection	1	1	—
Trochanteric bursitis	2	0	—
Preoperative Harris hip score	51.0 (30.3-78.0)	48.5 (30.2-83.8)	0.45
Postoperartive Harris hip score	85.6 (26.2-100)	82.9 (47.7-99.9)	0.54
Change in Harris hip score	36.2 (−9.5 to 88.6)	33.8 (−8 to 66)	0.64

Bold numerals indicate statistically significant.
THA indicates total hip arthroplasty.

intraoperative fracture (5), bleeding (1), and nerve injury (1), whereas no patients in the control group sustained major complications ($P = 0.017$).

Conclusions.—Retained pediatric implants removed at the time of THA were associated with increased operative time, length of stay, and risk of intraoperative fracture. This data supports routine removal of proximal femoral implants in pediatric patients with a high likelihood of future THA.

Level of Evidence.—III, case-control study (Table 2).

▶ I reviewed this article before I noticed it was from my home institution. A constant issue for us has been the one addressed here. Earlier data suggested an increased incidence of sepsis if hardware was removed at the time of total hip arthroplasty. This prompted the practice by some of my colleagues to remove the hardware at a separate prior procedure. Of interest, although the litany of complications is rather long, infection was not one of the complications seen with increased frequency (Table 2). I am not quite sure these data allow the conclusion of routine removal of hardware from the pediatric hip, but it is very clear that if there is a likelihood the child will have a bad hip in adulthood, the hardware should definitely be removed at an early age.

B. F. Morrey, MD

Changing Transfusion Practice in Total Hip Arthroplasty: Observational Study of the Reduction of Blood Use Over 6 Years

Robinson PM, Obi N, Harison T, et al (The Queen Elizabeth Hosp King's Lynn NHS Foundation Trust, Norfolk, UK)
Orthopedics 35:e1586-e1591, 2012

Patients undergoing primary total hip arthroplasty (THA) have historically been over transfused. In a district general hospital setting, the authors observed a significant downward trend in blood transfusion requirements in these patients over 6 years after a change in transfusion policy. The purpose of this study was to retrospectively analyze the change in transfusion practice and present the results of the restrictive transfusion policy.

All patients undergoing primary THA between January 2003 and December 2008 were identified from hospital records. Pre- and postoperative hemoglobin levels, transfusion trigger hemoglobin, blood transfusion requirements, patient age and sex, 30- day mortality, and length of stay data were analyzed for all patients. A total of 1169 primary THAs were performed. Annual allogeneic blood transfusion requirements reduced progressively from 151 units in 2003 to 90 units in 2008 despite an increase in the number of patients undergoing THA. During this period, the proportion of patients transfused decreased from 35% to 17%. A reduction of mean transfusion trigger hemoglobin from 79 to 73 g/L was observed over the study period. No patient experienced any significant complications as a result of undertransfusion.

The authors' institution has steadily restricted the use of blood transfusion in patients undergoing THA to those symptomatic of anemia. Increasing confidence among medical and nursing staff that reduced postoperative hemoglobin levels can be safely tolerated has resulted in a 55%

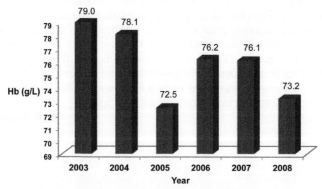

FIGURE 2.—Mean transfusion trigger hemoglobin (Hb) per year. (Reprinted from Robinson PM, Obi N, Harison T, et al. Changing transfusion practice in total hip arthroplasty: observational study of the reduction of blood use over 6 years. *Orthopedics.* 2012;35:e1586-e1591.)

reduction in blood transfusion in patients undergoing THA with no other change of practice (Fig 2).

▶ This study directly addresses the safety and cost-effectiveness direction in which our profession should be headed. In a large community hospital setting, the authors show a dramatic reduction from 35% to 17% in patients after hip replacement who have received a transfusion over the period 2003–2008. There were no associated increases in anemia-associated complications. The beauty of this study is that with such a complex subject, with so many variables, they were able to attribute the improvement to 1 practice change, which was the willingness to with-hold the transfusion based on clinical as well as laboratory findings. In so doing, the mean hemoglobin at the time of transfusion decreased from 7.9 to 7.3 g/L (Fig 2). One variable!! Well done.

B. F. Morrey, MD

B. F. Morrey, MD

8 Total Knee Arthroplasty

Introduction

The projected increased frequency with which the knee will be replaced is truly staggering. This reality places a tremendously increased burden on the orthopedic community "to get it right the first time." Society truly cannot bear the burden of unsuccessful knee joint replacement based on the projected volumes in the coming years. We are aware of this responsibility and have tried to reflect some of the more controversial issues and findings in this year's volume. Thus, whether or not the patella should be replaced in the primary procedure is reviewed along with the management of various complications, which will be seen with increasing frequency. In addition, we have attempted to focus on the importance of restoring function with the management of the complication of infection. This means that, going forward, we must consider function, not just eradicating the infection. This is a challenging time for us, because knee replacement will be the target of increased scrutiny from society. On the one hand, people will be demanding the procedure for themselves. On the other, they'll be questioning the cost to society of performing the procedure in such large numbers. Hopefully, this year's selections will provide some insight into these trends and direct our thought process and our practice appropriately.

Bernard F. Morrey, MD

Determinants of Direct Medical Costs in Primary and Revision Total Knee Arthroplasty
Maradit Kremers H, Visscher SL, Moriarty JP, et al (Mayo Clinic, Rochester, MN)
Clin Orthop Relat Res 471:206-214, 2013

Background.—TKA procedures are increasing rapidly, with substantial cost implications. Determining cost drivers in TKA is essential for care improvement and informing future payment models.

Questions/Purposes.—We determined the components of hospitalization and 90-day costs in primary and revision TKA and the role of demographics, operative indications, comorbidities, and complications as potential determinants of costs.

Methods.—We studied 6475 primary and 1654 revision TKA procedures performed between January 1, 2000, and September 31, 2008, at a single center. Direct medical costs were measured by using standardized, inflation-adjusted costs for services and procedures billed during the 90-day period. We used linear regression models to determine the cost impact associated with individual patient characteristics.

Results.—The largest proportion of costs in both primary and revision TKA, respectively, were for room and board (28% and 23%), operating room (22% and 17%), and prostheses (13% and 24%). Prosthesis costs were almost threefold higher in revision TKA than in primary TKA. Revision TKA procedures for infections and bone and/or prosthesis fractures were approximately 25% more costly than revisions for instability and loosening. Several common comorbidities were associated with higher costs. Patients with vascular and infectious complications had longer hospital stays and at least 80% higher 90-day costs as compared to patients without complications.

Conclusions.—High prosthesis costs in revision TKA represent a factor potentially amenable to cost containment efforts. Increased costs associated with demographic factors and comorbidities may put providers at financial risk and may jeopardize healthcare access for those patients in greatest need.

▶ This study was selected, not because it was done by my colleagues at the Mayo Clinic, but because it offers objective data to help understand a growing concern in our joint replacement practice: cost. The frequency of knee replacement is growing at a meteoric rate. Hence, it would be of value to understand the most common causes of failure and their associated costs. In a word: infection. Other problems certainly arise, but because of frequency and cost, infection after major replacement is and will be a major issue in the cost effective equation going forward.

B. F. Morrey, MD

Biomechanical effects of joint line elevation in total knee arthroplasty
Fornalski S, McGarry MH, Bui CNH, et al (VA Long Beach Healthcare System and Univ of California Irvine)
Clin Biomech 27:824-829, 2012

Background.—Inadequate restoration of the knee joint line after total knee arthroplasty may lead to a poor clinical outcome. The purpose of this study was to quantitatively assess the effects of joint line elevation following total knee arthroplasty with increased joint volume on patellofemoral contact kinematics.

Methods.—Six cadaveric specimens were tested. Patellofemoral contact area, contact pressure, and kinematics were measured following total knee arthroplasty with an anatomic joint line and after 4 and 8 mm of joint line

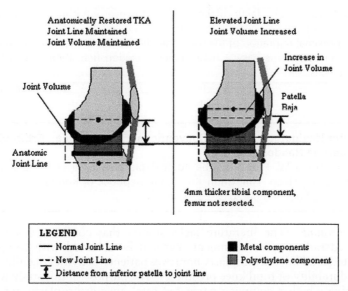

FIGURE 2.—Schematic of joint line elevation, which causes increased joint volume and a pseudo patella baja condition. (Reprinted from Clinical Biomechanics. Fornalski S, McGarry MH, Bui CNH, et al. Biomechanical effects of joint line elevation in total knee arthroplasty. *Clin Biomech*. 2012;27:824-829, Copyright 2012, with permission from Elsevier.)

elevation, at knee flexion angles of 0°, 30°, 60°, 90° and 120°. Repeated measures analysis of variance with a Tukey post hoc test with a significance level of 0.05 was used for statistical analyses.

Findings.—There was a decrease in contact area with joint line elevation at flexion angles of 60°, 90° and 120° ($P = 0.009-0.04$). There was a significant increase in contact pressure only at 30° of knee flexion with 8 mm of joint line elevation ($P = 0.004$). Three of the six specimens showed inferior edge loading of the patella component following 8 mm of joint line elevation at 120° of knee flexion. The sagittal plane patellofemoral angle increased significantly with joint line elevation except for 0° knee flexion ($P = 0.0002-0.02$).

Interpretation.—Knee joint line elevation with increased knee volume significantly affects patellofemoral contact area and kinematics and produced inferior edge loading/impingement between the patella and tibial components, this may result in loss of knee range of motion, postoperative pain, and premature component wear (Fig 2).

▶ As more and more total knee arthroplasty procedures are performed, the surgeon will be faced with more and more revisions. When faced with marked femoral bone loss, we are often forced to accept a strategy of altering the "nominal" joint line. It is very important to understand the theoretical implications of such a procedure. This study clearly documents the theoretical implications of a 4 and 8 mm proximal migration of the joint line (Fig 2). As noted, this does impose increased stress and potential for failure on the patellofemoral articulation. Hence, this could be a source of failure of the revision. However, what are the alternatives? During the real-time procedure, the surgeon must first be aware of the implications of proximal migration of the joint line, the technical alternatives, and then decide. For me this is easy: Obtain femoral fixation first, then deal with the consequences.

B. F. Morrey, MD

Computer-Navigated Versus Conventional Total Knee Arthroplasty: A Prospective Randomized Trial

Kim Y-H, Park J-W, Kim J-S (The Joint Replacement Ctr at Ewha Womans Univ MokDong Hosp, YangChun-Ku, Seoul, Republic of Korea)
J Bone Joint Surg Am 94:2017-2024, 2012

Background.—The literature lacks studies that confirm whether the improved radiographic alignment that can be achieved with computer-navigated total knee arthroplasty improves patients' activities of daily living or the durability of total knee prostheses. The purpose of this study was to determine whether computer-navigated total knee arthroplasty improves the clinical function, alignment, and survivorship of the components.

Methods.—We prospectively compared the results of 520 patients with osteoarthritis who underwent computer-navigated total knee arthroplasty for one knee and conventional total knee arthroplasty for the other. The assignment of the knee to navigation or not was done randomly. There were 452 women (904 knees) and sixty-eight men (136 knees) with a mean age of sixty-eight years (range, forty-nine to eighty-eight years) at the time of the index arthroplasty. The mean follow-up period was 10.8 years (range, ten to twelve years). The patients were assessed clinically and radiographically with the rating system of the Knee Society and with the Western Ontario and McMaster Universities Osteoarthritis Index (WOMAC) score at three months, one year, and annually thereafter.

Results.—Total knee scores, knee function scores, pain scores, WOMAC scores, knee motion, and activity scores did not show statistically significant

---

TABLE 1.—Demographic Data of the 1040 Total Knee Arthroplasties*

	Study Groups		
Parameters	PFC Sigma CR-Mobile-Bearing	NexGen LPS-Flex Fixed-Bearing	P Value
Number of patients (knees)	200 (400)	320 (640)	0.511
Number of males/females	30/170	38/282	0.468
Age* (yr)	67.4 (49-88)	68.7 (50-86)	0.897
Height* (cm)	151.3 (141-168)	151.2 (140-181)	0.498
Weight* (kg)	63.1 (41-91)	64.0 (38-108)	0.721
BMI* (kg/m²)	27.6 (21-32.3)	27.9 (19.4-32.9)	0.812
Diagnosis of osteoarthritis	400 knees	640 knees	0.125
Follow-up* (yr)	11.1 (10-12)	10.5 (10-12)	0.119

*Values are given as the mean, with the range in parentheses. BMI = body mass index.

TABLE 3.—Operative Data*

Parameters	Computer-Navigated Total Knee Arthroplasty (N = 520 Knees)	Conventional Total Knee Arthroplasty (N = 520 Knees)	P Value
Operative time (*min*)	88 (67 to 109)	76 (54 to 87)	<0.001
Tourniquet time (*min*)	59 (45 to 82)	42 (31 to 61)	<0.001
Mean length of incision (*cm*)			
Extension	14.8 (13 to 17.8)	12.8 (10 to 14)	0.823
Flexion	16.3 (14 to 18.6)	13.9 (12 to 16.7)	0.894
Intraoperative blood loss (*mL*)	241 (71 to 530)	238.6 (96 to 596)	0.812
Drainage volume (*mL*)	761.8 (140 to 1280)	718.6 (67 to 1390)	0.519
Drainage duration (*days*)	3.9 (2 to 5)	3.1 (3 to 6)	0.176
Volume of transfusion (*mL*)	1678.4 (150 to 2670)	1785.5 (190 to 2540)	0.078

*The values are given as the mean, with the range in parentheses.

TABLE 4.—Radiographic Results at a Mean of 10.8 Years of Follow-up*

	Computer-Navigated Total Knee Arthroplasty (N = 520)	Conventional Total Knee Arthroplasty (N = 520)	P Value
Mechanical axis (coronal plane)	5.3° of varus to 4.8° of valgus alignment	5.1° of varus to 5.1° of valgus alignment	0.912
Outliers (>3°)	57 (11%)	67 (13%)	0.673
Femoral angle (coronal plane)	92°-101°	90°-103°	0.746
Outliers (>3°)	48 (9%)	53 (10%)	0.704
Femoral angle (sagittal plane)	2.1° ± 1.9°	2.8° ± 2.1°	0.132
Outliers (>3°)	31 (6%)	47 (9%)	0.231
Tibial angle (coronal plane)	86°-93°	84°-95°	0.121
Outliers (>3°)	57 (11%)	78 (15%)	0.133
Tibial angle (sagittal plane)	75°-93°	74°-91°	0.379
Outliers (>3°)	68 (13%)	78 (15%)	0.496

*Outlier values are given as the number of knees, with the percentage of the 520 total knees in parentheses.

differences between the two groups preoperatively or at the time of the final follow-up. Alignment and the survivorship of the components were not significantly different between the two groups. The Kaplan-Meier survivorship with revision as the end point at 10.8 years was 98.8% (95% confidence interval [CI], 0.96 to 1.00) in the computer-navigated total knee arthroplasty group and 99.2% (95% CI, 0.96 to 1.00) in the conventional total knee arthroplasty group.

Conclusions.—Our data demonstrated no difference in clinical function or alignment and survivorship of the components between the knees that underwent computer-navigated total knee arthroplasty and those that underwent conventional total knee arthroplasty.

Level of Evidence.—Therapeutic <u>Level I</u>. See Instructions for Authors for a complete description of levels of evidence (Tables 1, 3 and 4).

▶ This is truly an outstanding study. The large sample of more than 500 procedures, with the patients serving as their own control and surveillance that exceeds

10 years, is impressive in its own right. Even more impressive is the exhaustive pre- and postoperative assessment, radiographically and with validated outcome tools. The authors document similar pathologic characteristics (Table 1). Operative variables reveal the statistically longer surgical time—as expected (Table 3). The extensive assessment of outcome includes no difference in the radiographic measurement of alignment (Table 4). Finally, the impressive 98% and 99% survival rate at more than 10 years demonstrates the skill and experience of these surgeons. So, for me, the conclusions are reinforcement of what is known: navigation takes longer, is of more value in the hands of less experienced surgeons, has not proven to improve outcomes, and with survival of 99% with conventional techniques, it never will. The only remaining questions are whether current, improved systems give different results, and will it or can it ever be proven to be cost-effective? My opinion: Maybe yes on the first question, but I doubt it on the second issue of cost-effectiveness.

B. F. Morrey, MD

Is Pain and Dissatisfaction After TKA Related to Early-grade Preoperative Osteoarthritis?

Polkowski GG II, Ruh EL, Barrack TN, et al (Univ of Connecticut Health Ctr, Farmington; Washington Univ School of Medicine, St Louis, MO)
Clin Orthop Relat Res 471:162-168, 2013

Background.—There is growing evidence to suggest many patients experience pain and dissatisfaction after TKA. The relationship between preoperative osteoarthritis (OA) severity and postoperative pain and dissatisfaction after TKA has not been established.

Questions/Purposes.—We explored the relationship between early-grade preoperative OA with pain and dissatisfaction after TKA by (1) determining the incidence of early-grade preoperative OA in painful TKAs with no other identifiable abnormality; and (2) comparing this incidence with the incidence of early-grade OA in three other cohorts of patients undergoing TKA.

Methods.—We evaluated all (n = 49) painful TKAs in a 1-year period that had no evidence of loosening, instability, malalignment, infection, or extensor mechanism dysfunction and classified the degree of preoperative OA according to the scale of Kellgren and Lawrence. For comparison, we identified three other cohorts of TKAs from the same center and classified their preoperative grade of OA: Group B (n = 100) was a consecutive series of primary TKAs performed for OA during the same year; Group C (n = 80) were asymptomatic TKAs from 1 to 4 years postoperatively; and Group D (n = 80) were TKAs with some degree of pain at 1 to 4 years postoperatively.

Results.—Patients in Group A had a higher incidence of early-grade OA is preoperatively (49%) compared with any of the comparison groups: Group B, 5%; Group C, 6%; and Group D, 10%.

Conclusions.—A high percentage of patients referred for unexplained pain after TKA had early-grade osteoarthritis preoperatively. Patients

TABLE 4.—Kellgren-Lawrence Grades of Preoperative OA for the Study Group (A) and the Comparison Groups (B, C, D) With Differences Among Groups in OA Grade Significant at a Level of $p < 0.001$ Using the Kruskal-Wallis Test

Patient Cohort	K-L OA Grade (1—4)	Number	Percent
A = painful TKA with no abnormality defined (n = 38)	1	7/38	18.4%
	2	12/38	31.6%
	3	11/38	29%
	4	8/38	21%
B = consecutive primary TKAs during the same year (n = 100)	1	2/100	2%
	2	3/100	3%
	3	31/100	31%
	4	64/100	64%
C = normal TKAs with no pain at followup (n = 80)	1	1/80	1.25%
	2	4/80	5%
	3	20/80	25%
	4	55/80	68.75%
D = normal TKAs with some pain at followup (n = 80)	1	2/80	2.5%
	2	6/80	7.5%
	3	30/80	37.5%
	4	42/80	52.5%

OA = osteoarthritis; K-L = Kellgren-Lawrence.

undergoing TKA for less than Grade 3 or 4 OA should be informed that they may be at higher risk for persistent pain and dissatisfaction (Table 4).

▶ I was really pleased to see this study because it confirmed what I have felt and what I have told residents and patients alike. I suspect virtually all orthopedic surgeons subscribe to the belief that the more pain before the procedure, the better the results, at least after a joint replacement. The corollary of this is the more severe the arthritis, the better the perceived benefit. These investigators have shown the latter perception to be a reality (Table 4). Hence, it is important to tell patients with mild disease they may not benefit or not benefit as much after replacement. Ideally, do not do the procedure on early grade disease.

B. F. Morrey, MD

Is patient reporting of physical function accurate following total knee replacement?

Hamilton DF, Gaston P, Simpson AHRW (Univ of Edinburgh, UK)
J Bone Joint Surg Br 94-B:1506-1510, 2012

The aim of this study was to determine the association between the Oxford knee score (OKS) and direct assessment of outcome, and to examine how this relationship varied at different time-points following total knee replacement (TKR). Prospective data consisting of the OKS, numerical rating scales for 'worst pain' and 'perceived mean daily pain', timed functional assessments (chair rising, stairs and walking ability), goniometry and lower limb power were recorded for 183 patients pre-operatively and at six, 26 and 52 weeks post-operatively. The OKS was influenced primarily by the patient's level of pain rather than objective functional assessments. The relationship between report of outcome and direct assessment changed over time: $R^2 = 35\%$ pre-operatively, 44% at six weeks, 57% at 26 weeks and 62% at 52 weeks.

The relationship between assessment of performance and report of performance improved as the patient's report of pain diminished, suggesting that patients' reporting of functional outcome after TKR is influenced more by their pain level than their ability to accomplish tasks.

▶ It is all about pain. I began my career being taught that we must objectively document outcomes, because we could not rely on subjective impressions (motives?) of the patient. Now all of this has changed. We are driven by subjective satisfaction, although we all know this is influenced by numerous irrelevant factors, and these vary over time. Hence, this clean and well-conducted study simply documents that the patient may be doing well but does not know it or accept it if he or she has pain (see Fig 2 in the original article). For me it underscores the problem of relying on patient opinion regarding outcome when so many variables come into play. This can include secondary gain.

B. F. Morrey, MD

Does obesity influence clinical outcome at nine years following total knee replacement?

Collins RA, Walmsley PJ, Amin AK, et al (Queen Margaret Hosp, Dunfermline, Kirkcaldy, UK; Victoria Hosp, Kirkcaldy, UK)
J Bone Joint Surg Br 94-B:1351-1355, 2012

A total of 445 consecutive primary total knee replacements (TKRs) were followed up prospectively at six and 18 months and three, six and nine years. Patients were divided into two groups: non-obese (body mass index (BMI) <30 kg/m^2) and obese (BMI ≥30 kg/m^2). The obese group was subdivided into mildly obese (BMI 30 to 35 kg/m^2) and highly obese (BMI ≥35 kg/m^2) in order to determine the effects of increasing obesity on outcome. The clinical data analysed included the Knee Society score, perioperative complications and implant survival. There was no difference in the overall complication rates or implant survival between the two groups.

Obesity appears to have a small but significant adverse effect on clinical outcome, with highly obese patients showing lower function scores than non-obese patients. However, significant improvements in outcome are sustained in all groups nine years after TKR. Given the substantial, sustainable relief of symptoms after TKR and the low peri-operative complication and revision rates in these two groups, we have found no reason to limit access to TKR in obese patients.

▶ I became interested in this subject after I became Editor of the YEAR BOOK. So many articles seemed only to confuse. However, the answer is becoming more and more clear. In fact, mild levels of obesity, body mass index (BMI) less than 35, do not have too much effect on complication or outcome. And, in fact, even BMI greater than 35 has only a mild effect. But, what is very clear is that patients of all BMI persuasions do benefit from the procedure. Knowing this, after a detailed discussion, I do operate on the markedly (morbid) obese patient—with reluctance and after considerable discussion and candor.

B. F. Morrey, MD

Have Bilateral Total Knee Arthroplasties Become Safer?: A Population-Based Trend Analysis
Memtsoudis SG, Mantilla CB, Parvizi J, et al (Weill Med College of Cornell Univ, NY; Mayo Clinic, Rochester, MN; Jefferson Univ, Philadelphia, PA)
Clin Orthop Relat Res 471:17-25, 2013

Background.—Studies suggest a trend in the selection of younger and healthier individuals to undergo bilateral TKAs in an attempt to diminish the incidence of complications. It remains unclear whether this development has reduced overall perioperative morbidity and mortality.

Questions/Purposes.—We investigated whether changes in demographics and comorbidity patterns of patients undergoing bilateral TKAs are detectable and coincide with changes in length and cost of hospitalization, incidence of perioperative complications, morbidity, and mortality.

Methods.—We accessed Nationwide Inpatient Survey data files between 1999 and 2008. One-year periods were created and changes in demographics, length of in-hospital stay, and perioperative morbidity and mortality were analyzed.

Results.—An estimated 258,524 bilateral TKAs were performed between 1999 and 2008 in the United States. The number of annual procedures increased from 19,288 to 33,679 (75%). Length of hospital stay decreased from 4.98 to 4.01 days. Absolute in-hospital mortality rates decreased at an average rate of 10% per year. The unadjusted percent and adjusted incidence per 1000 inpatient days decreased from 0.42% and 0.85 to 0.16% and 0.39. Although the unadjusted incidence of pneumonia, pulmonary embolism, and nonmyocardial infarction cardiac complications did not change, an increase with time was detectable after adjustment for length of stay. No changes in adjusted incidence were seen for other complications.

Conclusions.—Although a decreased incidence was seen for some major complications, others either remained unchanged or had an increased incidence when adjusted for length of stay. Future interventions should focus on reducing perioperative risk to improve patient safety.

▶ I must confess, because I still perform bilateral knee replacements under the same anesthetic, I have a special interest in this topic. That's my disclosure. Parvizi authored a definitive study showing the slight but statistically increased risk of bilateral simultaneous knee replacement. The key was the risk in the older patient with cardiac disease. The follow-up study could not definitively show the hypothesis that the complications would be fewer in younger patients that have subsequently been felt to be candidates for this procedure. What is known is patient preference seems to be driving this procedure (Table 1 in the original article). Also, in my practice, I use extramedullary alignment techniques. This issue has never been studied in this setting.

B. F. Morrey, MD

All-polyethylene Tibial Components are Equal to Metal-Backed Components: Systematic Review and Meta-Regression
Nouta KA, Verra WC, Pijls BG, et al (Leiden Univ Med Ctr, The Netherlands)
Clin Orthop Relat Res 470:3549-3559, 2012

Background.—Less than 1% of all primary TKAs are performed with an all-polyethylene tibial component, although recent studies indicate all-polyethylene tibial components are equal to or better than metal-backed ones.

Questions/Purposes.—We asked whether the metal-backed tibial component was clinically superior to the all-polyethylene tibial component in primary TKAs regarding revision rates and clinical functioning, and which modifying variables affected the revision rate.

Methods.—We systematically reviewed the literature for clinical studies comparing all-polyethylene and metal-backed tibial components used in primary TKAs in terms of revision rates, clinical scores, and radiologic parameters including radiostereometric analysis (RSA). Meta-regression techniques were used to explore factors modifying the observed effect. Our search yielded 1557 unique references of which 26 articles were included, comprising more than 12,500 TKAs with 231 revisions for any reason.

Results.—Meta-analysis showed no differences between the all-polyethylene and metal-backed components except for higher migration of the metal-backed components. Meta-regression showed strong evidence that the all-polyethylene design has improved with time compared with the metal-backed design.

Conclusions.—The all-polyethylene components were equivalent to metal-backed components regarding revision rates and clinical scores. The all-polyethylene components had better fixation (RSA) than the metal-backed components. The belief that metal-backed components are better than all-polyethylene ones seems to be based on studies from earlier TKAs. This might no longer be true for modern TKAs.

Level of Evidence.—Level II, therapeutic study. See Guidelines for Authors for a complete description of levels of evidence.

▶ I think this is a really important study. To be honest, this is partly because it supports a decision I made 20 years ago to go to an all-polyethylene tibial component. But, in fact, the data on revision for any reason, Fig 1 in the original article, and revision for loosening, Fig 2 in the original article, support this conclusion. The literature clearly demonstrates wear as a cause of failure of total knee arthroplasty, which became evident with modular implants. In addition, virtually every comparative study supports the all-polyethylene implant from virtually every perspective. Going forward, this is also the cost-effective option.

B. F. Morrey, MD

Differences in long-term fixation between mobile-bearing and fixed-bearing knee prostheses at ten to 12 years' follow-up: a single-blinded randomised controlled radiostereometric trial

Pijls BG, Valstar ER, Kaptein BL, et al (Leiden Univ Med Ctr, The Netherlands)
J Bone Joint Surg Br 94-B:1366-1371, 2012

This single-blinded randomised controlled trial investigated whether one design of mobile-bearing (MB) total knee replacement (TKR) has any advantage over a fixed-bearing (FB) design on long-term fixation as measured by radiostereometry. The amount of wear underneath the mobile bearing was also evaluated. A series of 42 knees was randomised to MB or FB tibial components with appropriate polyethylene inserts and followed for between ten and 12 years, or until the death of the patient. The polyethylene in the MB group was superior in that it was gamma-irradiated in inert gas and was calcium-stearate free; the polyethylene in the FB group was gamma-irradiated in air and contained calcium stearate. In theory this should be advantageous to the wear rate of the MB group. At final follow-up the

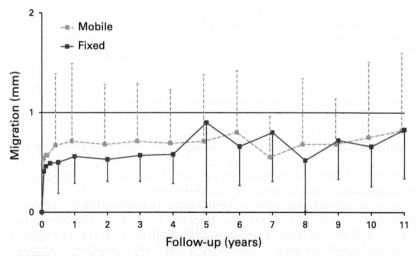

FIGURE 2.—Graph showing the mean migration in maximum total point motion (MTPM) according to the duration of follow-up in the mobile- and fixed-bearing groups. The groups do not differ significantly in MTPM ($p = 0.42$, GLMM). The error bars represent the standard deviation. (Reprinted from Pijls BG, Valstar ER, Kaptein BL, et al. Differences in long-term fixation between mobile-bearing and fixed-bearing knee prostheses at ten to 12 years' follow-up: a single-blinded randomised controlled radiostereometric trial. *J Bone Joint Surg Br.* 2012;94-B:1366-1371, with permission from British Editorial Society of Bone and Joint Surgery.)

overall mean migration was 0.75 mm (SD 0.76) in the MB group and 0.66 mm (SD 0.4) in the FB group, with the FB group demonstrating more posterior tilt and the MB group more internal rotation. In the FB group there was one revision for aseptic loosening, but none in the MB group. There were no significant differences in clinical or radiological scores.

For the MB group, the mean linear wear rate on the under-surface was 0.026 mm/year (SD 0.014). This was significantly smaller than the wear rate of 0.11 mm/year (SD 0.06) in the MB between femur and polyethylene ($p < 0.001$). Nevertheless, even in a best-case setting the mobile bearings of this TKR design had no apparent advantage in terms of fixation over the FB knee prosthesis at ten to 12 years. The wear underneath the mobile bearing was small and is unlikely to be clinically relevant (Fig 2).

▶ While the issue of mobile bearing knees was a hot subject a decade ago, there is little interest in this design today. The reason is that the data simply did not demonstrate an advantage. Functionally, the 2 concepts of fixed or mobile bearing show similar outcomes. This study was included to reinforce the reality of no real difference. The sample size is small, 42, but the question of back side wear is interesting and relevant. Given the minimum of 10-year surveillance, the finding of comparable wear and motion (Fig 2) offers further evidence of no difference in the 2 design philosophies.

B. F. Morrey, MD

Fixed flexion deformity and total knee arthroplasty
Su EP (Hosp for Special Surgery, NY)
J Bone Joint Surg Br 94-B:112-115, 2012

Fixed flexion deformities are common in osteoarthritic knees that are indicated for total knee arthroplasty. The lack of full extension at the knee results in a greater force of quadriceps contracture and energy expenditure. It also results in slower walking velocity and abnormal gait mechanics, overloading the contralateral limb. Residual flexion contractures after TKA have been associated with poorer functional scores and outcomes.

Although some flexion contractures may resolve with time after surgery, a substantial percentage will become permanent. Therefore, it is essential to correct fixed flexion deformities at the time of TKA, and be vigilant in the post-operative course to maintain the correction.

Surgical techniques to address pre-operative flexion contractures include: adequate bone resection, ligament releases, removal of posterior osteophytes, and posterior capsular releases. Post-operatively, extension can be maintained with focused physiotherapy, a specially modified continuous passive motion machine, a contralateral heel lift, and splinting.

▶ In spite of the huge success in the clinical performance of the total knee arthroplasty, residual flexion contracture remains a problem. Almost 5% have more than a 10° residual contracture, and the adverse impact of such a degree of contracture has been well recognized. Although it has been reported that some small contractures resolve with time, there is no question that the goal is to take the contracture out at the time of surgery. This article thus was included to remind us of the problem and the technical maneuvers to correct the problem. The 2 keys maneuvers are to strip the posterior capsule, especially the posterior cruciate ligament. If this is not adequate, it is helpful to know about a 10° improvement is realized with each additional 2 mm of distal femoral resection. Finally, just a reminder that a modest contracture of, say, greater than 20°, in a valgus knee is well known to be associated with peroneal palsy—so beware.

B. F. Morrey, MD

Does pre-coating total knee tibial implants affect the risk of aseptic revision?

Bini SA, Chen Y, Khatod M, et al (Kaiser Permanente, San Diego, CA)
Bone Joint J 95-B:367-370, 2013

We evaluated the impact of pre-coating the tibial component with poly-methylmethacrylate (PMMA) on implant survival in a cohort of 16 548 primary NexGen total knee replacements (TKRs) in 14 113 patients. In 13 835 TKRs a pre-coated tray was used while in 2713 TKRs the non-pre-coated version of the same tray was used. All the TKRs were performed between 2001 and 2009 and were cemented. TKRs implanted with a pre-coated tibial component had a lower cumulative survival than those with a non-pre-coated tibial component ($p = 0.01$). After adjusting for diagnosis, age, gender, body mass index, American Society of Anesthesiologists grade, femoral coupling design, surgeon volume and hospital volume, pre-coating was an independent risk factor for all-cause aseptic revision (hazard ratio 2.75, $p = 0.006$). Revision for aseptic loosening was uncommon for both pre-coated and non-pre-coated trays (rates of 0.12% and 0%, respectively). Pre-coating with PMMA does not appear to be protective of revision for this tibial tray design at short-term follow-up.

▶ I really liked the concept of studying (challenging?) an accepted tactic of knee replacement—covering the tibial tray with polymethylmethacrylate as a precoat. Quite frankly, I already use this technique. This nicely done study, with adequate numbers, is quite revealing. It does not matter, as shown in Fig 1 in the original article. On the other hand, what difference does it make either way? Precoating is not more expensive or time consuming, so to me it is an academic study of academic significance. The rate of tray loosening is very uncommon, period. But the concept of challenging accepted rituals is relevant (ie, use of drains?). Also of note, this is not a study from the Scandinavian registries—it is from the Kaiser group in the United States.

B. F. Morrey, MD

Comparison of patient-reported outcome measures following total and unicondylar knee replacement

Baker PN, Petheram T, Jameson SS, et al (Newcastle Univ, Newcastle upon Tyne, UK)

J Bone Joint Surg Br 94-B:919-927, 2012

Following arthroplasty of the knee, the patient's perception of improvement in symptoms is fundamental to the assessment of outcome. Better clinical outcome may offset the inferior survival observed for some types of implant. By examining linked National Joint Registry (NJR) and patient-reported outcome measures (PROMs) data, we aimed to compare PROMs collected at a minimum of six months post-operatively for total (TKR: n = 23 393) and unicondylar knee replacements (UKR: n = 505). Improvements in knee-specific (Oxford knee score, OKS) and generic (Euro-Qol, EQ-5D) scores were compared and adjusted for case-mix differences using multiple regression. Whereas the improvements in the OKS and EQ-5D were significantly greater for TKR than for UKR, once adjustments were made for case-mix differences and pre-operative score, the improvements in the two scores were not significantly different. The adjusted mean differences in the improvement of OKS and EQ-5D were 0.0 (95% confidence interval (CI) −0.9 to 0.9; $p = 0.96$) and 0.009 (95% CI −0.034 to 0.015; $p = 0.37$), respectively.

We found no difference in the improvement of either knee-specific or general health outcomes between TKR and UKR in a large cohort of registry patients. With concerns about significantly higher revision rates for UKR observed in worldwide registries, we question the widespread use of an arthroplasty that does not confer a significant benefit in clinical outcome (Table 3).

▶ The reader might notice a trend of the articles being selected for this year's publication and review. We see fewer and fewer case studies that seem to be of value and rather are drawn to analytic reviews of the literature, meta-analyses, or large database studies. This assessment is of interest because it studies a

TABLE 3.—Comparison of the Unadjusted Patient Reported Outcome Measures for Total Knee Replacement (TKR) and Unicondylar Knee Replacement (UKR)

Outcome Measure*	TKR	UKR	p-Value†
Mean OKS (95% CI)			
Pre-operative	18.9 (18.8 to 19.0)	21.5 (20.8 to 22.2)	<0.001
Post-operative	34.0 (33.9 to 34.2)	35.5 (34.5 to 36.4)	0.002
Change	15.1 (15.0 to 15.3)	13.9 (13.1 to 14.8)	0.007
Mean EQ-5D (95% CI)			
Pre-operative	0.407 (0.403 to 0.411)	0.470 (0.442 to 0.497)	<0.001
Post-operative	0.710 (0.707 to 0.714)	0.736 (0.711 to 0.760)	0.04
Change	0.303 (0.298 to 0.307)	0.266 (0.236 to 0.296)	0.02

*OKS, Oxford knee score; EQ-5D, EuroQol.
†Student's independent t-test.

controversial issue in knee replacement. It challenges, and, in my opinion, tends to refute the traditional logic and rationale for the unicompartment replacement, that is, trade off of superior function for a poorer survival likelihood. The documentation of poorer survival has been shown repeatedly, but this study of approximately 1300 procedures equally divided between the total versus the unireplacement reveal no functional differences (Table 3). The conclusion is based on validated outcome tools: the Oxford Knee Score and the Euro Qol - 5D system, which assesses 5 outcome domains. Hence, the numbers are adequate and the tools valid to support the conclusions—no difference in function between the 2 techniques. While I continue to do an occasional unireplacement, I will rethink my indications based on these data.

B. F. Morrey, MD

Differences in Short-Term Complications Between Spinal and General Anesthesia for Primary Total Knee Arthroplasty
Pugely AJ, Martin CT, Gao Y, et al (Univ of Iowa Hosps and Clinics, Iowa City)
J Bone Joint Surg Am 95:193-199, 2013

Background.—Spinal anesthesia has been associated with lower postoperative rates of deep-vein thrombosis, a shorter operative time, and less blood loss when compared with general anesthesia. The purpose of the present study was to identify differences in thirty-day perioperative morbidity and mortality between anesthesia choices among patients undergoing total knee arthroplasty.

Methods.—The American College of Surgeons National Surgical Quality Improvement Program (ACS NSQIP) database was searched to identify patients who underwent primary total knee arthroplasty between 2005 and 2010. Complications that occurred within thirty days after the procedure in patients who had been managed with either general or spinal anesthesia were identified. Patient characteristics, thirty-day complication rates, and mortality were compared. Multivariate logistic regression identified predictors of thirty-day morbidity, and stratified propensity scores were used to adjust for selection bias.

Results.—The database search identified 14,052 cases of primary total knee arthroplasty; 6030 (42.9%) were performed with the patient under spinal anesthesia and 8022 (57.1%) were performed with the patient under general anesthesia. The spinal anesthesia group had a lower unadjusted frequency of superficial wound infections (0.68% versus 0.92%; $p = 0.0003$), blood transfusions (5.02% versus 6.07%; $p = 0.0086$), and overall complications (10.72% versus 12.34%; $p = 0.0032$). The length of surgery (ninety-six versus 100 minutes; $p < 0.0001$) and the length of hospital stay (3.45 versus 3.77 days; $p < 0.0001$) were shorter in the spinal anesthesia group. After adjustment for potential confounders, the overall likelihood of complications was significantly higher in association with general anesthesia (odds ratio, 1.129; 95% confidence interval, 1.004 to 1.269). Patients with the highest number of preoperative comorbidities, as

TABLE 3.—Significant Risk Factors for Complications After Total Knee Arthroplasty as Determined with Multivariate Logistic Regression Analysis

Characteristic	P Value	Adjusted Odds Ratio*
Demographic data		
Age		
70 to 79 yr	<0.0001	1.531 (1.263 to 1.856)
≥80 yr	<0.0001	2.173 (1.725 to 2.737)
Sex		
Female versus male	0.0141	1.176 (1.033 to 1.338)
Race		
Black versus white	<0.0001	1.678 (1.346 to 2.092)
Laboratory values		
Creatinine	<0.0001	1.474 (1.243 to 1.748)
Operative variables		
ASA class	0.0112	1.204 (1.060 to 1.367)
Operative time	0.0007	1.003 (1.001 to 1.004)
General versus spinal anesthesia	0.0430	1.129 (1.004 to 1.269)

*The 95% confidence interval is given in parentheses.

defined by propensity score-matched quintiles, demonstrated a significant difference between the groups with regard to the short-term complication rate (11.63% versus 15.28%; $p = 0.0152$). Age, female sex, black race, elevated creatinine, American Society of Anesthesiologists class, operative time, and anesthetic choice were all independent risk factors of short-term complication after total knee arthroplasty.

Conclusions.—Patients undergoing total knee arthroplasty who were managed with general anesthesia had a small but significant increase in the risk of complications as compared with patients who were managed with spinal anesthesia; the difference was greatest for patients with multiple comorbidities. Surgeons who perform knee arthroplasty may consider spinal anesthesia for patients with comorbidities (Table 3).

▶ This is a really important study because we can immediately benefit from the findings. A question such as subtle differences in complications as a function of anesthesia type requires a massive number of patients studied. Hence the use of the large database with about 6000 patients (43%) in the spinal and 8000 (53%) in the general anesthesia groups. The statistical significance of more complications overall in the general anesthesia group may surprise some. The real value is the demonstration of the various comorbidities that all have a greater likelihood of generating a complication in the general anesthesia group (Table 3). Hence the simple recommendation of the authors would seem prudent: consider a spinal if your patient has these comorbidities.

B. F. Morrey, MD

Alternatives to revision total knee arthroplasty

Jones RE, Russell RD, Huo MH (Univ of Texas Southwestern Med Ctr, Dallas)
J Bone Joint Surg Br 94-B:137-140, 2012

Most problems encountered in complex revision total knee arthroplasty can be managed with the wide range of implant systems currently available. Modular metaphyseal sleeves, metallic augments and cones provide stability even with significant bone loss. Hinged designs substitute for significant ligamentous deficiencies. Catastrophic failure that precludes successful reconstruction can be encountered. The alternatives to arthroplasty in such drastic situations include knee arthrodesis, resection arthroplasty and amputation. The relative indications for the selection of these alternatives are recurrent deep infection, immunocompromised host, and extensive non-reconstructible bone or soft-tissue defects.

▶ This article reads more like an instructional course than a scientific contribution. I have included it for several reasons. It is always good to not just be aware of the salvage options, but also the expected results. I feel this article was misnamed. Fusion, resection, and amputation are NOT alternatives to revision; they are options when revision has failed, and as such, they are purely salvage options. The high rate of conversion from resection should be noted. And, the high rate of nonunion of attempted fusion, correlated with amount of bone loss should also be noted. In a word, these salvage operations can eradicate infection, but they are not very functional in outcome and have high complication rates in their own right.

B. F. Morrey, MD

Assessing the Gold Standard: A Review of 253 Two-Stage Revisions for Infected TKA

Mahmud T, Lyons MC, Naudie DD, et al (Univ of Western Ontario & London Health Sciences Centre, Ontario, Canada)
Clin Orthop Relat Res 470:2730-2736, 2012

Background.—Periprosthetic joint infection has been the leading cause of failure following TKA surgery. The gold standard for infection control has been a two-staged revision TKA. There have been few reports on mid- to long-term survivorship, functional outcomes, and fate of patients with a failed two-stage revision TKA.

Questions/Purposes.—Therefore, we determined (1) the mid-term survivorship of two-stage revision TKA, (2) the function of patients in whom infection was controlled, and (3) the outcome of patients with a failed two-stage revision due to recurrent infection.

Methods.—We retrospectively reviewed 239 patients who underwent 253 two-stage revision TKAs for periprosthetic infection. There were 239

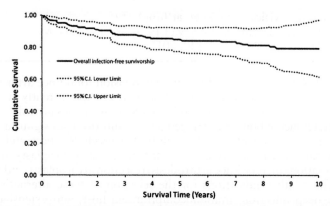

FIGURE 1.—The graph shows the overall infection-free survivorship for two-stage revision TKA. (With kind permission from Springer Science+Business Media: Mahmud T, Lyons MC, Naudie DD, et al. Assessing the gold standard: a review of 253 two-stage revisions for infected TKA. *Clin Orthop Relat Res.* 2012;470:2730-2736, with permission from The Association of Bone and Joint Surgeons.)

patients (253 knees), 104 men and 135 women, with a mean age of 70 ± 10 years at the time of two-stage revision and a mean BMI of 31.53 ± 6.74 kg/m². During followup, we obtained WOMAC and The Knee Society Clinical Rating Scores and radiographs. The minimum followup was 1 year (median, 4 years; range, 1–17 years).

Results.—Thirty-three patients experienced a failed two-staged TKA. Sixteen patients experienced failure due to recurrent sepsis. There were 17 failures for aseptic causes.

Conclusion.—The overall infection-free survivorship for two-stage revision TKA was 85% at 5 years and 78% at 10 years.

Level of Evidence.—Level IV, therapeutic study. See the Guidelines for Authors for a complete description of levels of evidence (Fig 1).

▶ I am always attracted to investigations that question traditional wisdom that is not well-founded on data. In this instance, the thorough assessment of 250 2-stage procedures reinforces what was already known. Two-staged replacement is effective, and if it is effective at 5 years, it will tend to be reliable ongoing (Fig 1). The reader should note that 50% of the 15% 5-year failure rate was not due to reinfection but rather to loosening or instability. My main disappointment is this article did not address the real issue—that is, the functional price paid for an infection. Although a reimplant may be possible, the functional result to the patient is not as good as an uncomplicated procedure. It's just the way it is.

B. F. Morrey, MD

Developing a strategy to treat established infection in total knee replacement: a review of the latest evidence and clinical practice
Vanhegan IS, Morgan-Jones R, Barrett DS, et al (Univ College London Hosp NHS Trust, UK)
J Bone Joint Surg Br 94-B:875-881, 2012

This review summarises the opinions and conclusions reached from a symposium on infected total knee replacement (TKR) held at the British Association of Surgery of the Knee (BASK) annual meeting in 2011. The National Joint Registry for England and Wales reported 5082 revision TKRs in 2010, of which 1157 (23%) were caused by infection. The diagnosis of infection beyond the acute post-operative stage relies on the identification of the causative organism by aspiration and analysis of material obtained at arthroscopy. Ideal treatment then involves a two-stage surgical procedure with extensive debridement and washout, followed by antibiotics. An articulating or non-articulating drug-eluting cement spacer is used prior to implantation of the revision prosthesis, guided by the serum level of inflammatory markers. The use of a single-stage revision is gaining popularity and we would advocate its use in certain patients where the causative organism is known, no sinuses are present, the patient is not immunocompromised, and there is no radiological evidence of component loosening or osteitis.

It is our opinion that single-stage revision produces high-quality reproducible results and will soon achieve the same widespread acceptance as it does in infected hip arthroplasty (Table 3).

▶ I think these kinds of studies can be game changers. We have published and practiced a stratified approach to managing the infected hip, knee, and elbow. However, I have never performed a single-staged revision, in spite of performing numerous-staged debridements. The data and rationale, however, are compelling. I have a personal relationship with the Endo-Klinik, the group that popularized this

TABLE 3.—Relative Contraindications to Attempting Singlestage Revision Surgery in Hip Replacement (Reproduced with permission from Oussedik et al[29])

Category	Compromising Factor
Local	Significant soft-tissue compromise
	Significant bone loss precluding cemented reconstruction
	Peripheral vascular disease
Host	Immunosuppression
	Concurrent sepsis
	Systemic disease
	Reinfection
Organism	Multiresistant organisms MRSA/MRSE*
	Polymicrobial infection
	Unusual commensals
	Unusual resistance profiles
	Unidentified infective organisms

Editor's Note: Please refer to original journal article for full references.
*MRSA, methicillin-resistant *Staphylococcus aureus*; MRSE, methicillin-resistant *Staphylococcus* epidermidis.

concept. I have absolute trust in their integrity and competency. I do believe that if we accept the contraindications reported for hip infection management (Table 3), this can be a very safe and cost-effective strategy for managing the infected knee. However, I would pay close attention to the virulence of the organism.

B. F. Morrey, MD

Evaluation of Centers of Excellence Program for Knee and Hip Replacement

Mehrotra A, Sloss EM, Hussey PS, et al (RAND Corporation, Pittsburgh, PA and Washington, DC; et al)
Med Care 51:28-36, 2013

Background.—Medicare and private plans are encouraging individuals to seek care at hospitals that are designated as centers of excellence. Few evaluations of such programs have been conducted. This study examines a large national initiative that designated hospitals as centers of excellence for knee and hip replacement.

Objective.—Comparison of outcomes and costs associated with knee and hip replacement at designated hospitals and other hospitals.

Research Design.—Retrospective claims analysis of approximately 54 million enrollees.

Study Population.—Individuals with insurance from one of the sponsors of this centers of excellence program who underwent a primary knee or hip replacement in 2007–2009.

Outcomes.—Primary outcomes were any complication within 30 days of discharge and costs within 90 days after the procedure.

Results.—A total of 80,931 patients had a knee replacement and 39,532 patients had a hip replacement of which 52.2% and 56.5%, respectively, were performed at a designated hospital. Designated hospitals had a larger number of beds and were more likely to be an academic center. Patients with a knee replacement at designated hospitals did not have a statistically significantly lower overall complication rate with an odds ratio of 0.90 ($P = 0.08$). Patients with hip replacement treated at designated hospitals had a statistically significant lower risk of complications with an odds ratio of 0.80 ($P = 0.002$). There was no significant difference in 90-day costs for either procedure.

Conclusions.—Hospitals designated as joint replacement centers of excellence had lower rates of complications for hip replacement, but there was no statistically significant difference for knee replacement. It is important to validate the criteria used to designate centers of excellence (Table 4).

▶ As may becoming evident, I am drawn to larger scope questions and studies. The issue of whether there is a measurable difference in outcomes between the high-volume, often academic, hospitals and community hospitals will emerge in the future to be less of academic and more of practical importance. As the orthopedic surgeon continues to lose control of our profession, we will see more and

TABLE 4.—Unadjusted Rates and Adjusted Odds Ratios for Selected Complication and Readmission Rates After Total Knee Replacements and Total Hip Replacements Performed in Designated Hospitals and Other Hospitals, July 2007–September 2009

| | Total Knee Replacement | | | | | Total Hip Replacement | | | | |
| | Designated Hospitals N=42,255 | | Other Hospitals N=38,676 | | | Designated Hospitals N=22,329 | | Other Hospitals N=17,203 | | |
Outcome Category	N	Rate (%)	N	Rate (%)	Odds Ratio (P)*	N	Rate (%)	N	Rate (%)	Odds Ratio (P)*
Any complication	778	2.17	1053	2.45	0.90 (0.08)	474	2.46	607	3.12	0.80 (0.00)
Acute myocardial infarction (within 7 d of admission)	39	0.11	65	0.15	0.79† (0.28)	29	0.15	18	0.09	1.51 (0.16)
Pneumonia (within 7 d of admission)	97	0.27	155	0.36	0.82 (0.15)	50	0.26	67	0.34	0.86 (0.42)
Sepsis/septicemia (within 7 d of admission)	144	0.40	188	0.44	0.90 (0.39)	34	0.18	67	0.34	0.50 (0.00)
Pulmonary embolism (within 30 d of admission)	252	0.70	283	0.66	1.05 (0.65)	62	0.32	70	0.36	1.08 (0.73)
Wound infection (within 30 d of admission)	69	0.19	125	0.29	0.70 (0.19)	39	0.20	75	0.38	0.54† (0.00)
Surgical-site bleeding (within 30 d of admission)	16	0.04	50	0.12	0.41 (0.00)	31	0.16	34	0.17	0.93† (0.78)
Mortality (within 30 d of admission)	19	0.05	18	0.04	1.25† (0.49)	4	0.02	7	0.04	0.43† (0.18)
Periprosthetic joint infection (within 90 d of admission)	105	0.29	137	0.32	0.93 (0.58)	77	0.40	72	0.37	0.95 (0.77)
Mechanical complication (within 90 d of admission)	118	0.33	146	0.34	1.03 (0.85)	202	1.05	264	1.36	0.80 (0.46)
Any readmission (within 30 d of discharge)	1149	3.20	1423	3.31	0.94 (0.18)	603	3.13	707	3.63	0.82 (0.00)

*For each complication among patients having a knee or hip replacement, this represents the odds ratio comparing designated hospitals to other hospitals. Models include: age, sex, and presence of 26 comorbidities.

†For this outcome, the odds ratios and P-values are based on a model with fewer covariates because initially the model did not converge. See Appendix for details.

more external regulation. Data such as presented here will be the kind used in the future to decide who does what. It is difficult to understand with certainty why there is no difference in knee replacement, but there is in hip replacement, depending on the type of hospital in which the surgery is performed (Table 4). I assume that it is either the knee replacement is less difficult, the increased frequency washes out subtle differences, or a combination of both. Regardless, we are alert to the fact that the information contained here will be used in the future to define access and reimbursement. Hopefully, I'll be fishing when this happens.

B. F. Morrey, MD

Articulating Spacers for the Treatment of Infected Total Knee Arthroplasty: Effect of Antibiotic Combinations and Concentrations

Nettrour JF, Polikandriotis JA, Bernasek TL, et al (Iowa Orthopaedic Ctr, Des Moines; Foundation for Orthopaedic Res and Education, Tampa, FL; Florida Orthopaedic Inst, Tampa)
Orthopedics 36:e19-e24, 2013

Performing 2-stage procedures using articulating antibiotic cement spacers to eradicate infection while providing pain relief and maintaining function has become common among many surgeons. Despite the efficacy of antibiotic cement spacers in the treatment of infected total knee arthroplasty, questions remain regarding the dosing of the antibiotic cement.

The authors assessed their experience with different antibiotic regimens and concentrations for the eradication of infection. Sixty-nine infected total knee arthroplasties with an average follow up of 31 months (range, 6-70 months) treated with articulating antibiotic spacers were retrospectively reviewed. Treatment groups were divided according to spacer antibiotic agents used and the amount of antibiotics added to the cement. Low-dose spacers were defined as those incorporating less than 4 g of antibiotic per 40-g bag of cement, and high-dose spacers were defined as those incorporating 4 g or more of antibiotic per 40-g bag of cement. High- vs low-dose spacers using a single or multiple antibiotic agents were compared.

TABLE 3.—Treatment Failures

Group	No. of Patients	No. (%) of Treatment Failures
All patients	69	8 (11.6)
One-agent spacers	33	4 (12.1)[a]
Low dose	18	3 (16.7)[b]
High dose	15	1 (6.7)[b]
Two-agent spacers	36	4 (11.1)
Low dose	14	0 (0.0)[c]
High dose	22	4 (18.2)[c]

[a]One-agent spacers vs 1-agent spacers; $P=.999$.
[b]One-agent low dose vs 1-agent high dose; $P=.607$.
[c]Two-agent low dose vs 2-agent high dose; $P=.141$.

TABLE 4.—Success Rate in Immune-Impaired Patients

Group	Success Rate in Immune-Impaired Patients, % (No.)
All patients	87.1 (27 of 31)
One-agent spacers	88.9 (8 of 9)[a]
Low dose	100 (5 of 5)[b]
High dose	75.0 (3 of 4)[b]
Two-agent spacers	86.4 (19 of 22)[a]
Low dose	100 (9 of 9)[c]
High dose	76.9 (10 of 13)[c]

[a]One-agent spacers vs 2-agent spacers; *P* =.999.
[b]One-agent low dose vs 1-agent high dose; *P* =.444.
[c]Two- agent low dose vs 2-agent high dose; *P* =.240.

The overall rate of infection eradication was 88%. Dose dependency was not detected for spacers that incorporated single or multiple antibiotic agents, and multiple-agent spacers produced comparable success rates despite more frequent use in patients with impaired immune function.

Further study of optimal combinations and concentrations of antibiotic agents incorporated into these spacers is needed to help minimize treatment failures while maximizing treatment efficacy (Tables 3 and 4).

▶ The use of low-friction articulated spacers is truly a major advance in the management of the infected knee. These surgeons report an impressive 88% infection-free outcome—recognizing the minimum surveillance is 6 months. Regardless, the question asked is important for the obvious reasons of developing resistant strains and cost. They do a nice job stratifying the outcome by immuno-competency (Tables 3 and 4). Although no statistical differences in regimens were found, for my part, low-dose, multiagent treatment appears to be effective in both groups.

B. F. Morrey, MD

A case-control study of spontaneous patellar fractures following primary total knee replacement

Seo JG, Moon YW, Park SH, et al (Sungkyunkwan Univ School of Medicine, Seoul, Korea)
J Bone Joint Surg Br 94-B:908-913, 2012

Peri-prosthetic patellar fracture following resurfacing as part of total knee replacement (TKR) is an infrequent yet challenging complication. This case-control study was performed to identify clinical, radiological and surgical factors that increase the risk of developing a spontaneous patellar fracture after TKR. Patellar fractures were identified in 74 patients (88 knees) from a series of 7866 consecutive TKRs conducted between 1998 and 2009. After excluding those with a previous history of extensor mechanism

TABLE 3.—Univariate Analysis of Surgical Variables

Parameter	Patient Group (n = 64)	Control Group (n = 64)	Odds Ratio (95% CI)	p-value
Previous surgeries (n, %)				
0	36 (56.3)	45 (70.3)	1.0	-
1	16 (25.0)	13 (20.3)	1.5 (0.6 to 3.9)	0.6025
<1	12 (18.7)	6 (9.4)	2.8 (0.9 to 5.6)	0.0386
Tibial component size (n, %)				
≤4	14 (21.9)	15 (23.4)	1.0	-
5 to 6	30 (46.9)	32 (50.0)	1.0 (0.4 to 2.4)	0.9921
≥7	20 (31.3)	17 (26.6)	0.8 (0.3 to 2.1)	0.6413
Femoral component size (n, %)				
≤4	8 (12.5)	10 (15.6)	1.0	-
5 to 6	27 (42.2)	36 (56.3)	1.1 (0.4 to 3.1)	0.9046
≥7	29 (45.3)	18 (28.1)	0.5 (0.2 to 1.5)	0.2123
Polyethylene thickness (n, %)				
<12 mm	2 (3.1)	6 (9.4)	1.0	-
12 mm	49 (76.6)	45 (70.3)	0.3 (0.1 to 1.6)	0.1599
>12 mm	13 (20.3)	13 (20.3)	0.3 (0.1 to 2.0)	0.2252
Patellar component size (n, %)				
3 mm	52 (81.3)	48 (75)	1.0	-
5 mm	12 (18.8)	16 (25)	1.2 (0.8 to 1.8)	0.3937
Lateral retinacular release (n, %)				
No	54 (84.4)	59 (82.2)	1.0	-
Yes	10 (15.6)	5 (7.8)	2.2 (0.7 to 6.8)	0.1771

realignment or a clear traumatic event, a metal-backed patella, any uncemented component or subsequent infection, the remaining 64 fractures were compared with a matched group of TKRs with an excellent outcome defined by the Knee Society score. The mean age of patients with a fracture was 70 years (51 to 81) at the time of TKR. Patellar fractures were detected at a mean of 13.4 months (2 to 84) after surgery. The incidence of patellar fracture was found to be strongly associated with the number of previous knee operations, greater pre-operative mechanical malalignment, smaller post-operative patellar tendon length, thinner postresection patellar thickness, and a lower post-operative Insall-Salvati ratio.

An understanding of the risk factors associated with spontaneous patellar fracture following TKR provides a valuable insight into prevention of this challenging complication (Table 3).

▶ I consider this a very important study for 4 reasons: This problem, when it occurs, is a disaster; very little is known about it, and even less has been documented regarding the risk factors; this effort provides insights for avoidance; avoidance is key because there is no good treatment for it when it occurs.

Although some of the risk factors are intuitive, these authors provide statistical evidence of a litany of preoperative correlations with subsequent fracture: A shorter patellar tendon and a thinner patellar resection are intuitive. The correlation with previous surgery and residual malalignment maybe less so (Table 3). For me, the variables in my control, and the insight to apply this knowledge, is in the patient with multiple prior knee procedures, especially with a shortened patellar tendon. In this instance, we should keep the resection to a minimum, or possibly not replace the patella at all unless it is clearly necessary.

B. F. Morrey, MD

Adjacent Segment Pathology Following Cervical Motion-Sparing Procedures or Devices Compared With Fusion Surgery: A Systematic Review
Harrod CC, Hilibrand AS, Fischer DJ, et al (Thomas Jefferson Univ and Hosps, Philadelphia, PA)
Spine 37:S96-S112, 2012

Study Design.—A systematic review.

Objective.—To critically review and summarize the literature comparing motion preservation devices to fusion in the cervical spine to determine whether the use of these devices decreases the development of radiographical (RASP) or clinical adjacent segment pathology (CASP) compared with fusion.

Summary of Background Data.—Historically, surgical treatment of symptomatic cervical disc disease presenting as radiculopathy and/or myelopathy with anterior cervical decompression and fusion has yielded excellent results. Controversy remains whether RASP and CASP requiring treatment is due to fusion-altered biomechanics and kinematics versus natural history.

Methods.—We conducted a systematic search in MEDLINE and the Cochrane Collaboration Library for literature published through February 2012 on human randomized control trials or cohort studies published in the English language containing abstracts to answer the following key questions: (1) Is there evidence that total disc replacement (TDR) is associated with a lower risk of RASP or CASP compared with fusion? (2) Is there evidence that other procedures that do not involve arthrodesis or other motion-sparing devices are associated with a lower risk of RASP or CASP compared with fusion? (3) Is one type of motion preservation device or procedure associated with a lower risk of RASP or CASP compared with others?

Results.—The initial literature search yielded 276 citations, of which 73 unique, potentially relevant citations that were evaluated against the inclusion/exclusion criteria set a *priori*. A total of 14 studies were selected for inclusion. For question 1, RASP was variably reported in studies that compared total disc replacement (TDR) to anterior cervical decompression and fusion (ACDF), and risk differences for reoperation due to CASP ranged from 1.0% to 4.8%, with no statistically significant differences between groups. For question 2, no studies comparing motion preservation devices to ACDF met our inclusion criteria. For question 3, one study comparing motion-sparing devices found the risk of RASP to be similar between groups.

Conclusion.—A paucity of high-quality literature comparing motion-preserving devices or treatment methods to fusion or other motion-preserving techniques or devices (with RASP and/or CASP as an outcome using consistent definitions) exists. Independently funded, blinded long-term follow-up prospective studies would be able to delineate the true effects regarding incidence of RASP and CASP and treatment of CASP.

Consensus Statement.—1. There is no significant difference in development of RASP and CASP after C-TDR versus ACDF at short- to mid-term follow-up.

Level of Evidence: Moderate.

Strength of Statement: Strong.

Recommendation 1: No recommendation can be made from comparative literature of nonarthroplasty motion preservation device or techniques compared with fusion regarding the risk of RASP or CASP.

Level of Evidence: Insufficient.

Strength of Statement: Strong.

Recommendation 2: No recommendation can be made from direct comparative literature of various motion preservation devices or techniques regarding the risk of RASP or CASP.

Level of Evidence: Insufficient.

Strength of Statement: Strong.

▶ This report from the Thomas Jefferson University Hospitals and Clinics and the Rothman Institute is a fine example of a systemic review of radiographic or clinical adjacent segment pathology comparing motion-preserving devices and techniques with cervical fusion. The strength of the publication comes from its rigid and systematic methodology and the measured but transparent statement of evidence in the conclusion. It acknowledges the potential of industry bias in the reporting of results in past motion-sparing device studies and correctly points out the lack of prospective studies comparing nonfusion techniques such as foraminotomy to artificial disc technology. The take-home point for all professional and casual spine surgeons should be there has yet to be shown any short-term to medium-term difference in anterior cervical decompression and fusion and motion-sparing devices in the prevention of symptomatic or asymptomatic adjacent segment disease. One of the challenges going forward will be to standardize a definition of adjacent segment pathology to bring all future clinical studies into alignment.

P. Huddleston, MD

9 Foot and Ankle

Introduction

Foot and ankle remains an interesting and challenging area for the orthopedic surgeon. The management of foot and ankle, of course, requires knowledge and competency to intervene in several dramatically different anatomic parts. The various selections this year have attempted to provide insight into all these anatomic areas with articles that are felt to be of significant value. As in previous years, we have also included articles that provide useful and practical insight into the management of the diabetic foot. With the explosion of this disease in our society, there are few areas of greater value than improving our management of the foot complications that result from this condition.

Bernard F. Morrey, MD

Age and Sex Differences Between Patient and Physician-Derived Outcome Measures in the Foot and Ankle

Baumhauer JF, McIntosh S, Rechtine G (Univ of Rochester School of Medicine and Dentistry, NY; Bay Pines VA Healthcare System, FL)
J Bone Joint Surg Am 95:209-214, 2013

Background.—Traditionally, physicians have identified which outcome factors are important to measure in order to determine the success or failure of treatment without any input from patients. The purpose of the present study was to ascertain the five outcome factors that are most important to the patient and the impact that age and sex have on these factors. These five most important patient-derived outcome factors were then compared with factors within two of the most commonly used outcome instruments for the foot and ankle.

Methods.—Informant interviews, pre-testing, consistency analysis, and pilot testing led to the construction of a twenty-item survey of outcome factors that patients identified as being important in the treatment of their foot or ankle problem. Subjects selected the top five factors and rank ordered them from 1 to 5 (with 1 representing extreme importance and 5 representing least importance). One thousand computer simulations identified the top five factors, and these were subsequently stratified for sex and age. Wilcoxon

TABLE 2.—Factor Ranking for Overall, Sex, and Age Groups

| | Factor Rank in Terms of Importance | | | | | Percentage of Patients Ranking Factor in Top Five in Terms of Importance | | | | | | |
| | | Sex | | Age | | | Sex | | | Age | | |
Factors	Overall	Male	Female	<55 Yrs	≥55 Yrs	Overall	Male	Female	P Value	<55 Yrs	≥55 Yrs	P Value
Activity-related pain	2	2	2	1	2	30.0%	32.5%	28.9%	0.49	31.6%	28.4%	0.88
Constant pain	3	3	3	3	3	21.2%	21.8%	20.9%	0.93	25.8%	16.6%	0.010*
Night pain	9	11	8	9	6	11.1%	9.1%	12.0%	0.36	11.2%	11.0%	0.90
Limp	14	9	16	16	14	8.4%	11.1%	7.2%	0.18	8.2%	8.7%	0.90
Stiffness	10	8	9	10	7	10.6%	11.1%	10.4%	0.89	10.0%	11.3%	0.90
Having to take a pill	15	14	15	14	15	8.6%	7.0%	9.3%	0.49	8.9%	8.2%	0.90
Walking aids	17	13	18	17	19	6.0%	7.8%	5.2%	0.27	7.7%	4.4%	0.13
Crooked foot/ankle/toes	16	18	13	13	16	8.2%	5.4%	9.4%	0.18	8.4%	7.9%	0.90
Fear of falling	11	10	10	11	8	10.7%	10.7%	10.7%	0.93	10.5%	11.0%	0.90
Loss of independence	12	12	12	12	12	8.7%	8.2%	8.9%	0.89	8.9%	8.4%	0.90
Difficulty fitting into shoes	7	16	4	8	4	15.6%	6.6%	19.6%	<0.05*	14.0%	17.1%	0.42
Inability to play sports	6	6	7	5	9	14.7%	18.1%	13.2%	0.18	19.1%	10.2%	0.005*
Inability to do job/housework	5	4	6	4	10	15.8%	20.6%	13.7%	0.06	21.4%	10.2%	0.000*
Prolonged standing	4	5	5	6	5	16.6%	20.6%	14.8%	0.18	19.6%	13.6%	0.13
Need for bracewear/orthotics	13	17	11	15	11	9.3%	6.6%	10.6%	0.18	8.4%	10.2%	0.85
Limit in walking	1	1	1	2	1	33.7%	34.2%	33.5%	0.77	32.7%	34.8%	0.78
Recurrent sores or infection	19	19	20	20	18	2.8%	4.5%	2.0%	0.18	1.3%	4.4%	0.0451*
Pain while driving	20	20	19	19	20	3.5%	2.5%	3.9%	0.49	3.8%	3.1%	0.90
Weakness	8	7	14	7	13	11.6%	16.5%	9.4%	0.04*	14.0%	9.2%	0.11
Numbness	18	17	17	18	17	6.3%	6.6%	6.1%	0.89	6.4%	6.1%	0.90

*Significant (p < 0.05).

rank-sum and Benjamini-Hochberg tests were used to compare the data between groups.

Results.—The survey was completed by 783 subjects. The five most important factors were limited walking ($p < 0.05$), activity-related pain ($p < 0.05$), constant pain ($p < 0.05$), difficulty with prolonged standing ($p = 0.754$), and inability to do one's job or housework ($p = 0.995$). Shoe-related issues and foot and ankle weakness were significantly different between the sexes. Constant pain, inability to play sports, inability to partic-ipate in a job or housework, and recurrent foot or ankle skin sores or infec-tions were significantly different between age groups. Between 38% and 50% of the outcome points found on two commonly used foot and ankle instruments included factors not of primary importance to the patient.

Conclusions.—There are sex and age-related differences regarding outcome factors following the treatment of disorders affecting the foot and ankle. As many as 50% of the factors in currently used foot and ankle outcome instruments are not of primary importance to patients (Table 2).

▶ With the advent of greater requirements to document outcomes, assessment of the legitimacy of the outcome measure is a worthwhile endeavor. This study took this question one step further and stratified the data by gender and age. The fact that we have a long way to go in developing measurement tools is well docu-mented in this study. As many as 50% of the issues considered important to the physician were not of interest to the patient. Additional concern is drawn to the fact that there are age and sex differences, implying a single measurement based on documented current deficiencies may well not be adequate unless it adjusts for these additional 2 variables.

B. F. Morrey, MD

Fixation of Ankle Syndesmotic Injuries: Comparison of Tightrope Fixation and Syndesmotic Screw Fixation for Accuracy of Syndesmotic Reduction

Naqvi GA, Cunningham P, Lynch B, et al (Our Lady of Lourdes Hosp, Drogheda, Ireland; et al)
Am J Sports Med 40:2828-2835, 2012

Background.—Ankle syndesmotic injuries are complex and require anatomic reduction and fixation to restore the normal biomechanics of the ankle joint and prevent long-term complications.

Purpose.—The aim of this study is to compare the accuracy and mainte-nance of syndesmotic reduction using TightRope versus syndesmotic screw fixation.

Study Design.—Cohort study; Level of evidence, 2.

Methods.—This cohort study included consecutive patients treated for ankle syndesmotic diastases between July 2007 and June 2009. Single slice axial computed tomography (CT) scans of both the ankles together were performed at the level of syndesmosis, 1 cm above the tibial plafond. A greater than 2-mm widening of syndesmosis compared with the untreated contralateral ankle was considered significant malreduction. Clinical outcomes were measured using the American Orthopaedics Foot and Ankle Society (AOFAS) and Foot and Ankle Disability Index (FADI) scores.

Results.—Forty-six of 55 eligible patients participated in the study; 23 patients were in the TightRope group and 23 in the syndesmotic screw group. The average age was 42 years in the TightRope and 40 years in the syndesmotic screw group, and the mean follow-up time was 2.5 years (range, 1.5-3.5 years). The average width of normal syndesmosis was 4.03 ± 0.89 mm. In the TightRope group, the mean width of syndesmosis was 4.37 mm (SD, ±1.12 mm) ($P=.30$, t test) compared with 5.16 mm (SD, ±1.92 mm) in the syndesmotic screw group ($P=.01$, t test). Five of 23 ankles (21.7%) in the syndesmotic screw group had syndesmotic malreduction, whereas none of the TightRope group showed malreduction on CT scans ($P=.04$, Fisher exact test). Average time to full weightbearing was 8 weeks in the TightRope group and 9.1 weeks in the syndesmotic screw group. There was no significant difference between the TightRope and syndesmotic screw groups in mean postoperative AOFAS score (89.56 and 86.52, respectively) or FADI score (82.42 and 81.22, respectively). Regression analysis confirmed malreduction of syndesmosis as the only independent variable that affected the clinical outcome (regression coefficient, -12.39; $t=-2.43$; $P=.02$).

Conclusion.—The results of this study indicate that fixation with TightRope provides a more accurate method of syndesmotic stabilization compared with screw fixation. Syndesmotic malreduction is the most important independent predictor of clinical outcomes; therefore, care should be taken to reduce the syndesmosis accurately (Fig 5).

▶ For whatever reason, I've always been attracted to the syndesmosis of the ankle. The issue of management has remained a source of controversy for my

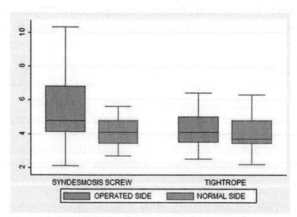

FIGURE 5.—Box plot comparing the syndesmotic width of the operated and contralateral ankles. Note the obvious wide range of syndesmotic width on the operated side in the syndesmotic screw group. (Reprinted from Naqvi GA, Cunningham P, Lynch B, et al. Fixation of ankle syndesmotic injuries: comparison of tightrope fixation and syndesmotic screw fixation for accuracy of syndesmotic reduction. *Am J Sports Med.* 2012;40:2828-2835, with permission from The Author(s).)

entire career. I was interested to see the tight rope technique did restore the anatomy better than prior efforts, such as the syndesmotic screw (Fig 5). The all-important correlation with clinical outcome, however, continues to be a little less convincing. Regardless, appropriate management of this important anatomic relationship does appear to be important. The so-called tight rope technique should be seriously considered.

B. F. Morrey, MD

Anatomic Lateral Ligament Reconstruction in the Ankle: A Hybrid Technique in the Athletic Population

Kennedy JG, Smyth NA, Fansa AM, et al (Hosp for Special Surgery, New York)
Am J Sports Med 40:2309-2317, 2012

Background.—Anatomic and checkrein tenodesis reconstruction techniques have been described as a means of treatment for chronic lateral ligament instability in the ankle. The current article describes a hybrid procedure using the most advantageous concepts of both techniques for use when insufficient normal ligament remains to fashion a direct repair of the anterior talofibular ligament (ATFL).

Purpose.—The authors report the results at a minimum 1-year follow-up of 57 patients who underwent a hybrid anatomic lateral ligament reconstruction technique in the ankle.

Study Design.—Case series; Level of evidence, 4.

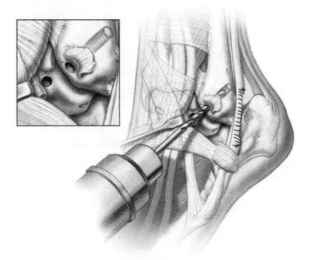

FIGURE 5.—Two drill holes at the native footprint of the anterior talofibular ligament are made to accommodate the tendon graft and interference screws. Illustration copyright J.G. Kennedy, MD; reproduced with permission. Reproduction without express written consent is prohibited. (Reprinted from Kennedy JG, Smyth NA, Fansa AM, et al. Anatomic lateral ligament reconstruction in the ankle: a hybrid technique in the athletic population. *Am J Sports Med.* 2012;40:2309-2317, with permission from The Author(s).)

Methods.—Fifty-seven patients underwent a hybrid anatomic lateral ligament reconstruction procedure under the care of the senior author. All patients were assessed preoperatively and postoperatively using the Foot and Ankle Outcome Score (FAOS) and Short Form—12 (SF-12) outcome score. The mean patient age at the time of surgery was 28 years (range, 17-65 years), including 39 male and 18 female patients. The mean follow-up time was 32 months (range, 12-47 months).

Results.—The FAOS improved from 58 points preoperatively to 89 points postoperatively ($P < .01$). The SF-12 score improved from 48 points before surgery to 80 points at final follow-up ($P < .01$). All patients achieved mechanical stability at final clinical follow-up; 7 patients (12%) demonstrated functional instability. Functional instability was found to significantly influence not returning to sport at the previous level.

Conclusion.—This hybrid anatomic lateral ligament reconstruction technique using a peroneus longus autograft to substitute the native ATFL provides an alternative to anatomic reconstruction when direct repair is not possible (Figs 5 and 6).

▶ Chronic ankle instability is not only disabling but can give rise to ankle arthritis. Not surprisingly, the Cochrane database concluded there is insufficient evidence

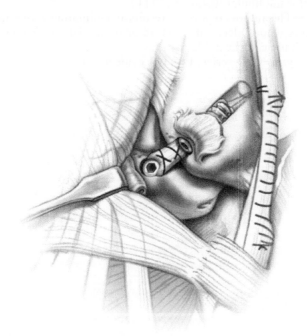

FIGURE 6.—After the first end of the tendon is docked in the talus, the graft is passed through the fibular drill hole, subsequently tensioned, and held with an interference fit using a bioabsorbable screw. Illustration copyright J.G. Kennedy, MD; reproduced with permission. Reproduction without express written consent is prohibited. (Reprinted from Kennedy JG, Smyth NA, Fansa AM, et al. Anatomic lateral ligament reconstruction in the ankle: a hybrid technique in the athletic population. *Am J Sports Med.* 2012;40:2309-2317, with permission from The Author(s).)

to make a comment about the treatment of this condition. I was attracted to the simplicity of the technique using a peroneus longus autograft as reported by the authors (Figs 5 and 6). The fact that 7 of 57 (12%) had functional instability is worthy of note. Further, the minimum follow-up is only 1 year, so these are probably the best results to be expected with deterioration in the future. But, it seems as good as the alternatives.

B. F. Morrey, MD

Comparison of the Calcaneo-Cuboid-Cuneiform Osteotomies and the Calcaneal Lengthening Osteotomy in the Surgical Treatment of Symptomatic Flexible Flatfoot

Moraleda L, Salcedo M, Bastrom TP, et al (Hospital Universitario la Paz, Madrid, Spain; Rady Children's Hosp and Health Ctr, San Diego, CA)
J Pediatr Orthop 32:821-829, 2012

Background.—Surgery is indicated in symptomatic flatfoot when conservative treatment fails to relieve the symptoms. Osteotomies appear to be the best choice for these painful feet. The purpose of this study was to compare the clinical and radiographic outcome of the calcaneo-cuboid-cuneiform osteotomies (triple C) and the calcaneal-lengthening osteotomy in the treatment of children with symptomatic flexible flatfoot.

Methods.—The surgeries were performed by senior surgeons who preferred either triple C or calcaneal lengthening. The results were graded by an orthopaedic surgeon uninvolved with the cases. The clinical and radiographic outcome was evaluated in 30 feet (21 patients) with a triple C osteotomy and 33 feet (21 patients) with a calcaneal-lengthening osteotomy. We used the American College of Foot and Ankle Surgeons (ACFAS) score (flatfoot module) for clinical assessment, which contains a subjective and objective test. We measured and compared 12 parameters on the anteroposterior and lateral weight-bearing radiographs. The effect of additional procedures (Kidner procedure, medial reefing of the talonavicular capsule, tendo-Achilles lengthening, peroneous brevis lengthening and, in the calcaneal-lengthening group, a medial cuneiform osteotomy) on the clinical and radiographic result was also evaluated.

Results.—Average age at the time of surgery was similar (triple C: 11.2 ± 3 y, calcaneal lengthening: 11.6 ± 2.5 y, $P = 0.51$). Average follow-up was 2.7 ± 2.2 years in the triple C group and 5.3 ± 4 years in the calcaneal-lengthening group. There were no significant differences in the clinical outcome measured by the ACFAS subjective test in the calcaneal-lengthening group ($P = 0.003$). There were no significant differences in the ACFAS score, both the subjective test (triple C: 43.3 ± 6.1, calcaneal lengthening: 44.7 ± 7.6, $P = 0.52$) and the ACFAS objective test (triple C: 28.6 ± 2, calcaneal lengthening: 25.9 ± 7, $P = 0.13$). We found significant differences in 2 of the 12 radiographic measurements: anteroposterior talo-first metatarsal angle (triple C: 15.5 ± 11.1, calcaneal lengthening: 7.4 ± 7.3, $P = 0.001$) and talonavicular coverage (triple C: 28 ± 14.7,

TABLE 1.—Additional Procedures Performed in Both Triple C Patients and Calcaneal-lengthening Patients

Additional Procedures	Triple C (n = 30) (%)	Calcaneal Lengthening (n = 33) (%)
Kidner procedure	13 (43.3)	10 (30.3)
Medial reefing	6 (20)	7 (21.2)
TAL	29 (96.7)	11 (33.3)
Peroneous brevis lengthening	19 (63.3)	6 (18.2)
Medial cuneiform osteotomy	—	6 (18.2)
Calcaneo-cuboid fixation	—	12 (36.4)

Triple C indicates calcaneo-cuboid-cuneiform osteotomies.

TABLE 2.—Preoperative and Postoperative Alignment of the Foot in Both the Groups According to 12 Parameters Measured on Anteroposterior and Lateral Weight-bearing Radiographs

	Normal Values	Preoperative Radiographs			Postoperative Radiographs		
		Triple C	CLO	P	Triple C	CLO	P
AP talo-first MTT angle	−20 to 15	21.8 ± 9.3	19.3 ± 8.6	0.299	15.5 ± 11.1	7.44 ± 7.3	0.001*
AP talocalcaneal angle	10 to 56	30.1 ± 12.7	31.8 ± 9.3	0.537	27.3	23 ± 10.2	0.162
Talonavicular coverage	5 to 39	41 ± 9.2	38.6 ± 9.9	0.334	28 ± 14.7	13.7 ± 12.4	<0.001*
AP talo-fifth MTT angle	N/A	40.1 ± 11.5	37.3 ± 8.3	0.278	32.5 ± 12.1	28.5 ± 8.5	0.136
L talo-first MTT angle	1 to 35	25.3 ± 12.2	23.4 ± 9.9	0.513	16.1 ± 10.25	13.7 ± 6.2	0.268
L talocalcaneal angle	15 to 60	49.1 ± 8.6	48.7 ± 7.2	0.875	50.1 ± 6.9	50.8 ± 7.3	0.692
Talohorizontal angle	−15 to 55	37.9 ± 10.4	37 ± 7.35	0.692	32.8 ± 8.6	31.1 ± 5	0.354
Calcaneal pitch	11 to 38	11.1 ± 5.4	11.8 ± 5.2	0.650	17.2 ± 5.2	19.7 ± 5.5	0.073
L calcaneo-fifth MTT angle	N/A	18.8 ± 5.8	21 ± 6.6	0.171	24.3 ± 6.2	27.4 ± 6.7	0.064
L first-fifth MTT angle	N/A	5.6 ± 4.6	5 ± 3.8	0.562	10.4 ± 3.8	10 ± 4.2	0.655
Naviculocuboid overlap (%)	22 to 85	84.1 ± 20.1	78.3 ± 16.4	0.221	63.1 ± 19.9	64.4 ± 19.3	0.786
Talocalcaneal index	45 to 103	79.1 ± 17.7	80.6 ± 10.6	0.699	77.4 ± 16.4	73.4 ± 11.5	0.269

Editor's Note: Please refer to original journal article for full references.
Both groups were similar preoperatively. Postoperatively, there were significant differences in the anteroposterior talo-first MTT angle and the talonavicular coverage.
Normal values described in the literature are provided.[16,19]
CLO indicates calcaneal lengthening osteotomy; MTT, metatarsal.
*Differences are statistically significant.

calcaneal lengthening: 13.7 ± 12.4, P < 0.001). None of the additional procedures improved the clinical outcome. There were 3 (10%) complications in the triple C group and 6 (18%) complications in the calcaneal-lengthening group. Also, calcaneocuboid subluxation was present in 17 (51.5%) feet of the calcaneal-lengthening group.

Conclusions.—Both techniques obtain good clinical and radiographic results in the treatment of symptomatic idiopathic flexible flatfoot in a pediatric population. The calcaneal-lengthening osteotomy achieves better improvement of the relationship of the navicular to the head of the talus but it is associated with more frequent and more severe complications. Additional soft-tissue procedures have not proven to improve clinical or radiographic results.

Level of Evidence.—Level III, retrospective comparative study (Tables 1 and 2).

▶ Although this is a case-control study, it was very well done and addressed an important and controversial question and, thus, was included in our review. The study was performed at the well-recognized San Diego Children's Hospital, which further enhances its value and the credibility of the findings. The sample size of those undergoing flatfoot correction by way of calcaneo-cuboid-cuneiform osteotomy and calcaneal-lengthening osteotomy was similar, as were the patient and pathologic characteristics. The assessment also included numerous associated procedures (Table 1). The conclusion is that both achieved good clinical results based on an array of postoperative measurements (Table 2). However, 3 important observations should be considered: (1) Calcaneal osteotomy provided a better talo-navicular relationship, (2) calcaneal osteotomy had a higher complication rate, and (3) the additional soft tissue procedures did not influence the observations. It would seem these findings would add refinement to our approach to the management of the flatfoot needing surgical correction.

B. F. Morrey, MD

Diffuse pigmented villonodular synovitis (diffuse-type giant cell tumour) of the foot and ankle

Stevenson JD, Jaiswal A, Gregory JJ, et al (Robert Jones & Agnes Hunt Hosp, Oswestry, UK)
Bone Joint J 95-B:384-390, 2013

Pigmented villonodular synovitis (PVNS) is a rare benign disease of the synovium of joints and tendon sheaths, which may be locally aggressive. We present 18 patients with diffuse-type PVNS of the foot and ankle followed for a mean of 5.1 years (2 to 11.8). There were seven men and 11 women, with a mean age of 42 years (18 to 73). A total of 13 patients underwent open or arthroscopic synovectomy, without post-operative radiotherapy. One had surgery at the referring unit before presentation with residual tibiotalar PVNS. The four patients who were managed non-operatively remain symptomatically controlled and under clinical and radiological surveillance. At final follow-up the mean Musculoskeletal Tumour Society score was 93.8% (95% confidence interval (CI) 85 to 100), the mean Toronto Extremity Salvage Score was 92 (95% CI 82 to 100) and the mean American Academy of Orthopaedic Surgeons foot and ankle score was 89 (95% CI 79 to 100). The lesion in the patient with residual PVNS resolved radiologically without further intervention six years after surgery. Targeted synovectomy without adjuvant radiotherapy can result in excellent outcomes, without recurrence. Asymptomatic patients can be successfully managed non-operatively. This is the first series to report clinical outcome scores for patients with diffuse-type PVNS of the foot and ankle.

▶ This case study is worthwhile to review because it addresses an uncommon and vexing problem of the foot and ankle and also of other joints. Pigmented villonodular synovitis has a deserved reputation as a "bad actor" that can cause joint stiffness and destroy articular cartilage. Hence, this study showing that subtotal synovectomy can result in very reliable 90% control at 5 years is interesting. Of greatest interest is the documentation that, in fact, this condition can also spontaneously resolve, without treatment (see Fig 2 in the original article)! This small sample case study can and should have an impact on the optimum management of this condition at the foot and ankle.

B. F. Morrey, MD

Functional Outcomes After Ankle Arthrodesis in Elderly Patients
Strasser NL, Turner NS III (Mayo Clinic, Rochester, MN)
Foot Ankle Int 33:699-703, 2012

Background.—Ankle arthrodesis has been the gold standard operative treatment for ankle arthritis refractory to nonoperative treatment. Although multiple studies have evaluated the outcomes after ankle fusion, none has focused on outcomes in elderly patients. The purpose of this study was to evaluate outcomes of ankle fusion in patients over the age of 70.
Methods.—Thirty patients (30 ankles) over the age of 70 who underwent ankle fusion were identified. Average age at the time of surgery was 74.5 years (± 3.7). The Foot and Ankle Ability Measure (FAAM) was obtained postoperatively in 22 of the 23 patients still living. Radiographs were followed until union with an average followup of 2.2 years.
Results.—Union was achieved in 27 of 30 ankles (90%). Postoperative radiographs showed 11 (36.6%) patients had progression of subtalar arthritis. The average postoperative FAAM score was 81.5 (± 18.3) with an average followup of 8.5 years (± 1.7). Subjectively, when asked to compare present function with their prearthritic state, the average response was 75.1% (± 19.6). The average American Orthopaedic Foot and Ankle Society hindfoot score was 73.0 (± 11.5). Complications included nonunion, deep infection, and adjacent joint arthritis.
Conclusions.—In this clinical cohort, ankle fusion was found to be effective in the treatment of ankle arthritis. Functional outcome was satisfactory and the rate of union was comparable with that previously reported in the literature for younger patients. Although total ankle arthroplasty is becoming increasingly popular, ankle arthrodesis is an effective surgical treatment option in an elderly patient population.

▶ Because I have written several articles on this subject, I am, not surprisingly, drawn to the topic. More importantly, this still is, regardless of all the total replacement hype, the gold standard. Also of interest, this article does not offer anything new but reinforces what we know. Arthrodesis is successfully attained in about 90% instances. When this occurs, patients do well. The issue of adjacent joint arthritis is real. However, in the final analysis, this is, in fact, a reasonable salvage procedure. As an aside, this may be the only article I reviewed that had no tables or figures in the text!!

B. F. Morrey, MD

Clinical Outcome and Gait Analysis of Ankle Arthrodesis

Fuentes-Sanz A, Moya-Angeler J, López-Oliva F, et al (Hosp FREMAP, Majadahonda, Madrid, Spain; Fundacion Jimenez Diaz, Madrid, Spain; Univ CEU- San Pablo, Madrid, Spain)
Foot Ankle Int 33:819-827, 2012

Background.—The purpose of our study was to describe and analyze the functional outcomes of mid-term followup patients with ankle arthrodesis.

Methods.—Twenty patients who had an isolated ankle arthrodesis were followed for a mean of 3 years after surgery. We performed physical and functional examination, radiographic examination and CT scan. Each completed standardized, self-reported outcome questionnaires SF-36, AOFAS and Mazur scores. All subjects were evaluated with a kinetic and kinematic gait analysis and a plantar pressure study.

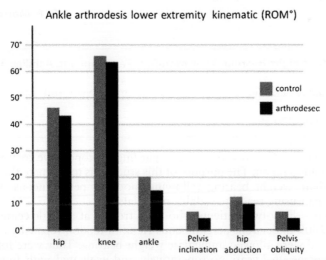

FIGURE 3.—Arthrodesis and contralateral foot ROM (degrees), during walking. We did not observe differences in ROM (degrees) of joints of the arthrodesis foot and contralateral healthy side. (Reprinted from Fuentes-Sanz A, Moya-Angeler J, López-Oliva F, et al. Clinical outcome and gait analysis of ankle arthrodesis. *Foot Ankle Int.* 2012;33:819-827, Copyright © 2012, by the American Orthopaedic Foot and Ankle Society, Inc, originally published in Foot & Ankle International and reproduced here with permission.)

Results.—Only one patient used a cane and seven patients required an insole to walk. We observed no relation between the scores obtained. Most of the patients showed good functional results and poor life quality scores. The joints that were significantly more degenerated were the Chopart and the subtalar joints, which were affected in 16 patients in the fused limb. The kinematic parameters showed compensatory motion in the neighboring joints and the kinetic parameters studied were similar in the arthrodesis limb and the control limb. There was no significant difference between the arthrodesis limb and the contralateral limb for plantar pressures.

Conclusion.—Although ankle arthrodesis will help to relieve pain and to improve overall function, it is considered to be a salvage procedure that causes persistent alterations in gait, with the possible development of symptomatic osteoarthritis in the other joints of the foot. Patients and treating physicians should also expect overall pain and functional limitations to increase over time (Fig 3).

▶ In an age in which we expect to effectively reconstruct all diseased joints, assessment of nonreplacement salvage option outcomes are of great value. This assessment is of value, as it carefully analyzes the functional outcome of ankle arthrodesis. What is of interest and of some surprise is the finding that ipsilateral joint motion is less in the arthrodesed side (Fig 3). This refutes the assumption that compensatory motion occurs in the operated extremity. The major disappointment is the demonstration with very short surveillance that joints distal to the fusion show early arthrosis. Hence, once again, fusion is a salvage procedure, and the orthopedic world awaits a reliable replacement as the first level of treatment for end-stage ankle arthrosis.

B. F. Morrey, MD

Immediate Weight Bearing After Modified Percutaneous Achilles Tendon Repair

Chandrakant V, Lozano-Calderon S, McWilliam J (New York Med College, Harrison)
Foot Ankle Int 33:1093-1097, 2012

Background.—Controversy exists regarding postoperative treatment of Achilles tendon repair. The purpose of this study was to evaluate the results of immediate weight bearing following modified percutaneous Achilles tendon repair using readily available materials.

Methods.—Fifty-two patients who were treated at a single center from 2000 to 2009 underwent percutaneous Achilles tendon repair by a single surgeon and were allowed immediate weight bearing. They were followed for on average of 2 years postoperatively and evaluated with functional and subjective outcomes.

Results.—The average American Orthopaedic Foot and Ankle Society ankle-hindfoot scale was 96 points (range, 81 to 100), with 95% confidence interval ranging from 89.1 to 102.9. Subjective evaluation demonstrated that 47 patients (90%) were able to return to a desired level of activity, with an overall complication rate of 11.5%.

Conclusion.—Immediate weight bearing after percutaneous Achilles tendon repair had a low overall complication rate with good clinical and functional outcomes.

▶ This is an interesting series, as it documents the problems and success with percutaneous repair of ruptured Achilles tendon. Because the direction of patient expectation is limited, invasive, rapid recovery efforts to accommodate these expectations are understandable. With more than 50 patients, the authors show the utility of the percutaneous technique. As expected, the sural nerve is the most vulnerable to injury (7%). However, the low frequency of wound problems, less than 4%, would justify this technique or one similar to it.

B. F. Morrey, MD

Comparison of Arthroscopic and Magnetic Resonance Imaging Findings in Osteochondral Lesions of the Talus

Bae S, Lee HK, Lee K, et al (Armed Forces Capital Hosp, Gyeonggi, Republic of Korea; et al)
Foot Ankle Int 33:1058-1062, 2012

Background.—Magnetic resonance imaging (MRI) is widely used for diagnosing osteochondral lesions in the talus. The purpose of this study was to directly compare the MRI with the arthroscopic findings.

Materials and Methods.—MR images of 42 ankles were retrospectively reviewed during a period of 67 months. The osteochondral lesions were evaluated by both MRI (0, normal; 1, subchondral trabecular compression and marrow edema; 2A, subchondral cyst; 2B incomplete separation fragment; 3, unattached, nondisplaced fragment with synovial fluid surrounding it; 4, displaced fragment) and arthroscopy (A, smooth and intact, but soft and ballottable cartilage; B, rough surfaces; C, fibrillations or fissures; D, flap present or bone exposed; E, loose, undisplaced fragment; F, displaced fragment). Arthroscopic grade A was considered to be equivalent to MR grade 1, B and C to MR grade 2A, D to 2B, E to 3, and F to 4.

Results.—Of the 44 lesions in 42 ankles, 29 lesions marked the same grade on both MRI and arthroscopy (65.9%). Nine lesions were upgraded on arthroscopy (20.5%), and six were downgraded (13.6%). MR grade 3 lesions showed the best correlation (83.3%) and MR grade 1 and 2B lesions showed the worst (50.0 and 55.6%). Arthroscopic grade A and F showed good correlation (80 and 100%). Grade C and E showed poor (25.0%) and intermediate correlation (66.7%), respectively.

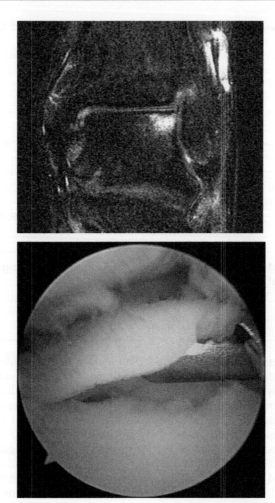

FIGURE 2.—Only marrow edema with intact overlying cartilage was seen on MRI of a 21-year-old man. After 2 months, he was taken to arthroscopy because of severe pain nonresponsive to conservative treatment. On arthroscopy, a large flap of cartilage was noticed (arthroscopic grade D). (Reprinted from Bae S, Lee HK, Lee K, et al. Comparison of arthroscopic and magnetic resonance imaging findings in osteochondral lesions of the talus. *Foot Ankle Int.* 2012;33:1058-1062, Copyright © 2012, by the American Orthopaedic Foot and Ankle Society, Inc, originally published in Foot & Ankle International and reproduced here with permission.)

Conclusion.—The MRI grading of osteochondral lesions in the talus was useful and showed a fairly good correlation with arthroscopic classification (Fig 2).

▶ As we continue to rely on magnetic resonance imaging (MRI) as a tool to assist in diagnosis, I have observed the worrisome trend that we have also allowed it to replace our judgment, including indications for surgery. This study suffers from some issues of methodology, relatively small numbers, and retrospective assessment of the MRI. However, the message is clear: There was relatively poor overall correlation between the MRI and arthroscopic findings (Fig 2). So what does this mean? In general, I avoid MRI if the findings will not change my intention to scope or perform open procedure. Both these modalities are expensive, and I fear we will not be afforded the luxury of doing both going forward.

B. F. Morrey, MD

Arthroscopic Synovectomy of the Ankle in Rheumatoid Arthritis
Choi WJ, Choi GW, Lee JW (Yonsei Univ College of Medicine, Seoul, South Korea; Seoul Veterans Hosp, South Korea)
Arthroscopy 29:133-140, 2013

Purpose.—To evaluate the outcome of arthroscopic synovectomy of the ankle joint in patients with early-stage rheumatoid arthritis (RA).

Methods.—Between 2005 and 2009, 18 consecutive patients with RA involving the ankle underwent arthroscopic synovectomy. Pain was measured using a visual analog scale (VAS), and clinical outcome was determined by calculating the American Orthopaedic Foot and Ankle Society (AOFAS) Ankle-Hindfoot Scale score with a mean follow-up of 5 years (60 months). Assessments were performed preoperatively, at 6 and 12 months postoperatively, and then yearly thereafter. Clinical success was defined as the absence of synovitis symptoms or when patients demonstrated good or excellent outcomes (AOFAS Ankle-Hindfoot Scale score ≥80) with >50% improvement in VAS score for pain. Demographic,

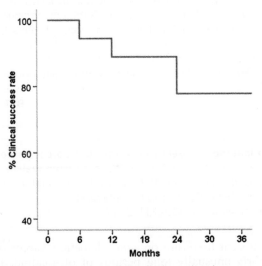

FIGURE 2.—Kaplan-Meier survival curve of the cumulative clinical success rate. (Reprinted from Choi WJ, Choi GW, Lee JW. Arthroscopic synovectomy of the ankle in rheumatoid arthritis. *Arthroscopy.* 2013;29:133-140, with permission from the Arthroscopy Association of North America.)

TABLE 4.—Preoperative and Postoperative Clinical Outcomes

Clinical Outcomes	Before Surgery	6 Months	1 Year	2 Years	Final Follow-up*	P Value[†]
VAS	5.6 ± 0.7	2.0 ± 0.6	1.2 ± 1.1	1.6 ± 1.5	2.2 ± 1.4	<.0001[‡]
AOFAS score	65.2 ± 4.4	84.8 ± 2.1	87.6 ± 5.6	86.3 ± 6.6	85.7 ± 6.7	<.0001[‡]
ROM (°)	60.0 ± 9.8	62.0 ± 9.4	62.5 ± 8.5	61.5 ± 9.2	61.1 ± 9.7	.279

VAS, visual analog scale; AOFAS, American Orthopaedic Foot and Ankle Society; ROM, range of motion in degrees.
*Mean follow-up of 5 years (range: 2–8.6 years).
[†]P value for final follow-up versus before surgery.
[‡]Statistically significant (P < .05).

laboratory, and radiological variables were evaluated to determine possible factors predicting clinical outcome.

Results.—VAS and AOFAS scores were significantly improved at the final follow-up (60 months; P < .0001). The greatest improvements in clinical scores were observed after 12 months; thereafter, they steadily declined. Of the 18 patients examined, 14 (77.8%) were considered to have had clinical success with no reintervention. Variables predictive of clinical success were short duration of symptoms (P = .042) and minimal radiographic changes based on the Larsen grading system (P = .030).

Conclusions.—Arthroscopic synovectomy is a safe and successful procedure in ankle joints affected by RA. The best clinical outcomes are achieved when the procedure is performed early in the disease course and when there is no evidence of cartilage degeneration.

Level of Evidence.—Level IV, prognostic case series (Fig 2, Table 4).

▶ As is noted, with the advent of disease-remitting agents, the need for synovectomy has been dramatically reduced for all joints. In fact, it is virtually never needed at the elbow in the United States today. Although the sample size is rather small at 18, and the surveillance is rather short, averaging 5 years, the findings are similar to prior studies in other joints. As expected, marked improvement in pain and function is noted (Table 4). Unfortunately, the benefit deteriorates rather rapidly (Fig 2). Regardless, because there are few really good options at the ankle, it is a worthwhile option to consider in the properly selected patient.

B. F. Morrey, MD

Duration of off-loading and recurrence rate in Charcot osteo-arthropathy treated with less restrictive regimen with removable walker
Christensen TM, Gade-Rasmussen B, Pedersen LW, et al (Univ of Copenhagen, Denmark; Steno Diabetes Ctr, Gentofte, Denmark)
J Diabetes Complications 26:430-434, 2012

Objective.—Recent literature on acute diabetic Charcot osteoarthropathy (CA) reports unusually long periods of off-loading. Data suggest that this might increase the re-currence rate. Subsequently we evaluated the influence of duration of off-loading on the risk of required re-casting.

Research Design and Methods.—In this retrospective consecutive series from 2000 to 2005, 56 people with diabetes and an acute Charcot foot were included. The inclusion criteria were an initial persistent temperature difference more than 2°C between the two feet, oedema, and typical hot spots on a bone scintigram, radiology, and a typical clinical course. Treatment was off-loading in a removable cast and 2 crutches. In-door walking was allowed. Gradually augmented weight bearing was prescribed when the skin temperature difference had decreased to a level less than 2°C and edema had subsided. Re-casting was required for immediate exacerbation during re-load as well as for recurrence — defined as new swelling and skin temperature difference of more than 2°C in the same foot occurring after a stable interval of at least one month after full weight bearing.

Results.—The duration of off-loading for all patients was 141 ± 21 days (mean ± SD). Three patients (5%) were re-casted immediately for exacerbation after re-load and 7 patients (12 %) after recurrence of the CA. Duration of re-casting was 79 ± 44 days. The primary period of off-loading was not statistically significantly different for those not requiring versus those requiring re-casting: 142 ± 24 days compared to 134 ± 41 days. Neither were the differences in demographic data, metabolic regulation, BMI or localization of CA.

Conclusions.—Patients with risk of exacerbation or recurrence of CA could not be identified in the present study and there was no relation to the duration of off-loading. Nevertheless off-loading periods with immobilisation should be kept as short as possible, due to other side effects. This can be obtained by early gradual augmented re-loading.

▶ As diabetes continues its relentless march to become a dominant disease of all societies, efforts to combat the consequences assume greater relevance. The traditional wisdom for managing the Charcot joint is "protect." For the foot, this means immobilization and crutch or ambulatory assist. This effort to document the effectiveness of this regimen followed a mean of 144 days; unfortunately, it did not reveal an ability to avoid recurrence of symptoms. In spite of this result, we really have nothing better than to protect. One key message is that the use of the air cast type of removable immobilizer does decrease the likelihood of complications seen with traditional casting.

B. F. Morrey, MD

Angiosome-targeted infrapopliteal endovascular revascularization for treatment of diabetic foot ulcers
Söderström M, Albäck A, Biancari F, et al (Helsinki Univ Central Hosp, Finland; Oulu Univ Hosp, Finland)
J Vasc Surg 57:427-435, 2013

Objective.—Because of the prolonged healing time of diabetic foot ulcers, methods for identifying ways to expedite the ulcer healing process

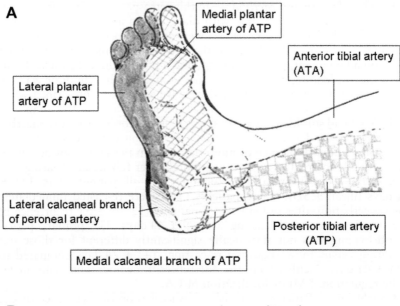

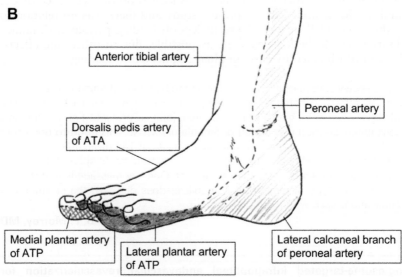

FIGURE 1.—A and B, The medial calcaneal, medial plantar, and lateral plantar and the arteries angiosomes are derived from the posterior tibial artery (*ATP*) and cover the lateral heel and the plantar surface of the foot. The dorsalis pedis artery angiosome, which prolongs the anterior tibial artery (*ATA*), nourishes the dorsum of the foot, the toes, and the upper anterior perimalleolar area. The lateral calcaneal artery from the peroneal artery supplies the lateral and plantar aspects of the heel. Modified with permission from Alexandrescu V, Söderström M, Venermo M. Angiosome theory: fact or fiction? *Scand J Surg* 2012;101:125-31. (Reprinted from the Journal of Vascular Surgery. Söderström M, Albäck A, Biancari F, et al. Angiosome-targeted infrapopliteal endovascular revascularization for treatment of diabetic foot ulcers. *J Vasc Surg.* 2013;57:427-435, Copyright 2013, with permission from the Society for Vascular Surgery.)

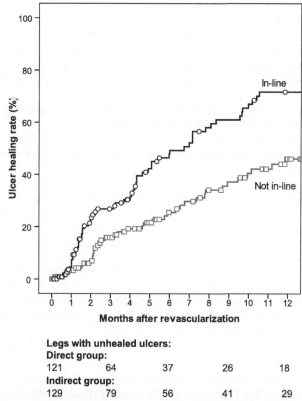

FIGURE 2.—Ulcer healing rates in patients with direct and those with indirect perfusion to the foot ulcer after endovascular revascularization in the overall series (log-rank test, *P* < .001). (Reprinted from the Journal of Vascular Surgery. Söderström M, Albäck A, Biancari F, et al. Angiosome-targeted infrapopliteal endovascular revascularization for treatment of diabetic foot ulcers. *J Vasc Surg*. 2013;57:427-435, Copyright 2013, with permission from the Society for Vascular Surgery.)

are needed. The angiosome concept delineates the body into three-dimensional blocks of tissue fed by specific source arteries. The aim of this study was to evaluate the benefit of infrapopliteal endovascular revascularization guided by an angiosome model of perfusion in the healing process of diabetic foot ulcers.

Methods.—A total of 250 consecutive legs with diabetic foot ulcers in 226 patients who had undergone infrapopliteal endovascular revascularization in a single center were evaluated. Patient records and periprocedural leg angiograms were reviewed. The legs were divided into two groups depending on whether direct arterial flow to the site of the foot ulcer based on the angiosome concept was achieved (direct group) or not achieved (indirect group). Ulcer healing time was compared between the two groups. A propensity score was used for adjustment of differences in pretreatment covariables in multivariate analysis and for 1:1 matching.

Results.—Direct flow to the angiosome feeding the ulcer area was achieved in 121 legs (48%) compared with indirect revascularization in 129 legs. Foot ulcers treated with angiosome-targeted infrapopliteal percutaneous transluminal angioplasty healed better. The ulcer healing rate was mean (standard deviation) 72% (5%) at 12 months for the direct group compared with 45% (6%) for the indirect group ($P < .001$). When adjusted for propensity score, the direct group still had a significantly better ulcer healing rate than the indirect group (hazard ratio, 1.97; 95% confidence interval, 1.34-2.90; $P = .001$).

Conclusions.—Attaining a direct arterial flow based on the angiosome model of perfusion to the foot ulcer appears to be important for ulcer healing in diabetic patients (Figs 1 and 2).

▶ This is really an important article for those involved in the management of the diabetic foot. Because it can be found within the vascular surgical literature and the study was performed in Finland, the concept may not be too familiar to the orthopedic surgeon. The concept of specifically revascularizing the vessel or vessels responsible for perfusing the area of the ulcer, the angiosome, is somewhat new (Fig 1). The study involved a large sample of 250 patients and clearly demonstrated the statistical advantage ($P = .001$) of the so-called infrapopliteal endovascular revascularization, also termed direct revascularization, compared with those in which this was not attained (Fig 2). I was duly impressed and found this to be a truly encouraging development.

B. F. Morrey, MD

A Reliable Method for Treatment of Nonhealing Ulcers in the Hindfoot and Midfoot Region in Diabetic Patients: Reconstruction With Abductor Digiti Minimi Muscle Flap

Altindas M, Ceber M, Kilic A, et al (Istanbul Univ Cerrahpasa Med Faculty, Turkey; Namik Kemal Univ Med Faculty, Tekirdag, Turkey; SEKA State Hosp, Kocaeli, Turkey)
Ann Plast Surg 70:82-87, 2013

The foot has a unique anatomic composition and a perfect architecture, which is necessary for mobilization. However, this complex structure is also responsible for healing problems in foot reconstruction. After 25 years of experience in diabetic foot surgery practice, we observed that some hindfoot ulcers are like an iceberg in that they have much more involvement in the plantar fat pad than the skin, and the lateral midfoot region is a common site for ulcer formation. Also the fifth tarsometatarsal joint region is a prominent anatomic structure vulnerable to repetitive trauma and ulcer formation that may easily spread to other parts of the foot. These ulcers should be reconstructed with well-vascularized tissues such as muscle flaps after debridement. Between 2003 and 2010, 17 diabetic patients with foot ulcers, involving bone and joint, were reconstructed with abductor digiti minimi muscle flap. When it is needed, the flap is covered with a small

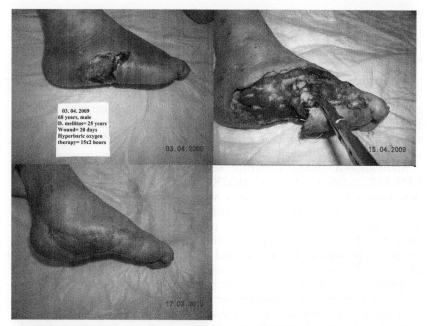

FIGURE 4.—Above, left, An acute infection that started on the fifth tarsometatarsal joint resulted in extensive and progressive necrosis of soft tissues. Above, right, Debridement of the necrotic tissues revealed the exact involvement of the underlying bones and joints. Below, left, The 1-year follow-up demonstrated that there was a durable coverage. (Reprinted from Altindas M, Ceber M, Kilic A, et al. A reliable method for treatment of nonhealing ulcers in the hindfoot and midfoot region in diabetic patients: reconstruction with abductor digiti minimi muscle flap. *Ann Plast Surg*. 2013;70:82-87, with permission from Lippincott Williams & Wilkins.)

split-thickness skin graft. In all cases, complete healing was achieved. The muscle flap functioned well as a versatile and shock absorbent coverage without recurrence of the ulcer during a mean follow-up period of around 2 years. Diabetic foot ulcers should be evaluated and treated individually depending on their location and affected tissue composition. The most appropriate reconstructive option should be selected for each lesion. The abductor digiti minimi muscle flap is extremely useful for the reconstruction of small-to moderate-sized defects that have exposed bone, joint, or tendons in the hindfoot and lateral plantar midfoot (Fig 4).

▶ Management of the diabetic foot ulcer is problematic, to say the least. Those ulcers over the lateral aspect of the foot often require surgery and, importantly, if local measures are not successful, amputation is required. To make matters worse, the burden of this disease increases exponentially. These authors have documented a reliable (17/17) salvage for the problematic ulcer, thus avoiding amputation. As they document, more than half (9) had bone or joint infection and some had significant soft tissue involvement (Fig 4). That all were successfully managed with the abductor digiti minimi would suggest such patients be referred to the surgeon capable of this surgery before amputation is carried out.

B. F. Morrey, MD

A Systematic Review of Skin Substitutes for Foot Ulcers

Felder JM, Goyal SS, Attinger CE (Georgetown Univ Hosp, Washington, DC)
Plast Reconstr Surg 130:145-164, 2012

Background.—Bioengineered and allograft-derived skin substitutes are increasingly available and marketed for use in the healing of chronic wounds. Plastic surgeons should have evidence-based information available to guide their use of these products. The authors systematically reviewed the literature to determine the published outcomes and effectiveness of different skin substitutes for healing chronic foot ulcers.

Methods.—A broad literature search of the MEDLINE, EBSCO, EMBASE, and the Cochrane Central Register of Controlled Trials databases was undertaken. Relevant studies were selected by three independent reviewers to include randomized controlled trials or systematic reviews examining the use of skin substitutes on foot ulcers. Results were narrowed further by the application of predetermined inclusion and exclusion criteria. Studies were assessed for quality and data were extracted regarding study characteristics and objective outcomes.

Results.—Of an initial 271 search results, 15 randomized controlled trials, one prospective comparative study, and five systematic reviews were included in the systematic review. Most of the included clinical studies were of moderate to low quality by objective standards, and reported results using cell-based skin substitutes. The primary outcome examined, success rate of complete healing, was equivalent to or better than that of standard therapy for all skin substitutes examined.

Conclusions.—A convincing body of evidence supports the effectiveness of living cell-based skin substitutes as an adjunctive therapy for increasing

TABLE 2.—Inclusion and Exclusion Criteria

Inclusion criteria
    Primary data from randomized controlled trials, systematic reviews/meta-analyses, comparative prospective cohort studies
    Human studies
    Studies that include results for patients with chronic diabetic (neuropathic), angiopathic, venous stasis, pressure-induced, or infected ulcers of the foot
    Studies that stratify patients based on wound cause or characteristics and provide comparable outcome measures for groups treated with skin substitutes or control methods
Exclusion criteria
    Review, technique, retrospective, case series, or case report articles; prospective studies lacking a comparison or control group
    Studies in which subjects are selected based on outcome (e.g., assessing only healed ulcers)
    Animal studies
    Studies with fewer than 20 total patients with foot ulcers
    Studies of acute foot wounds
    Studies specific to leg ulcers that do not include foot ulcers
    Studies without well-defined patient or wound groups
    Studies with nonstandard skin substitute or wound care techniques
    Studies with no extractable outcomes
    Articles focused solely on children (<18 yr)
    Traumatic wounds

the rate of complete healing in chronic foot ulcers when basic tenets of wound care are also being implemented. Acellular skin substitutes also show some promise for treatment of foot wounds but require further study (Table 2).

▶ Chronic foot ulcers are a major and growing problem with the increasing incidence of diabetes. The topic and findings of this study are, therefore, worthy of note. While I have noted the dearth of high-quality orthopedic studies, this analysis of largely plastic surgery literature finds the same limitation.

The authors reviewed 271 articles, and, applying strict inclusion and exclusion standards (Table 2) were able to use only 15 in their analysis. Hence, based on legitimate studies, the utility of cell-based grafts seems to be established. The literature is simply not adequate to know if non—cell-based grafts might not also be effective.

B. F. Morrey, MD

Geographic variation in Medicare spending and mortality for diabetic patients with foot ulcers and amputations
Sargen MR, Hoffstad O, Margolis DJ (Univ of Pennsylvania Perelman School of Medicine, Philadelphia)
J Diabetes Complications 27:128-133, 2013

Aims.—The purpose of this study was to identify the presence or absence of geographic variation in Medicare spending and mortality rates for diabetic patients with foot ulcers (DFU) and lower extremity amputations (LEA).

Methods.—Diabetic beneficiaries with foot ulcers (n = 682,887) and lower extremity amputations (n = 151,752) were enrolled in Medicare Parts A and B during the calendar year 2007. We used ordinary least squares (OLS) regression to explain geographic variation in per capita Medicare spending and one-year mortality rates.

Results.—Health care spending and mortality rates varied considerably across the nation for our two patient cohorts. However, higher spending was not associated with a statistically significant reduction in one-year patient mortality ($P = .12$ for DFU, $P = .20$ for LEA). Macrovascular complications for amputees were more common in parts of the country with higher mortality rates ($P < .001$), but this association was not observed for our foot ulcer cohort ($P = .12$). In contrast, macrovascular complications were associated with increased per capita spending for beneficiaries with foot ulcers ($P = .01$). Rates of hospital admission were also associated with higher per capita spending and increased mortality rates for individuals with foot ulcers ($P < .001$ for health spending and mortality) and lower extremity amputations ($P < .001$ for health spending, $P = .01$ for mortality).

Conclusions.—Geographic variation in Medicare spending and mortality rates for diabetic patients with foot ulcers and amputations is associated

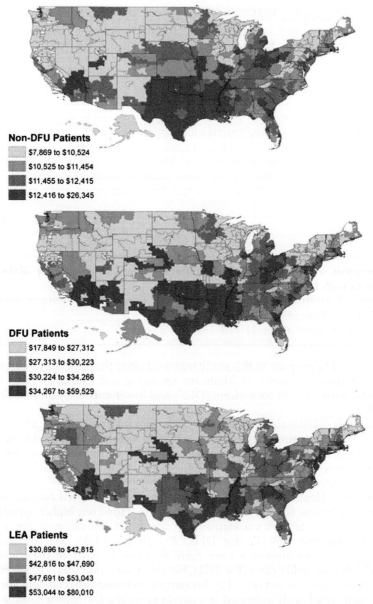

Non-DFU Patients
- $7,869 to $10,524
- $10,525 to $11,454
- $11,455 to $12,415
- $12,416 to $26,345

DFU Patients
- $17,849 to $27,312
- $27,313 to $30,223
- $30,224 to $34,266
- $34,267 to $59,529

LEA Patients
- $30,896 to $42,815
- $42,816 to $47,690
- $47,691 to $53,043
- $53,044 to $80,010

FIGURE 1.—Quartile Map of Medicare Reimbursements for Non-Diabetic Foot Ulcer, Diabetic Foot Ulcer, and Lower Extremity Amputation Cohorts, 2007. Fig. 1 illustrates Medicare reimbursements by hospital referral region for diabetic patients without foot ulcers, diabetic patients with foot ulcers, and diabetic patients with lower extremity amputations. We used CMS (Centers for Medicare and Medicaid Services) geographic adjustment factors (GAF) to adjust for regional differences in Medicare reimbursement rates. For each patient cohort, there exists significant geographic variation in treatment costs. Reimbursements were significantly increased for all three cohorts in parts of Texas, Oklahoma, and Louisiana. (Reprinted from Sargen MR, Hoffstad O, Margolis DJ. Geographic variation in Medicare spending and mortality for diabetic patients with foot ulcers and amputations. *J Diabetes Complications.* 2013;27:128-133, with permission from Elsevier.)

with regional differences in the utilization of inpatient services and the prevalence of macrovascular complications (Fig 1).

▶ The analysis and methodology are much more complex than the title of this article would suggest. It can come as no surprise that these areas with the greatest use of procedures are associated with the highest per capita spending. What should be explained is the rather dramatic national variation on procedures and costs (Fig 1).

The single most important observation is that the increased procedures and spending did not decrease mortality. This study does underscore the problem of variation, for which there is growing awareness and concern.

B. F. Morrey, MD

10 Sports Medicine

Introduction

In the past, I have always mentioned that I have tried to avoid having this section be synonymous with ACL surgery, and this year is no exception. It is well known, of course, that ACL in its various expressions, frequency, gender specificity, associated injuries, surgical techniques, long-time outcomes, and functional implications have all been addressed on a regular and repetitive basis. We have attempted to select primarily ACL as it relates to the implications for subsequent arthritis, focusing on selection and the associated concurrent injury of the meniscus. It is felt that these represent the most significant issues going forward, at least in our opinion. However, we have also provided selections from other anatomic parts and have, as always, attempted to balance this section for the orthopedic surgeon who is required to care for the full spectrum of sports injuries. In this context, we have high-lighted the growing awareness of managing the head-injured patient. We are all well aware of the secular interest in the consequences of head injury in professional and non-professional athletes. This growing and relevant topic is specifically highlighted in this year's section.

Bernard F. Morrey, MD

American Medical Society for Sports Medicine position statement: concussion in sport
Harmon KG, Endorsed by the National Trainers' Athletic Association and the American College of Sports Medicine (Univ of Washington, Seattle; et al)
Br J Sports Med 47:15-26, 2013

Definition.—▶ Concussion is defined as a traumatically induced transient disturbance of brain function and involves a complex pathophysiological process. Concussion is a subset of mild traumatic brain injury (MTBI) which is generally self-limited and at the less-severe end of the brain injury spectrum.

Pathophysiology.—▶ Animal and human studies support the concept of postconcussive vulnerability, showing that a second blow before the brain has recovered results in worsening metabolic changes within the cell.

▶ Experimental evidence suggests the concussed brain is less responsive to usual neural activation and when premature cognitive or physical activity occurs before complete recovery the brain may be vulnerable to prolonged dysfunction.

Incidence.—▶ It is estimated that as many as 3.8 million concussions occur in the USA per year during competitive sports and recreational activities; however, as many as 50% of the concussions may go unreported.

▶ Concussions occur in all sports with the highest incidence in football, hockey, rugby, soccer and basketball.

'Sideline' Evaluation and Management.—▶ Any athlete suspected of having a concussion should be stopped from playing and assessed by a licenced healthcare provider trained in the evaluation and management of concussions.

▶ Recognition and initial assessment of a concussion should be guided by a symptoms checklist, cognitive evaluation (including orientation, past and immediate memory, new learning and concentration), balance tests and further neurological physical examination.

▶ While standardised sideline tests are a useful framework for examination, the sensitivity, specificity, validity and reliability of these tests among different age groups, cultural groups and settings is largely undefined. Their practical usefulness with or without an individual baseline test is also largely unknown.

▶ Balance disturbance is a specific indicator of a concussion, but not very sensitive. Balance testing on the sideline may be substantially different than baseline tests because of differences in shoe/cleat-type or surface, use of ankle tape or braces, or the presence of other lower extremity injury.

▶ Imaging is reserved for athletes where intracerebral bleeding is suspected.

▶ There is no same day RTP for an athlete diagnosed with a concussion.

▶ Athletes suspected or diagnosed with a concussion should be monitored for deteriorating physical or mental status.

Return to Play.—▶ Concussion symptoms should be resolved before returning to exercise.

▶ A RTP progression involves a gradual, step-wise increase in physical demands, sports-specific activities and the risk for contact.

▶ If symptoms occur with activity, the progression should be halted and restarted at the preceding symptom-free step.

▶ RTP after concussion should occur only with medical clearance from a licenced healthcare provider trained in the evaluation and management of concussions.

Short-Term Risks of Premature RTP.—▶ The primary concern with early RTP is decreased reaction time leading to an increased risk of a repeat concussion or other injury and prolongation of symptoms.

Long-Term Effects.—▶ There is an increasing concern that head impact exposure and recurrent concussions contribute to long-term neurological sequelae.

▶ Some studies have suggested an association between prior concussions and chronic cognitive dysfunction. Large-scale epidemiological studies are needed to more clearly define risk factors and causation of any long-term neurological impairment.

Education.—▶ Greater efforts are needed to educate involved parties, including athletes, parents, coaches, officials, school administrators and healthcare providers to improve concussion recognition, management and prevention.

▶ Physicians should be prepared to provide counselling regarding poten tial long-term consequences of a concussion and recurrent concussions.

▶ This article is difficult to summarize, but its relevance is clear. This football season I cared for 2 athletes who sustained concussions during high school football games. It is essential to recognize a few points about this common injury— with 3.8 million episodes a year—as a very serious injury. Return to sport before the damage has resolved is associated with increased risk of reinjury, with increased seriousness. The simple definition is posttraumatic alteration of cognitive function. A thoughtful sideline assessment most critically includes assessment of cognitive function, especially memory. Without question, a player who has sustained a concussion during a game or practice must be held out of the competition until a formal recovery process has been accomplished. The key features of this are restoration of cognitive function to base line and absence of symptoms with sequential return to full activity. In all instances, return is supervised and ultimately provided by the knowledgeable medical caregiver.

B. F. Morrey, MD

Cognitive effects of one season of head impacts in a cohort of collegiate contact sport athletes
McAllister TW, Flashman LA, Maerlender A, et al (Dartmouth Med School, Lebanon; et al)
Neurology 78:1777-1784, 2012

Objective.—To determine whether exposure to repetitive head impacts over a single season negatively affects cognitive performance in collegiate contact sport athletes.

Methods.—This is a prospective cohort study at 3 Division I National Collegiate Athletic Association athletic programs. Participants were 214 Division I college varsity football and ice hockey players who wore instrumented helmets that recorded the acceleration-time history of the head following impact, and 45 noncontact sport athletes. All athletes were assessed prior to and shortly after the season with a cognitive screening battery (ImPACT) and a subgroup of athletes also were assessed with 7 measures from a neuropsychological test battery.

Results.—Few cognitive differences were found between the athlete groups at the preseason or postseason assessments. However, a higher percentage of the contact sport athletes performed more poorly than predicted postseason on a measure of new learning (California Verbal Learning

Test) compared to the noncontact athletes (24% vs 3.6%; $p < 0.006$). On 2 postseason cognitive measures (ImPACT Reaction Time and Trails 4/B), poorer performance was significantly associated with higher scores on several head impact exposure metrics.

Conclusion.—Repetitive head impacts over the course of a single season may negatively impact learning in some collegiate athletes. Further work is needed to assess whether such effects are short term or persistent.

▶ This is a well-conducted, sophisticated study with a reasonable sample and sound methodology. This methodology is less familiar to the orthopedic community. The reason to include it is to simply provide an example of the growing body of evidence of the measurable and negative impact of head injury on cognitive function. This contribution complements the prior report discussing the American Medical Society for Sports Medicine guidelines for return to play after concussion.

B. F. Morrey, MD

An evidence-based review: Efficacy of safety helmets in the reduction of head injuries in recreational skiers and snowboarders

Haider AH, on behalf of the Eastern Association for the Surgery of Trauma Injury Control/Violence Prevention Committee (Johns Hopkins School of Medicine, Baltimore, MD; et al)
J Trauma Acute Care Surg 73:1340-1347, 2012

Background.—Approximately 600,000 ski- and snowboarding-related injuries occur in North America each year, with head injuries accounting for up to 20% of all injuries. Currently, there are no major institutional recommendations regarding helmet use for skiers and snowboaders in the United States, in part owing to previous conflicting evidence regarding their efficacy. The objective of this review was to evaluate existing evidence on the efficacy of safety helmets during skiing and snowboarding, particularly in regard to head injuries, neck and cervical spine injuries, and risk compensation behaviors. These data will then be used for potential recommendations regarding helmet use during alpine winter sports.

Methods.—The PubMed, Cochrane Library, and EMBASE databases were searched using the search string *helmet* OR *head protective devices* AND (*skiing* OR *snowboarding* OR *skier* OR *snowboarder*) for articles on human participants of all ages published between January 1980 and April 2011. The search yielded 83, 0, and 96 results in PubMed, Cochrane Library, and EMBASE, respectively. Studies published in English describing the analysis of original data on helmet use in relation to outcomes of interest, including death, head injury, severity of head injury, neck or cervical spine injury, and risk compensation behavior, were selected. Sixteen published studies met a priori inclusion criteria and were reviewed in detail by authors.

Results.—Level I recommendation is that all recreational skiers and snowboarders should wear safety helmets to reduce the incidence and severity of head injury during these sports. Level II recommendation/observation is that helmets do not seem to increase risk compensation behavior, neck injuries, or cervical spine injuries among skiers and snowboarders. Policies and interventions to increase helmet use should be promoted to reduce mortality and head injury among skiers and snowboarders.

Conclusion.—Safety helmets clearly decrease the risk and severity of head injuries in skiing and snowboarding and do not seem to increase the risk of neck injury, cervical spine injury, or risk compensation behavior. Helmets are strongly recommended during recreational skiing and snowboarding.

▶ This study complements the guidelines for management of concussion previously reviewed. Using evidence-based literature review techniques, the authors conclude the use of helmets does significantly decrease the incidence of serious head injury to skiers and snowboarders. It should be noted that head injuries do account for 20% of the 600 000 injuries reported each year occurring from these 2 sports. Of particular note is the review also assessed the possibility of the unintended consequence of increased incidence of neck injury with helmets. Association does not exist was not found.

B. F. Morrey, MD

'Batter's Shoulder': Can Athletes Return to Play at the Same Level After Operative Treatment?

Wanich T, Dines J, Dines D, et al (Montefiore Med Ctr, Bronx, NY; Hosp for Special Surgery, NY; et al)
Clin Orthop Relat Res 470:1565-1570, 2012

Background.—Batter's shoulder has been defined as posterior subluxation of the lead shoulder during the baseball swing. However, it is unclear whether or how frequently patients may return to play after treatment of this uncommon condition.

Questions/Purposes.—We therefore determined the rate of return to play after operative treatment for Batter's shoulder and whether ROM was restored.

Methods.—We retrospectively reviewed the records of 14 baseball players diagnosed with Batter's shoulder. Four played professionally, six were in college, and four were in varsity high school. The average age was 20.3 years (range, 16—33 years). All had physical examinations and MRI findings consistent with posterior labral tears involving the lead shoulder. Treatment involved arthroscopic posterior labral repair (n = 10), débridement (n = 2), or rehabilitation (n = 2). The minimum followup was 18 months (average, 2.8 years; range, 18—64 months).

Results.—Eleven of 12 surgically treated patients returned to their previous level of batting at an average of 5.9 months after surgery. The one patient who was unable to return to play also had an osteochondral lesion of the glenoid identified at surgery. Players typically returned to

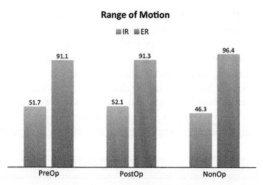

Range of Motion

■ IR ■ ER

FIGURE 2.—Average preoperative and postoperative ROM is demonstrated. IR = internal rotation; ER = external rotation. (With kind permission from Springer Science+Business Media: Wanich T, Dines J, Dines D, et al. 'Batter's shoulder': can athletes return to play at the same level after operative treatment? *Clin Orthop Relat Res.* 2012;470:1565-1570, with permission from The Association of Bone and Joint Surgeons®.)

hitting off a tee at 3 months and to facing live pitching at 6 months postoperatively. All patients regained full internal and external ROM as compared with preoperative data.

Conclusions.—Batter's shoulder is an uncommon form of posterior instability in hitters affecting their lead shoulder. Most athletes are able to return to play at the same level after arthroscopic treatment of posterior capsulolabral lesions.

Level of Evidence.—Level IV, case series. See Guidelines for Authors for a complete description of levels of evidence (Fig 2).

▶ The interesting feature of this article is that it serves not as a basis of recommendation for the affected athlete, but more importantly for me, it also shows some pathology can be accurately diagnosed and treated in a manner that reliably and quickly returns the high-level athlete to his or her former level of function. I was impressed at the accuracy of diagnosis, with the assistance of magnetic resonance imaging. I was also struck by the technical effectiveness and reliability of the intervention as well as the ability to stabilize and not alter range of motion (Fig 2). In summary, it is a nice example of the progress we have made in upper extremity sports injury.

B. F. Morrey, MD

Iliotibial Band Syndrome in Runners: A Systematic Review
van der Worp MP, van der Horst N, de wijer A, et al (Univ of Applied Sciences Utrecht, the Netherlands; et al)
Sports Med 42:969-992, 2012

Background.—The popularity of running is still growing and, as participation increases, the incidence of running-related injuries will also rise.

Iliotibial band syndrome (ITBS) is the most common injury of the lateral side of the knee in runners, with an incidence estimated to be between 5% and 14%. In order to facilitate the evidence-based management of ITBS in runners, more needs to be learned about the aetiology, diagnosis and treatment of this injury.

Objective.—This article provides a systematic review of the literature on the aetiology, diagnosis and treatment of ITBS in runners.

Search Strategy.—The Cochrane Library, MEDLINE, EMBASE, CINAHL, Web of Science, and reference lists were searched for relevant articles.

Selection Criteria.—Systematic reviews, clinical trials or observational studies involving adult runners (>18 years) that focused on the aetiology, diagnosis and/or treatment of ITBS were included and articles not written in English, French, German or Dutch were excluded.

Data Collection and Analysis.—Two reviewers independently screened search results, assessed methodological quality and extracted data. The sum of all positive ratings divided by the maximum score was the percentage quality score (QS). Only studies with a QS higher than 60% were included in the analysis. The following data were extracted: study design; number and characteristics of participants; diagnostic criteria for ITBS; exposure/treatment characteristics; analyses/outcome variables of the study; and setting and theoretical perspective on ITBS.

Main Results.—The studies of the aetiology of ITBS in runners provide limited or conflicting evidence and it is not clear whether hip abductor weakness has a major role in ITBS. The kinetics and kinematics of the hip, knee and/or ankle/foot appear to be considerably different in runners with ITBS to those without. The biomechanical studies involved small samples, and data seem to have been influenced by sex, height and weight of participants. Although most studies monitored the management of ITBS using clinical tests, these tests have not been validated for this patient group. While the articles were inconsistent regarding the treatment of ITBS, hip/knee coordination and running style appear to be key factors in the treatment of ITBS. Runners might also benefit from mobilization, exercises to strengthen the hip, and advice about running shoes and running surface.

Conclusion.—The methodological quality of research into the management of ITBS in runners is poor and the results are highly conflicting. Therefore, the study designs should be improved to prevent selection bias and to increase the generalizability of findings.

▶ The salient point of this article has been made by many others—the orthopedic literature is very poor when subjected to systematic review. Hence, we are faced with the equally disappointing conclusion for this condition that plagues about 10% of all runners: The methodology and quality of literature regarding iliotibial band syndrome is poor and results in highly conflicting conclusions. Better study design and execution is required to address the diagnosis and treatment of this condition. The study design is shown in Fig 1 in the original article. Of the 209 articles reviewed on this subject, only 36 were adequate to assess in detail. Hip abductor weakness and alterations in classic running style were most often implicated but not proven as potential causes. No conclusion regarding treatment specifics could be recommended, but time and therapy, of some sort, seemed beneficial.

Oh my, enough said. Seems we know nothing about this condition?

B. F. Morrey, MD

Accuracy of Magnetic Resonance Imaging in Grading Knee Chondral Defects

Zhang M, Min Z, Rana N, et al (First Affiliated Hosp of Xi'an Jiaotong Univ, China)

Arthroscopy 29:349-356, 2013

Purpose.—To determine the accuracy of routine magnetic resonance imaging (MRI) in the grading of knee cartilage lesions through a meta-analysis.

Methods.—A search of English-language literature published before February 2012 was carried out in PubMed. Articles using arthroscopy as a gold standard, a 6−knee region dividing method, and a 5-level grading system were included in our meta-analysis. After data extraction, a bivariate mixed-effects model and hierarchical weighted symmetric summary receiver operating curve were used to pool the results of diagnostic tests. A sensitivity analysis was conducted to explore the potential sources of heterogeneity.

Results.—Overall, 8 studies were included in the meta-analysis. The overall sensitivity, specificity, diagnostic odds ratio, positive likelihood ratio, and negative likelihood ratio were 75% (95% confidence interval [CI], 62% to 84%), 94% (95% CI, 89% to 97%), 47 (95% CI, 18 to 122), 12.5 (95% CI, 6.5 to 24.2), and 0.27 (95% CI, 0.17 to 0.42), respectively. There was substantial heterogeneity among the results. Sensitivity analysis showed the inconsistency of 2 studies. However, eliminating the 2 studies had no significant impact on the overall results.

Conclusions.—Our results showed that MRI was effective in discriminating normal morphologic cartilage from disease but was less sensitive in detecting knee chondral lesions (higher than grade 1). The negative results of MRI should not prevent a diagnostic arthroscopy.

Level of Evidence.—Level II, meta-analysis of Level I and II studies (Fig 1, Table 2).

▶ As I have admitted many times, I am drawn to these types of studies. The authors have asked an important question—does the magnetic resonance image (MRI) accurately diagnose chondral lesions. The simple answer is yes, but the details are worth noting. The study outline might be considered (Fig 1). It is noteworthy that only 8 studies contributed to the analysis and conclusion. The results are well summarized in Table 2. Most authors found the same thing. MRI is both sensitive and specific to diagnose chondral injury but not very good at discriminating the severity. We would concur with the simple conclusion,

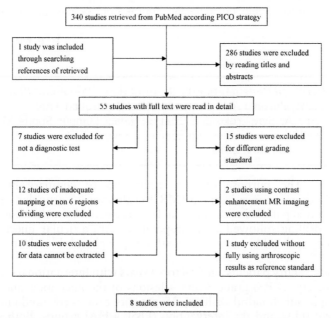

FIGURE 1.—Flowchart of search results. (MR, magnetic resonance.) (Reprinted from Arthroscopy: The Journal of Arthroscopic and Related Surgery. Zhang M, Min Z, Rana N, et al. Accuracy of magnetic resonance imaging in grading knee chondral defects. *Arthroscopy*. 2013;29:349-356, with permission from the Arthroscopy Association of North America.)

TABLE 2.—Primary Outcomes and QUADAS

Study	Sensitivity (%)	Specificity (%)	Level of Evidence	QUADAS* 1	2	4	5	8	10	11	3, 6, 7, 9, 12-14
Bredella et al.[17]	89.7	99.0	I	U	N	Y	N	Y	Y	Y	Y
Sonin et al.[18]	65.4	89.2	I	U	Y	U	N	Y	Y	U	U
Mohr[19]	44.4	95.1	I	U	Y	Y	N	Y	Y	Y	Y
von Engelhardt et al.[20]	91.2	85.2	I	U	Y	Y	N	Y	Y	U	U
Duc et al.[21]	57.3	89.1	II	U	Y	Y	N	N	U	Y	Y
Mathieu et al.[22]	70.0	98.1	I	U	Y	Y	N	Y	U	U	U
Galea et al.[23]	83.0	94.3	II	U	Y	Y	N	Y	U	Y	Y
Li et al.[24]	72.0	87.8	I	U	Y	N	Y	Y	Y	Y	Y

Editor's Note: Please refer to original journal article for full references.

N, no; U, unclear; Y, yes.

*The QUADAS criteria were as follows: (1) Was the spectrum of patients representative of the patients who will receive the test in practice? (2) Were selection criteria clearly described? (3) Was the reference standard likely to correctly classify the target condition? (4) Was the time period between reference standard and index test short enough to be reasonably sure that the target condition did not change between the 2 tests? (5) Did the whole sample or a random selection of the sample receive verification using a reference standard of diagnosis? (6) Did patients receive the same reference standard regardless of the index test result? (7) Was the reference standard independent of the index test (i.e., the index test did not form part of the reference standard)? (8) Was the execution of the index test described in sufficient detail to permit replication of the test? (9) Was the execution of the reference standard described in sufficient detail to permit its replication? (10) Were the index test results interpreted without knowledge of the results of the reference standard? (11) Were the reference standard results interpreted without knowledge of the results of the index test? (12) Were the same clinical data available when test results were interpreted as would be available when the test is used in practice? (13) Were uninterpretable/intermediate test results reported? (14) Were withdrawals from the study explained?

the MRI findings should not deter an arthroscopic examination if clinically indicated.

B. F. Morrey, MD

Articular Cartilage Regeneration With Autologous Peripheral Blood Stem Cells Versus Hyaluronic Acid: A Randomized Controlled Trial
Saw K-Y, Anz A, Siew-Yoke Jee C, et al (Kuala Lumpur Sports Medicine Centre, Malaysia; Andrews Res and Education Inst, Gulf Breeze, FL; et al)
Arthroscopy 29:684-694, 2013

Purpose.—The purpose of this study was to compare histologic and magnetic resonance imaging (MRI) evaluation of articular cartilage regeneration in patients with chondral lesions treated by arthroscopic sub-chondral drilling followed by postoperative intra-articular injections of hyaluronic acid (HA) with and without peripheral blood stem cells (PBSC).

Methods.—Fifty patients aged 18 to 50 years with International Cartilage Repair Society (ICRS) grade 3 and 4 lesions of the knee joint underwent arthroscopic subchondral drilling; 25 patients each were randomized to the control (HA) and the intervention (PBSC + HA) groups. Both groups received 5 weekly injections commencing 1 week after surgery. Three additional injections of either HA or PBSC + HA were given at weekly intervals 6 months after surgery. Subjective IKDC scores and MRI scans were obtained preoperatively and postoperatively at serial visits. We performed second-look arthroscopy and biopsy at 18 months on 16 patients in each group. We graded biopsy specimens using 14 components of the International Cartilage Repair Society Visual Assessment Scale II (ICRS II) and a total score was obtained. MRI scans at 18 months were assessed with a morphologic scoring system.

Results.—The total ICRS II histologic scores for the control group averaged 957 and they averaged 1,066 for the intervention group ($P = .022$). On evaluation of the MRI morphologic scores, the control group averaged 8.5 and the intervention group averaged 9.9 ($P = .013$). The mean 24-month IKDC scores for the control and intervention groups were 71.1 and 74.8, respectively ($P = .844$). One patient was lost to follow-up. There were no notable adverse events.

Conclusions.—After arthroscopic subchondral drilling into grade 3 and 4 chondral lesions, postoperative intra-articular injections of autologous PBSC in combination with HA resulted in an improvement of the quality of articular cartilage repair over the same treatment without PBSC, as shown by histologic and MRI evaluation.

Level of Evidence.—Level II, randomized controlled trial (RCT) (Fig 3).

▶ Prospective randomized studies are difficult to design and execute. This study was successfully completed with a modest number of patients (25) in each of 2 arms: with and without peripheral blood stem cells as an adjunct to drilling for full

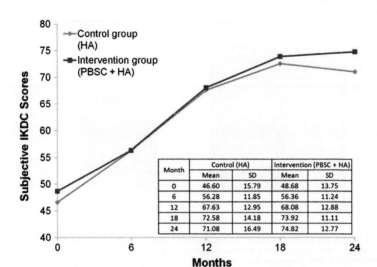

FIGURE 3.—Subjective IKDC outcomes. (SD, standard deviation.) (Reprinted from Arthroscopy: The Journal of Arthroscopic and Related Surgery. Saw K-Y, Anz A, Siew-Yoke Jee C, et al. Articular cartilage regeneration with autologous peripheral blood stem cells versus hyaluronic acid: a randomized controlled trial. *Arthroscopy.* 2013;29:684-694, Copyright 2013, with permission from the Arthroscopy Association of North America.)

thickness cartilage lesions. The findings at 18 months reveal significant differences in the histologic appearance and the MRI findings. However, clinically, the results are the same (Fig 3). Enhancing accepted treatment modalities with some expression of growth enhancement is an important and ongoing source of intense investigation. I feel this is going in the right direction.

B. F. Morrey, MD

Fresh osteochondral allograft is a suitable alternative for wide cartilage defect in the knee

Giorgini A, Donati D, Cevolani L, et al (Modena Policlinic, Italy; Rizzoli Orthopaedic Inst, Bologna, Italy)

Injury 44:S16-S20, 2013

Introduction.—There are several surgical options to restore a wide osteochondral defect in the knee. Fresh osteochondral allografts are usually considered a poor alternative due to their difficulties in surgical application. The aim of this work is first to present our experience including the surgical technique and the functional results of patients receiving fresh osteochondral allograft to restore major knee lesions, then, to compare our results with other results presented in literature.

Methods.—Between 2006 and 2011, we treated 11 patients with osteochondral lesion of the knee (Outerbridge IV°). The average lesion size was

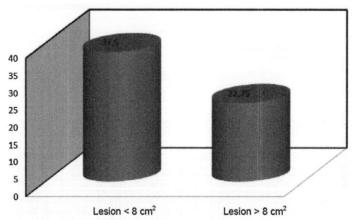

FIGURE 2.—Improvement of IKDC scores. (Reprinted from Giorgini A, Donati D, Cevolani L, et al. Fresh osteochondral allograft is a suitable alternative for wide cartilage defect in the knee. *Injury.* 2013;44:S16-S20, with permission from Elsevier.)

10.3 cm^2 (range 3–20 cm^2). The average age was 34 years (range 18–66). Patients were followed from 12 to 55 months (average of 26.5) through clinical examination, X-ray film and MRI every 3 months for the first year, then every 6 months.

Results.—The treatment was successful in 10 patients showing pain regression and mean IKDC subjective score improvements from 27.3 to 58.7. The IKDC objective score also improved of at least one class for each patient except the who failed. The radiographs show good osteointegration in all cases but one.

Conclusions.—Fresh allograft is an effective therapy for osteochondral defects repair because it allows functional recovery in a considerable number of patients. This technique obtains better results in lesion smaller than 8 cm^2. However larger lesion show good results.

Level of Evidence.—Therapeutic study, Level IV (Fig 2).

▶ Although the sample is only 11 patients, and the surveillance is only 12 months in some patients, I have included this study because it addresses a major problem: managing the knee with a larger, 8 cm^2 cartilage loss. These authors report on the use of a technique not in as much favor as autologous options: osteoarticular allografts. The technique is carefully described. The assessment is also carefully done with objective studies, magnetic resonance imaging, and subjective assessment. The overall standardized, International Knee Documentation Committee score was considered a success in 10 of 11 patients. As expected, the smaller lesions did better than the larger ones (Fig 2). Although not definitive, it is worthy of awareness.

B. F. Morrey, MD

Do Cartilage Repair Procedures Prevent Degenerative Meniscus Changes?:
Longitudinal $T_{1\rho}$ and Morphological Evaluation With 3.0-T MRI
Jungmann PM, Li X, Nardo L, et al (Univ of California-San Francisco)
Am J Sports Med 40:2700-2708, 2012

Background.—Cartilage repair (CR) procedures are widely accepted for treatment of isolated cartilage defects in the knee joint. However, it is not well known whether these procedures prevent degenerative joint disease.

Hypothesis.—Cartilage repair procedures prevent accelerated qualitative and quantitative progression of meniscus degeneration in individuals with focal cartilage defects.

Study Design.—Cohort study; Level of evidence, 2.

Methods.—Ninety-four subjects were studied. Cartilage repair procedures were performed on 34 patients (osteochondral transplantation, n = 16; microfracture, n = 18); 34 controls were matched. An additional 13 patients received CR and anterior cruciate ligament (ACL) reconstruction (CR and ACL), and 13 patients received only ACL reconstruction. Magnetic resonance imaging at 3.0- tesla with $T_{1\rho}$ mapping and sagittal fat-saturated intermediate-weighted fast spin echo (FSE) sequences was performed to quantitatively and qualitatively analyze menisci (Whole-Organ Magnetic Resonance Imaging Score [WORMS] assessment). Patients in the CR and CR and ACL groups were examined 4 months (n = 34; n = 13), 1 year (n = 21; n = 8), and 2 years (n = 9; n = 5) after CR. Control subjects were scanned at baseline and after 1 and 2 years, ACL patients after 1 and 2 years.

Results.—At baseline, global meniscus $T_{1\rho}$ values (mean ± SEM) were higher in individuals with CR (14.2 ± 0.5 ms; $P =.004$) and in individuals with CR and ACL (17.1 ± 0.9 ms; $P < .001$) when compared with controls (12.8 ± 0.6 ms). After 2 years, there was a statistical difference between $T_{1\rho}$ at the overlying meniscus above cartilage defects (16.4 ± 1.0 ms) and $T_{1\rho}$ of the subgroup of control knees without cartilage defects (12.1 ± 0.8 ms; $P < .001$) and a statistical trend to the CR group (13.3 ± 1.0 ms; $P =.09$). At baseline, 35% of subjects with CR showed morphological meniscus tears at the overlying meniscus; 10% of CR subjects showed an increase in the WORMS meniscus score within the first year, and none progressed in the second year. Control subjects with (without) cartilage defects showed meniscus tears in 30% (5%) at baseline; 38% (19%) increased within the first year, and 15% (10%) within the second year.

Conclusion.—This study demonstrated more severe meniscus degeneration after CR surgery compared with controls. However, progression of $T_{1\rho}$ values was not observed from 1 to 2 years after surgery. These results suggest that CR may prevent degenerative meniscus changes (Fig 3).

▶ Because knee injuries typically occur in the young, and because the protective function of the meniscus is well demonstrated, efforts to assure meniscus integrity after injury are critical. This nicely performed study has several useful findings. The first is that efforts to preserve or restore cartilage function actually lessen the

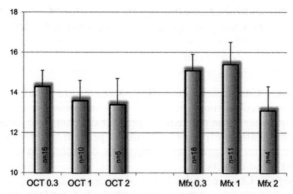

FIGURE 3.—The $T_{1\rho}$ values of the overlying meniscus above the repair region in subjects with osteochondral transplantation (OCT) and subjects with microfracture procedure (Mfx) 0.3, 1, and 2 y after surgery. Differences between the groups were not significant ($P > .05$). (Reprinted from Jungmann PM, Li X, Nardo L, et al. Do cartilage repair procedures prevent degenerative meniscus changes?: longitudinal $T_{1\rho}$ and morphological evaluation with 3.0-T MRI. *Am J Sports Med.* 2012;40:2700-2708, with permission from The Author(s).)

likelihood of meniscus degeneration. This is an important and clinically relevant observation. But, as was shown by another article in this section, the impact of the cartilage restoration technique was not important in demonstrating the protective effect (Fig 3). Hence, if there is a localized cartilage defect, it should be treated for several reasons, including the protective effect on the meniscus.

B. F. Morrey, MD

Adverse Outcomes Associated With Elective Knee Arthroscopy: A Population-Based Cohort Study

Bohensky MA, deSteiger R, Kondogiannis C, et al (Univ of Melbourne, Australia; Epworth Hosp, Richmond, Australia; Melbourne Health, Australia)
Arthroscopy 29:716-725, 2013

Purpose.—The aims of this study were to quantify the frequency of adverse outcomes after elective knee arthroscopies in Victoria, Australia, and to identify risk factors associated with adverse outcomes.

Methods.—We performed a retrospective, longitudinal cohort study of elective orthopaedic admissions using the Victorian Admitted Episodes database, a routinely collected public and private hospital episodes database linked to death registry data, from July 1, 2000, to June 30, 2009. Adverse outcome measures included pulmonary embolism (PE), deep vein thrombosis (DVT), hemarthrosis, effusion and synovitis, cellulitis, wound infection, synovial fistula, acute renal failure, myocardial infarct, stroke, and death. Patients were excluded if they had an additional procedure performed during the arthroscopy admission. We identified complications during the admission and within readmissions up to 30 days after the procedure. PE, DVT, and death within 90 days of the arthroscopy episode were

TABLE 3.—Frequency of Adverse Outcomes in Hospital and Within Readmissions

Episodes With Identified Complications Based on Previous Literature Reports or Death	In Hospital n	%	Median LOS (25th-75th Quartile)	Episodes With Any 30-d Hospital Readmission Including Identified Complications or Death	Readmissions n	%	Total Patients (In Hospital and Readmissions)	Rate per 1,000 Procedures
Total	59	0.03	3 (1-7)	Total	1,100*	0.61	1,159	6.4
Thromboembolism								
DVT	19	0.01	6 (4-9)	30-d DVT	556	0.31	579	3.2
PE	2	<0.01	2.5 (2-4)	30-d PE	138	0.08	147	0.8
Joint complications								
Hemarthrosis	14	0.01	3.5 (3-9)	30-d hemarthrosis	124	0.07	134	0.7
Effusion and synovitis	8	<0.01	3 (1.5-5)	30-d effusion and synovitis	146	0.08	154	0.9
Cellulitis	1	<0.01	4 (4-4)	30-d cellulitis	59	0.03	60	0.4
Wound infection	0	<0.01		30-d wound infection	62	0.02	62	0.2
Synovial fistula	0	<0.01		30-d synovial fistula	4	<0.01	4	0.0
Other major complications								
Acute renal failure	1	<0.01	2	30-d acute renal failure	18	0.01	19	0.1
Myocardial infarct	3	<0.01	3 (2-9)	30-d myocardial infarct	33	0.02	36	0.2
Stroke	3	<0.01	3 (2-4)	30-d stroke	37	0.02	40	0.2
In-hospital mortality	10	0.01	2 (2-3)	30-d mortality (all natural causes)	45	0.02	55	0.3

LOS, length of stay.
*One hundred twenty-two episodes contained multiple complications.

also examined. We used logistic regression analysis to identify risk factors associated with complications.

Results.—After we excluded 16,807 patients (8.5%) with an additional procedure during their admission, there were 180,717 episodes involving an elective arthroscopy during the period studied. The most common adverse outcomes within 30 days were DVT (579, 0.32%), effusion and synovitis (154, 0.09%), PE (147, 0.08%), and hemarthrosis (134, 0.07%). The 30-day orthopaedic readmission rate was 0.77%, and there were 55 deaths (0.03%). Within 90 days of arthroscopy, we identified 655 events of DVT (0.36%) and 179 PE events (0.10%). Logistic regression analysis identified that potential risk factors for complications were older age, presence of comorbidity, being married, major mechanical issues, and having the procedure performed in a public hospital.

Conclusions.—Our study found 6.4 adverse outcomes per 1,000 elective knee arthroscopy procedures (0.64%), with the 3 most common complications being DVT, effusion and synovitis, and PE. We have also identified risk factors for adverse outcomes, particularly chronic kidney disease, myocardial infarction, cerebrovascular accident, and cancer.

Level of Evidence.—Level III, retrospective cohort study (Table 3).

▶ This is an impressive study based on the sheer number of patients studied: greater than 180 000. The question is also relevant. I clearly remember the first complication of a deep vein thrombosis (DVT) I had after knee arthroscopy; of course the patient was an attorney! Hence, when we do offer the most commonly performed orthopedic procedure in the world, it is good to know that while the complication rate is very low, 6 in 1000, the impact can be considerable and unexpected. Two of the 3 most common problems involve pulmonary embolism and DVT; both are worthy of note (Table 3).

B. F. Morrey, MD

Disability, Impairment, and Physical Therapy Utilization After Arthroscopic Partial Meniscectomy in Patients Receiving Workers' Compensation
Di Paola J (Occupational Orthopedics, LLC, Tualatin, OR)
J Bone Joint Surg Am 94:523-530, 2012

Background.—The treatment of meniscal tears in injured workers is associated with less favorable outcomes and higher utilization of clinical services. It was hypothesized that patients receiving Workers' Compensation who undergo arthroscopic meniscectomy can have excellent outcomes with physical therapy utilization below the national best-practices benchmarks.

Methods.—The records of 155 injured workers who had undergone 164 primary arthroscopic meniscectomies were reviewed at least one year following claim closure. The time to release to unrestricted full work duty and the number of postoperative physical therapy visits were compared between the study group (managed with a protocol-driven, independent

TABLE 1.—Description of Results

Factor	Study Group (N = 94)	Control Group (N = 70)	Combined Group (N = 164)	P Value
No. of weeks to light duty				0.17*
Median	2.0	2.0	2.0	
Mean	2.2	2.6	2.2	
No. of weeks to full duty[†]				0.76*
Median	9.5	9.0	9.0	
Mean	10.9	11.5	11.2	
No. of weeks to closure				0.45*
Median	15.0	15.0	15.0	
Mean	16.6	20.3	18.2	
Permanent partial disability rate (%)	0%	4.3%	1.8%	0.08[‡]

*Wilcoxon rank-sum test.
[†]N = 161 (excludes three meniscectomies that resulted in permanent partial disability).
[‡]Fisher exact test.

TABLE 4.—Median Number of Physical Therapy Visits (N = 164 Meniscectomies)

Characteristic	Study Group (N = 94)*	Control Group (N = 70)*	Test	P Value
Protocol	6 ± 0.5	10 ± 0.8	$t_{162} = 4.20$	<0.001
Sex				
Male	6 ± 0.6	10 ± 0.9	$t_{160} = 3.58$	<0.001
Female	7 ± 1.9	6 ± 1.8	$t_{160} = 0.38$	0.71
Age at surgery			$t_{161} = 4.02$	<0.001
30 to <40 yr	6 ± 0.8	10 ± 1.1		
40 to <50 yr	6 ± 1.0	10 ± 1.1		
50 to <60 yr	6 ± 1.0	10 ± 1.1		
Physical therapy provider			$t_{161} = 3.98$	<0.001
Major	6 ± 0.6	10 ± 0.9		
Minor	6 ± 1.1	10 ± 1.1		
U.S. Department of Labor job classification			$t_{157} = 3.39$	0.001
Sedentary	2 ± 1.2	6[†]		
Light	4 ± 2.8	8 ± 2.7		
Medium	6 ± 1.2	10 ± 1.4		
Heavy	6 ± 0.8	10 ± 1.1		
Very heavy	7 ± 1.5	11 ± 1.6		
Body mass index			$t_{161} = 4.03$	<0.001
<25 kg/m^2	6 ± 1.6	10 ± 1.7		
≥25 kg/m^2	6 ± 0.6	10 ± 0.8		

*The values are given as the median number of physical therapy visits and the standard error.
[†]The standard error could not be reliably estimated for this value.

exercise program) and the control group (managed with traditional outpatient physical therapy). The traditional therapy regimen was implemented by means of a written referral stating general goals (knee range of motion, strength, and function) and recommending a range or a maximum number of visits to be attended. Patients in the study group received a written referral specifying the exact number of visits that were approved, a kit containing exercise equipment with a booklet illustrating twenty-five exercises, and a prescribed rehabilitation protocol outlining the philosophy, expected subjective and functional outcomes, and specific objective weekly goals.

Results.—The median number of physical therapy visits per patient was 40% lower in the study group than in the control group (six compared with ten; $p < 0.001$). There was no difference between the study group and the control group with regard to the permanent partial disability rate (0% compared with 4.3%; $p = 0.076$). Following arthroscopic meniscectomy, there was no significant difference between the study group and the control group in terms of the time to release to light duty, the time to release to full duty, the time to claim closure, or the rate of impairment.

Conclusions.—The implementation of a structured, independent exercise protocol appears promising as a method to reduce physical therapy utilization to levels below the national best-practices benchmarks without negatively impacting impairment and disability rates for patients receiving Workers' Compensation who undergo arthroscopic meniscectomy (Tables 1 and 4).

▶ I was attracted to this study because it was rather straightforward and relevant. We all know the confounding effect of worker's compensation on morbidity and outcome after ____. You fill in the blank. So to demonstrate that individuals with similar problems and treatment will realize similar outcomes based on expectations and explanations is quite impressive (Tables 1 and 4). If nothing else, this study does emphasize that as surgeons, we can influence outcome, even with those on compensation, based on our approach and interaction with the patient.

B. F. Morrey, MD

Does Obesity Negatively Affect the Functional Results of Arthroscopic Partial Meniscectomy? A Retrospective Cohort Study

Erdil M, Bilsel K, Sungur M, et al (Bezmialem Vakif Univ, Turkey; et al)
Arthroscopy 29:232-237, 2013

Purpose.—The purpose of this study was to evaluate the impact of body mass index (BMI) on early functional results of patients who undergo isolated partial meniscectomy.

Methods.—The functional results for 1,090 patients who underwent partial meniscectomy, in 2 different orthopaedic clinics, were evaluated retrospectively. The study includes cases with arthroscopic partial meniscectomy for isolated meniscal tears; patients with concomitant knee pathology were excluded. Three hundred forty-one (31%) patients with isolated lateral meniscal tears, 628 (58%) patients with isolated medial meniscal tears, and 121 (11%) patients with both medial and lateral meniscal tears underwent arthroscopic partial meniscectomy. We divided these patients into 3 sub-groups on the basis of their BMI; <26, between 26 and 30, ≥30. Preoperative

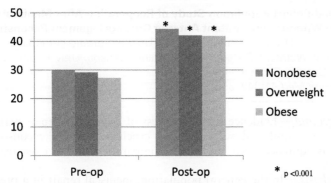

FIGURE 1.—Preoperative and postoperative Oxford Knee Scoring System scores for 3 body mass index (BM) subgoups: N (BMI <26), OW (BMI between 26 and 30), and OB (BMI >30). (Reprinted from Erdil M, Bilsel K, Sungur M, et al. Does obesity negatively affect the functional results of arthroscopic partial meniscectomy? A retrospective cohort study. *Arthroscopy.* 2013;29:232-237, with permission from the Arthroscopy Association of North America.)

functional results were compared with 1-year postoperative follow-up results using the International Knee Documentation Committee (IKDC), Lysholm Knee Scale, and Oxford Scoring System scores.

Results.—According to all 3 knee scales, age, side of lesion, and tear type had no effect on functional outcome. When compared with the group with BMI <26, the patients with BMI between 26 and 30 and the patients with BMI ≥30 had significantly worse outcomes as measured by the IKDC, Oxford Scoring System, and Lysholm Knee Scale scores. Patients with BMI between 26 and 30 and ≥30 did not have significantly different functional outcomes.

Conclusions.—Short-term outcomes after arthroscopic partial menisectomy reflect significant improvement in subjective outcome. However, patients with moderate or significant obesity (BMI >26) have inferior short-term outcomes compared with nonobese patients.

Level of Evidence.—Level IV, therapeutic case series (Fig 1).

▶ These authors have derived similar conclusions as were drawn from a study of the effects of obesity joint arthroplasty. The threshold body mass index of 26 is usually reached before a difference is generally seen. As with joint replacement, the obese patient realizes a significant improvement after arthroscopic partial meniscectomy. However, unlike with joint replacement, where the improvement tends to be greater in the obese patient, this is not so with a partial meniscectomy (Fig 1). I would love to see a study on the longer-term effects and whether the anticipated poorer survival free of additional procedures could be documented. Bottom line, do not withhold the procedure on obese patients, but do warn them of the negative effects obesity could have.

B. F. Morrey, MD

A Matched-Cohort Population Study of Reoperation After Meniscal Repair With and Without Concomitant Anterior Cruciate Ligament Reconstruction

Wasserstein D, Dwyer T, Gandhi R, et al (Univ of Toronto Orthopaedic Sports Medicine at Women's College Hosp, Ontario, Canada; Univ Health Network, Toronto, Ontario, Canada; et al)
Am J Sports Med 41:349-355, 2013

Background.—Evidence for the success of a meniscal repair performed alone versus combined with anterior cruciate ligament reconstruction (ACLR) is equivocal. No large-scale comparative studies exist regarding this issue.

Hypothesis.—In the general population, meniscal repair in a presumed stable knee has the same rate of reoperation as meniscal repair performed with ACLR.

Study Design.—Cohort study; Level of evidence, 3.

Methods.—All meniscal repairs performed with ACLR in Ontario, Canada, between July 2003 and March 2008 in patients aged 15 to 60 years were identified using administrative billing, diagnostics, and procedural coding. This cohort was matched 1:1 for sex, age, and calendar year of surgery with a cohort of patients who underwent meniscal repair alone. The McNemar test of matched pairs was used to compare reoperation rates (debridement or repair) within 2 years of the index procedure. Conditional logistic regression analysis was used to identify potential risk factors for reoperation among unmatched patient (socioeconomic status surrogate, comorbidity) and provider (surgeon volume, academic hospital status) factors.

Results.—Of 1332 patients who underwent meniscal repair and ACLR, 1239 (93%) were matched with patients who underwent meniscal repair alone. The rate of meniscal reoperation was 9.7% in the combined cohort compared with 16.7% in the repair alone cohort ($P < .0001$). In the regression analysis, only ACLR was protective against meniscal reoperation (odds ratio, 0.57; $P < .0001$). Surgeon volume of meniscal repair did not influence outcome.

TABLE 1.—Inclusion/Exclusion Criteria for the Development of the Case Cohort[a]

	n
Knee ligament reconstruction (CCI procedural + OHIP fee code)	14,908
Exclusion criteria	
Revision ACLR	450
Age ≤14 y or ≥60 y	155
Non-Ontario resident	17
Hospital admission through emergency room	153
Multiple ligament codes from same admission	2
ICD-10 code for posterior cruciate ligament injury	106
Net ACLR	14,025
ACLR (as above) + OHIP fee code for meniscal repair	1332
Matched (age + sex + year) cases	1239

[a]CCI, Canadian Classification of Health Interventions; OHIP, Ontario Health Insurance Plan; ACLR, anterior cruciate ligament reconstruction; ICD-10, International Classification of Diseases, Tenth Revision.

Conclusion.—A meniscal repair performed in conjunction with ACLR carries a 7% absolute and 42% relative risk reduction of reoperation after 2 years compared with isolated meniscal repair (Table 1).

▶ This is a signature study because it answers a clinically relevant question—is anterior cruciate ligament (ACL) reconstruction protective of a concurrent meniscus tear?

This is a central question because it relates to the subsequent development of arthritis. In addition to the importance of the question and the clarity of the findings, ACL reconstruction is statistically significantly protective at avoiding retear at 2 years.

This study is also included as an excellent example of the emerging health science research using large cohorts and sophisticated statistical analysis. The methodology Table 1 is important to provide credibility to the conclusions.

B. F. Morrey, MD

Cumulative Incidence of ACL Reconstruction After ACL Injury in Adults: Role of Age, Sex, and Race

Collins JE, Katz JN, Donnell-Fink LA, et al (Brigham and Women's Hosp, Boston, MA)
Am J Sports Med 41:544-549, 2013

Background.—Anterior cruciate ligament (ACL) injuries are common and potentially disabling and frequently prompt surgical reconstruction. The utilization of ACL reconstruction among ACL-injured patients has not been examined rigorously.

Purpose.—This study reports the 3-year cumulative incidence of ACL reconstruction among adults with ACL injury and compares demographic and clinical characteristics of ACL-injured patients who do and do not go on to undergo ACL reconstruction.

Study Design.—Cohort study; Level of evidence, 3.

Methods.—A tertiary health care system patient data repository was used to identify patients diagnosed with an ACL injury between January 1, 2001, and December 31, 2007. Follow-up data were obtained to determine how many patients with ACL injury underwent ACL reconstruction within 3 years of ACL injury diagnosis. Stratified analyses were used to examine incidence rates separately by sex, age, race, primary language, socioeconomic status (SES), and health insurance status. Multivariable logistic regression models were built to examine the association of patient characteristics with utilization of ACL reconstruction.

Results.—There were 2304 patients, with a mean age of 47 years, diagnosed with an ACL injury between 2001 and 2007. The 3-year cumulative incidence of ACL reconstruction after ACL injury diagnosis was 22.6% (95% CI, 20.9%-24.3%). Eighty-six percent of patients undergoing reconstruction did so within 6 months of injury diagnosis, while 94% underwent

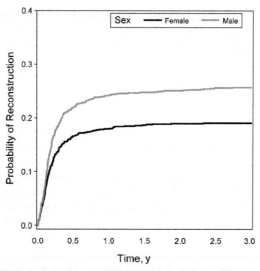

FIGURE 2.—Kaplan-Meier curves depicting the probability of ACL reconstruction for patients with ACL injury stratified by sex. Each line represents the probability of undergoing reconstruction by time since first documentation of ACL injury stratified by sex (dark line for women, light line for men). The log-rank P value for a difference in the survival curves is $< .001$. (Reprinted from Collins JE, Katz JN, Donnell-Fink LA, et al. Cumulative incidence of ACL reconstruction after ACL injury in adults: role of age, sex, and race. *Am J Sports Med.* 2013;41:544-549, with permission from The Author(s).)

TABLE 2.—ACL Reconstruction Status (in Percentages) by Patient Characteristic

Characteristic	No Reconstruction	Reconstruction
Sex		
Male	74.3	25.7
Female	80.9	19.1
Age group, y		
20-29	54.7	45.3
30-39	67.9	32.1
40-49	74.1	25.9
50-59	86.9	13.1
60-69	92.5	7.5
70+	97.3	2.7
Race		
Nonwhite	83.6	16.4
White	77.0	23.0
Unknown	73.6	26.4
Language		
English	76.5	23.5
Spanish	92.2	7.8
Other	83.6	16.4
Socioeconomic status		
High	76.1	23.9
Medium	75.8	24.2
Low	80.4	19.6
Insurance		
Private insurance	73.3	26.7
Medicare	92.3	7.7
Other	72.4	27.6
Free care	85.5	14.5
Self-pay	83.1	16.9

reconstruction within 1 year. In multivariable models, several patient features were independently associated with a higher adjusted odds of undergoing ACL reconstruction, including male sex (adjusted odds ratio [aOR], 1.4; 95% CI, 1.1-1.7), younger age (aOR per decade, 1.8; 95% CI, 1.7-2.0), white race (aOR, 1.4; 95% CI, 0.94-1.9), higher SES (aOR, 1.4; 95% CI, 1.04-1.8 for high vs low SES; aOR, 1.3; 95% CI, 1.02-1.8 for medium vs low SES), and private health insurance versus self-pay (aOR, 1.9; 95% CI, 1.04-3.5).

Conclusion.—Less than a quarter of patients with a diagnosed ACL injury underwent ACL reconstruction in the 3 years after diagnosis. The odds of having surgery were higher for men, whites, younger patients, patients with higher SES, and patients with private health insurance (Fig 2, Table 2).

▶ This somewhat elaborate study confirms what we might suspect when asked to characterize the most likely candidate to undergo anterior cruciate ligament reconstruction: young white male in an upper socioeconomic category with a recent injury (Table 2, Fig 2). Does anything more need to be said?

So why include this article? Hopefully it will draw attention to the emerging issue of bias in judgment or indications and a possible realization of recognition of improved outcomes based on the very same factors.

B. F. Morrey, MD

Comparison of Osteochondral Autologous Transplantation, Microfracture, or Debridement Techniques in Articular Cartilage Lesions Associated With Anterior Cruciate Ligament Injury: A Prospective Study With a 3-Year Follow-up
Gudas R, Gudaitė A, Mickevičius T, et al (Univ of Health Sciences Kaunas Clinics, Lithuania; Lithuanian Univ of Health Sciences, Kaunas, Lithuania; et al)
Arthroscopy 29:89-97, 2013

Purpose.—To compare the concomitant treatment of articular cartilage damage in the medial femoral condyle with osteochondral autologous transplantation (OAT), microfracture, or debridement procedures at the time of anterior cruciate ligament (ACL) reconstruction.

Methods.—Between 2006 and 2009, 102 patients with a mean age of 34.1 years and with an ACL rupture and articular cartilage damage in the medial femoral condyle of the knee were randomized to undergo OAT, microfractures, or debridement at the time of ACL reconstruction. A matched control group was included, comprising 34 patients with intact articular cartilage at the time of ACL reconstruction. There were 34 patients in the OAT-ACL group, 34 in the microfracture (MF)—ACL group, 34 in the debridement (D)—ACL group, and 34 in the control group with intact artic-ular cartilage (IAC-ACL group). The mean time from ACL injury to opera-tion was 19.32 ± 3.43 months, and the mean follow-up was 36.1 months (range, 34 to 37 months). Patients were evaluated with the International

TABLE 5.—Time From Surgery to Return to Sports

	OAT-ACL Patients (n = 34)	MF-ACL Patients (n = 34)	D-ACL Patients (n = 34)	IAC-ACL Patients (n = 34)
Time from surgery to return to sports				
6-8 mo	3	1	2	16
8-10 mo	12	11	9	10
10-12 mo	13	12	12	6
>12 mo	2	4	4	0
Mean return time (mo)	10.2	11.1	11.5	7.8
Did not return	4	6	7	2

Knee Documentation Committee (IKDC) score, Tegner activity score, and clinical assessment.

Results.—Of 102 patients, 97 (95%) were available for the final follow-up. According to the subjective IKDC score, all 4 groups fared significantly better at the 3-year follow-up than preoperatively ($P < .005$). The OAT-ACL group's IKDC subjective knee evaluation was significantly better than that of the MF-ACL group ($P = .024$) and D-ACL group ($P = .018$). However, the IKDC subjective score of the IAC-ACL group was significantly better than the OAT-ACL group's IKDC evaluation ($P = .043$). There was no significant difference between the MF-ACL and D-ACL groups' IKDC subjective scores ($P = .058$). Evaluation of manual pivot-shift knee laxity according to the IKDC knee examination form showed similar findings for the 4 groups immediately postoperatively and at 3-year follow-up, and the findings were rated as normal or nearly normal (IKDC grade A or B) in 29 of 33 patients (88%) in the OAT-ACL group, 28 of 32 patients (88%) in the MF-ACL group, 27 of 32 patients (84%) in the D-ACL group, and 31 of 34 patients (91%) in the IAC-ACL group.

Conclusions.—Our study shows that intact articular cartilage during ACL reconstruction yields more favorable IKDC subjective scores compared with any other articular cartilage surgery type. However, if an articular defect is present, the subjective IKDC scores are significantly better for OAT versus microfracture or debridement after a mean period of 3 years. Anterior knee stability results were not significantly affected by the different articular cartilage treatment methods.

Level of Evidence.—Level II, prospective comparative study (Table 5).

▶ The generic topic is really important. The most important single question with an anterior cruciate ligament (ACL) injury is what is the prognosis. This question has 2 parts: return to sport and the long-term effect. Because a high percent of patients have cartilage injury, management of this confounding variable is important. I was, quite frankly, surprised the osteochondral autologous transplantation (OATS) procedure was better than microfracture. But, as is noted in Table 5, none of the adjunct procedures to address cartilage deficiency approaches the quality of outcome of the intact cartilage. Regardless, this helps define treatment course. If there is a cartilage lesion concurrent with ACL injury, OATs is the best reconstructive option; at least, based on this experience.

B. F. Morrey, MD

Current Treatments of Isolated Articular Cartilage Lesions of the Knee Achieve Similar Outcomes
Lim H-C, Bae J-H, Song S-H, et al (Korea Univ Med Ctr, Guro-gu, Seoul)
Clin Orthop Relat Res 470:2261-2267, 2012

Background.—Many surgical techniques, including microfracture, periosteal and perichondral grafts, chondrocyte transplantation, and osteochondral grafts, have been studied in an attempt to restore damaged articular cartilage. However, there is no consensus regarding the best method to repair isolated articular cartilage defects of the knee.

Questions/Purposes.—We compared postoperative functional outcomes, followup MRI appearance, and arthroscopic examination after microfracture (MF), osteochondral autograft transplantation (OAT), or autologous chondrocyte implantation (ACI).

Methods.—We prospectively investigated 30 knees with MF, 22 with OAT, and 18 with ACI. Minimum followup was 3 years (mean, 5 years; range, 3–10 years). We included only patients with isolated cartilage defects and without other knee injuries. The three procedures were compared in terms of function using the Lysholm knee evaluation scale, Tegner activity scale, and Hospital for Special Surgery (HSS) score; modified Outerbridge cartilage grades using MRI; and International Cartilage Repair Society (ICRS) repair grade using arthroscopy.

Results.—All three procedures showed improvement in functional scores. There were no differences in functional scores and postoperative MRI grades among the groups. Arthroscopy at 1 year showed excellent or good results in 80% after MF, 82% after OAT, and 80% after ACI. Our study did not show a clear benefit of either ACI or OAT over MF.

Conclusions.—Owing to a lack of superiority of any one treatment, we believe MF is a reasonable option as a first-line therapy given its ease and affordability relative to ACI or OAT.

Level of Evidence.—Level II, therapeutic study. See Guidelines for Authors for a complete description of levels of evidence (Table 2).

▶ This is yet another excellent study originating from Korea. The subject is very timely, with numerous options becoming available commercially for the management of the isolated cartilage defect in the knee. The reasonable sample size of each of the 3 groups studied, the minimum surveillance of 3 years, and the careful postoperative assessment, including the Lysholm, Hospital for Special Surgery, and Tegner scores and arthroscopy, all provide credence to the findings. There is simply no difference in the efficacy of microfracture, of osteoarticular graft, or of autogenous cartilage implants (Table 2).

TABLE 2.—Overall Clinical Scores at 5 Years Postoperative

Procedures (number of knees)	Lysholm Scale (mean ± SD) Preoperative	Postoperative	p Value	Tegner Scale (mean ± SD) Preoperative	Postoperative	P Value	HSS Scores (mean ± SD) Preoperative	Postoperative	P Value
MF (25)	51.2 ± 6.2	85.6 ± 6.8	$p < 0.001$	2.8 ± 1.4	5.1 ± 1.5	$p < 0.001$	78.22 ± 9.12	87.60 ± 4.56	$p < 0.001$
OAT (22)	53.2 ± 7.2	84.8 ± 5.5	$p < 0.001$	2.7 ± 1.5	5.3 ± 1.2	$p < 0.001$	78.66 ± 7.23	88.12 ± 4.15	$p < 0.001$
ACI (18)	52.4 ± 6.4	84.6 ± 6.1	$p < 0.001$	2.9 ± 1.8	5.2 ± 1.3	$p < 0.001$	77.52 ± 8.16	87.51 ± 4.58	$p < 0.001$
p value		0.432			0.213			0.516	

MF = microfracture; OAT = osteochondral autograft transplantation; ACI = autologous chondrocyte implantation; HSS = Hospital for Special Surgery.

Fortunately, in the properly selected patient, they are all about 80% successful. This isn't too bad, but can be improved on, which is what all the effort is about. This study serves as a very nice benchmark for further studies of this issue.

B. F. Morrey, MD

Cartilage Status In Relation to Return to Sports After Anterior Cruciate Ligament Reconstruction

Van Ginckel A, Verdonk P, Victor J, et al (Ghent Univ, Belgium; et al)
Am J Sports Med 41:550-559, 2013

Background.—Osteoarthritis after anterior cruciate ligament (ACL) reconstruction receives much attention in orthopaedic science. Anterior cruciate ligament reconstruction is related to increased joint fluid volumes, bone marrow edema, and cartilage biochemical and morphological changes believed to cause fragile joint conditions. These joint conditions may not be able to adequately counter the imposed loads during sports.

Hypothesis.—At 6 months after surgery, knee cartilage displays inferior quality in ACL-reconstructed knees when compared with controls. This inferior quality is influenced by the time to return to sports and/or by the time to surgery.

Study Design.—Cross-sectional study; Level of evidence, 3.

Methods.—Fifteen patients treated with isolated ACL reconstruction were compared with 15 matched controls. In all participants, a 3-T magnetic resonance imaging cartilage evaluation was performed entailing quantitative morphological characteristics (3-dimensional volume/thickness), biochemical composition (T2/T2* mapping), and function (after a 30-minute run: in vivo deformation including recovery). Nonparametric statistics were executed reporting median (95% CI).

Results.—No volume and thickness between-group differences existed. In patients, medial femur (FM) T2 was higher (45.44 ms [95% CI, 40.64-51.49] vs 37.19 ms [95% CI, 34.67-40.39]; $P = .028$), whereas T2* was lower in the FM (21.81 ms [95% CI, 19.89-22.74] vs 24.29 ms [95% CI, 22.70-26.26]; $P = .004$), medial tibia (TM) (13.81 ms [95% CI, 10.26-16.78] vs 17.98 ms [95% CI, 15.95-18.90]; $P = .016$), and lateral tibia (TL) (14.69 ms [95% CI, 11.71-16.72] vs 18.62 ms [95% CI, 17.85-22.04]; $P < .001$). Patients showed diminished recovery at 30 minutes after a 30-minute run in the FM (-1.60% [95% CI, -4.82 to -0.13] vs 0.01%[95% CI, -0.34 to 1.23]; $P = .040$) and at 30 (-3.76% [95% CI, -9.29 to -1.78] vs 0.04% [95% CI, -1.52 to -0.72]; $P = .004$) and 45 minutes after exercise (-1.86% [95% CI, -4.66 to -0.40] vs 0.43% [95% CI, -0.91 to 0.77]; $P = .024$) in the TL. Eight patients returned to sports at 6 months or earlier. Return before 5 months (3/8 patients) was associated with increased cartilage thickness (in TM, TL, and lateral femur [FL]), deformation (in FL), and delayed recovery after running (in FL and FM). Median surgical delay was 10 weeks (range, 5-17 weeks). Surgery within 10 weeks (9/15 patients) was also associated with delayed cartilage recovery (in FL and FM). For the other parameters, no significant relationships could be established for either return to sports or surgical delay.

Conclusion.—At 6 months after surgery, cartilage in patients with ACL reconstruction shows diminished quality and in vivo resiliency compared with controls. Caution is advised in an early return to sports especially when dealing with patients who received prompt surgery. Possibly, high impacts on this qualitatively diminished cartilage might play a role in the development of osteoarthritis in ACL reconstruction. Replication in larger samples and follow-up are warranted.

▶ This interesting study really does advance our understanding of the anterior cruciate ligament—injured knee. It must be cautioned that the conclusions are predicated on the validity of the MRI findings to accurately reflect cartilage health and damage. The study was well constructed, and if the imaging assessment is a valid one, then the conclusions are really important to the practicing sports physician. Henceforth, I will proceed somewhat slower than in the past in allowing an athlete to return to aggressive activity. This study thus implies we need an additional tool to assess cartilage health before allowing return to activity.

B. F. Morrey, MD

Anterior Cruciate Ligament Reconstruction in Skeletally Immature Patients With Transphyseal Tunnels

Redler LH, Brafman RT, Trentacosta N, et al (Columbia Univ Med Ctr, NY)
Arthroscopy 28:1710-1717, 2012

Purpose.—Our purpose was to evaluate the results of transphyseal anterior cruciate ligament (ACL) reconstruction with hamstring autograft in skeletally immature patients.

Methods.—Eighteen knees in 18 skeletally immature pubescent patients with a mean chronologic age of 14.2 years underwent transphyseal ACL reconstruction with hamstring autograft between 2002 and 2007. Concurrent meniscal surgery was performed in 9 knees. The final patient evaluation occurred at a mean of 43.4 months (range, 24.0 to 86.6 months) and included physical examination, KT-1000 arthrometry testing (MEDmetric, San Diego, CA), and functional outcome instruments, including the International Knee Documentation Committee subjective knee form, the Lysholm knee score, and the Tegner knee activity scale.

Results.—At the latest follow-up, the mean International Knee Documentation Committee subjective knee score was 92.4 ± 10, the mean Lysholm knee score was 94.3 ± 8.8, and the mean Tegner activity scale score was 8.5 ± 1.4. Lachman and pivot-shift testing were negative in all knees. No restriction in knee range of motion of 5° or greater when compared with the contralateral knee was observed in any patient. The mean manual maximum side-to-side difference with KT-1000 testing was 0.29 ± 1.07 mm, and no patients had a difference greater than 3 mm. No angular

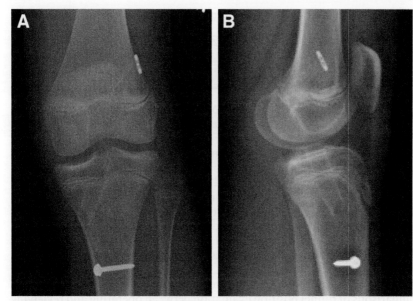

FIGURE 1.—(A) Anteroposterior and (B) lateral postoperative radiographs showing tunnel location and fixation devices. (Reprinted from Redler LH, Brafman RT, Trentacosta N, et al. Anterior cruciate ligament reconstruction in skeletally immature patients with transphyseal tunnels. *Arthroscopy.* 2012;28:1710-1717, Copyright 2012, with permission from the Arthroscopy Association of North America.)

deformities were noted, and all leg-length measurements were symmetric bilaterally on clinical examination. No patients had traumatic graft disruption or underwent revision ACL reconstruction, whereas 3 patients sustained an ACL injury in the contralateral leg while participating in sports.

Conclusions.—Transphyseal ACL reconstruction with autogenous quadrupled hamstring graft with metaphyseal fixation in skeletally immature pubescent patients yielded excellent functional outcomes in a high percentage of patients without perceived clinical growth disturbance.

Level of Evidence.—Level IV, therapeutic case series (Fig 1).

▶ Of the numerous studies related to anterior cruciate ligament reconstruction, this one is important because it addresses a controversial question: How do you handle the skeletally immature patient? Using transepiphyseal tunnels, as with a mature patient (Fig 1), the authors were not able to detect any growth disturbance. The sample size included only patients younger than 16 years of age, and hence is understandably small at 18 patients. My one concern is that the radiographic follow-up is only 6 months, and critical measurements such as leg length disturbances were only measured clinically. It would seem reasonable to follow this cohort for a longer period to prove this is a safe and effective technique.

B. F. Morrey, MD

Arthroscopic Agreement Among Surgeons on Anterior Cruciate Ligament Tunnel Placement

McConkey MO, Amendola A, Ramme AJ, et al (The Univ of Iowa, Iowa City; et al)
Am J Sports Med 40:2737-2746, 2012

Background.—Little is known about surgeon agreement and accuracy using arthroscopic evaluation of anterior cruciate ligament (ACL) tunnel positioning.

Purpose.—To investigate agreement on ACL tunnel position evaluated arthroscopically between operating surgeons and reviewing surgeons. We hypothesized that operating and evaluating surgeons would characterize tunnel positions significantly differently.

Study Design.—Controlled laboratory study.

Methods.—Twelve surgeons drilled ACL tunnels on 72 cadaveric knees using transtibial (TT), medial portal (MP), or 2-incision (TI) techniques and then completed a detailed assessment form on tunnel positioning. Then, 3 independent blinded surgeon reviewers each arthroscopically evaluated tunnel position and completed the assessment form. Statistical comparisons of tunnel position evaluation between operating and reviewing surgeons were completed. Three-dimensional (3D) computed tomography (CT) scans were performed and compared with arthroscopic assessments. Arthroscopic assessments were compared with CT tunnel location criteria.

Results.—Operating surgeons were significantly more likely to evaluate femoral tunnel position (92.6% vs 69.2%; $P = .0054$) and femoral back wall thickness as "ideal" compared with reviewing surgeons. Tunnels were judged ideal by reviewing surgeons more often when the TI technique was used compared with the MP and TT techniques. Operating surgeons were more likely to evaluate tibial tunnel position as ideal (95.5% vs 57.1%; $P < .0001$) and "acceptable" compared with reviewers. The ACL tunnels drilled using the TT technique were least likely to be judged as ideal on the tibia and the femur. Agreement among surgeons and observers was poor for all parameters ($\kappa = -0.0053$ to 0.2457). By 3D CT criteria, 88% of femoral tunnels and 78% of tibial tunnels were placed within applied criteria.

Conclusion.—Operating surgeons are more likely to judge their tunnels favorably than observers. However, independent surgeon reviewers appear to be more critical than results of 3D CT imaging measures. When subjectively evaluated arthroscopically, the TT technique yields more subjectively poorly positioned tunnels than the TI and MP techniques. Surgeons do not agree on the ideal placement for single-bundle ACL tunnels.

Clinical Relevance.—This study demonstrates that surgeons do not currently uniformly agree on ideal single-bundle tunnel placement and that the TT technique may yield more poorly placed tunnels (Table 1).

▶ This study is reviewed because it is so clever. The question is whether the operating surgeon or an independent observer is more critical regarding accuracy of

TABLE 1.—Comparison Between Surgeon and Observer Assessments of Femoral Tunnel Positions[a]

	Femoral Tunnel Position Assessment, n (%) Agreement				
	Ideal	Too Anterior	Too Horizontal	Too Posterior	Too Vertical
Surgeon (n = 68)	63 (92.65)	0 (0)	1 (1.47)	2 (2.94)	2 (2.94)
Observer (n = 198)	137 (69.19)	11 (5.56)	10 (5.05)	20 (10.10)	20 (10.10)

[a]$P = .003$ (Fisher exact test). Frequency (n) distributions among staff by femoral tunnel position are different.

tunnel placement for anterior cruciate ligament reconstruction. This cadaver study revealed what we might expect: We as surgeons are less critical of our work than an independent reviewer (Table 1).

What is of additional and maybe of greater importance is that the 2-incision technique was associated with the highest frequency of optimum placement judgments, and the transtibial technique had the lowest rating. But, one confounding factor is that, there was no statistical agreement as to what truly constitutes ideal tunnel placement. Oh me. This after hundreds of articles on the subject!

B. F. Morrey, MD

11 Trauma and Amputation

Introduction

In this year's rather large group of selections, the trend is toward a greater number of clinical trials, meta-analyses, and registry analyses. These clinical research designs have a much greater relevance to the practicing orthopedist who treats patients with fractures. The pediatric orthopedic community has been very active, and there are a large number of selections related to optimum management of femur, forearm, and elbow fractures in children and adolescents. These contributions will help all orthopedic surgeons who provide urgent and emergent care for these patients. The hip fracture selections continue to focus on optimum management decisions in terms of implant selection as well as the current issue of the effects of bisphosphonates on fracture healing. The one disappointment for this year is the relative paucity of high-quality manuscripts that relate to amputee care. It is my hope that this is only a temporary situation and that 2013 will see a rebound so that we can continue to improve care to this segment of our patient population.

Marc F. Swiontkowski, MD

Amputation Surgery: Technical Issues/Prosthetic Related Amputation Issues

Skin Grafts Provide Durable End-bearing Coverage for Lower-extremity Amputations With Critical Soft Tissue Loss

Kent T, Yi C, Livermore M, et al (Univ of Colorado School of Medicine, Denver)
Orthopedics 36:132-135, 2013

Lower-extremity amputations in the presence of soft tissue loss represent an unresolved conundrum because surgeons must consider sacrificing bone length to obtain adequate soft tissue coverage. Local flaps and microvascular soft tissue transfers are established strategies for maintaining residual limb length. However, the use of skin grafts remains controversial due to the presumed inferiority compared with flaps with regard to enabling prosthetic fitting and full weight bearing. The current study was designed to test

TABLE 1.—Demographic Data of 9 Patients With Lower-extremity Amputations Managed by Split-thickness Skin Grafting

Patient Sex/Age, y	Cause of Limb Loss	Length of Stay, d	No. of Surgeries Until STSG	No. of Complications Related to STSG	STSG Until Prosthetic Fitting, d	Last Follow-up After STSG, d
M/28	Gustilo-Anderson type IIIC open tibia fracture	28	5	0	65	130[a]
M/33	Frostbite gangrene	34	8	0	50	190
M/17	Traumatic amputation	21	9	0	58	197
M/61	Gustilo-Anderson type IIIB open ankle fracture– dislocation	34	11	0	125	331
F/67	Chronic infection, peripheral vascular disease	57	8	0	69	62
F/40	Gustilo-Anderson type IIIB open tibia fracture, infected nonunion	8	2	0	52	57
M/39	Frostbite gangrene	37	7	0	45	169
M/36	Frostbite gangrene	27	4	0	39	130
F/63	Chronic diabetic gangrene	34	8	0	48	150

Abbreviation: STSG, split-thickness skin graft.
[a]At another hospital.

the hypothesis that split-thickness skin grafts represent a safe and feasible option to preserve bone length in lower-extremity amputations with critical soft tissue loss (Table 1).

▶ There is very little available in the published literature about the outcome of split-thickness skin graft (STSG) for coverage of the terminal ends of residual limb length after amputation. Although this is a simple outcome study, retrospective in design, it does confirm that the use of STSG on terminal limb surfaces to preserve limb length for posttraumatic amputation is a viable solution. Rather than convert below-knee level amputation length to above- or through-knee level because of the lack of skin coverage, STSG should be attempted and has a high chance of success.

M. F. Swiontkowski, MD

An experimental study of the interface pressure profile during level walking of a new suspension system for lower limb amputees

Eshraghi A, Abu Osman NA, Gholizadeh H, et al (Univ of Malaya, Kuala Lumpur, Malaysia; Univ of Calgary, Canada)
Clin Biomech 28:55-60, 2013

Background.—Different suspension systems that are used within prosthetic devices may alter the distribution of pressure inside the prosthetic

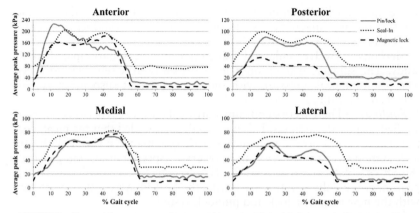

FIGURE 3.—Pattern of pressure acceptance over four sensor sites with three suspension systems during one gait cycle. (Reprinted from Clinical Biomechanics. Eshraghi A, Abu Osman NA, Gholizadeh H, et al. An experimental study of the interface pressure profile during level walking of a new suspension system for lower limb amputees. *Clin Biomech*. 2013;28:55-60, Copyright 2013, with permission from Elsevier.)

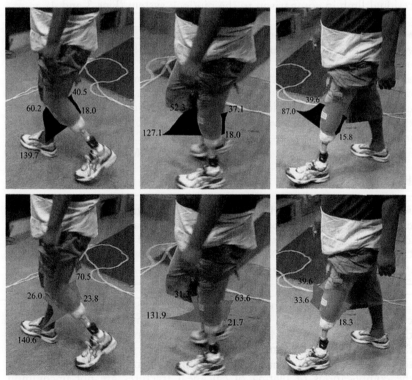

FIGURE 4.—Pressure profile with new magnetic lock (top) and pin/lock systems (bottom) during stance; right to left: early stance, mid stance, late stance. All values (average peak pressure) are in kPa. (Reprinted from Clinical Biomechanics. Eshraghi A, Abu Osman NA, Gholizadeh H, et al. An experimental study of the interface pressure profile during level walking of a new suspension system for lower limb amputees. *Clin Biomech*. 2013;28:55-60, Copyright 2013, with permission from Elsevier.)

socket in lower limb amputees. This study aimed to compare the interface pressure of a new magnetic suspension system with the pin/lock and Seal-In suspension systems.

Methods.—Twelve unilateral transtibial amputees participated in the study. The subjects walked on a level walkway at a self-selected speed. The resultant peak pressure with the three different suspension systems was recorded using F-socket transducers.

Findings.—There were significant statistical differences between the three studied suspension systems. Pair-wise analyses revealed that the mean peak pressure (kPa) was lower with the magnetic system than it was with the pin/lock system over the anterior and posterior aspects during one gait cycle (89.89 vs. 79.26 and 47.22 vs. 26.01, respectively). Overall, the average peak pressure values were higher with the Seal-In system than they were with the new magnetic lock and pin/lock system.

Interpretation.—The new magnetic system might reduce the pressure within the prosthetic socket in comparison to the pin/lock and Seal-In system during one gait cycle. This is particularly important during the swing phase of gait and may reduce the pain and discomfort at the distal residual limb in comparison to the pin/lock system (Figs 3 and 4).

▶ Continued innovation in prosthetic suspension systems is necessary and welcome. The ideal suspension system would have low peak skin pressure in all phases of gait with no slippage or shear on the skin, be very lightweight, and be durable. The research described in this report may serve as a future standard for how innovation in suspension systems will be evaluated. Although there are potential issues with detection bias with this experimental design, it looks as if the magnetic suspension system has potential and should be further evaluated in more clinical-based outcomes research.

M. F. Swiontkowski, MD

Foot and Ankle

A comparison of absorbable screws and metallic plates in treating calcaneal fractures: A prospective randomized trial

Zhang J, Ebraheim N, Lausé GE, et al (Sixth Hosp of Ningbo, Zhejiang, China; Univ of Toledo Med Ctr, OH)
J Trauma Acute Care Surg 72:E106-E110, 2012

Background.—Intra-articular calcaneal fractures are more likely to suffer consequences in terms of pain and disability. Many studies have suggested that operative treatment for these fractures may result in better outcomes than nonoperative treatment. The metallic screws and plates are among the most common alternatives to stabilize calcaneal fractures. However, the complications of plating of calcaneal fractures are not uncommon. Complications such as infection, poor wound healing, and soft tissue irritation exist. With the advent of bioabsorbable screws, many reports have demonstrated favorable results in treating intra-articular fractures with these screws. The comparative outcomes of operative treatment of calcaneal fractures stabilized with plates and absorbable screws are rarely reported. The purpose of this study is to compare the clinical outcomes and complications related to fracture stabilization with plates and absorbable screws.

Methods.—Ninety-seven patients with intra-articular calcaneal fractures were managed at our institution between February 2007 and March 2009. In this prospective, randomized study, the plates were used in 52 cases (group A), and the absorbable screws were used in 47 cases (group B). There were 71 men and 26 women who had a mean age of 41 years (range, 19–67 years). The clinical outcome and complications were assessed and compared. The adjusted American Orthopaedic Foot and Ankle Society Ankle-Hindfoot Scale (subjective component only), Foot Function Index, and the calcaneal fracture scoring system were used to assess the results.

Results.—The patients were followed up at an average of 23 months (range, 15–32 months). Radiographically, there were no nonunions in either group. One year after operation, in group A and B, the mean adjusted American Orthopaedic Foot and Ankle Society Ankle-Hindfoot Score were 71.6 ± 12.5 and 72.3 ± 17.4, respectively ($p > 0.05$); the mean Foot Function Index score were 21.4 ± 6.6 and 22.7 ± 5.2, respectively ($p > 0.05$); and the mean calcaneal fracture scoring system score were 73.5 ± 8.3 and 75.1 ± 6.9, respectively ($p > 0.05$). In group A, there were six cases of poor wound healing, one case of deep infection, and four cases of peroneal tendon irritation. In group B, there was one case of superficial infection, and no deep infection and soft tissue irritation.

Conclusions.—In this report, the outcomes of operative treatment with absorbable screws are comparable with the outcomes of operative treatment with plates. Both plates and absorbable screws showed favorable results in the surgical treatment of calcaneal fractures. However, the metallic plates were associated with increased complications. The stabilizations of displaced intra-articular calcaneal fractures with bioabsorbable screws are reasonable with advantages of fewer complications and without the need for screw removal (Tables 1-3).

▶ This seems to be a reasonably well-done controlled trial comparing the use of bioabsorbable and metal implants in the open management of calcaneus fractures. The groups are comparable with regard to fracture classification and other patient attributes, as one would expect with a randomized design. The

TABLE 1.—Patient Demographic Data ($p > 0.05$)

	Group A	Group B
No. patients	52	47
Median age (yr)	40 (19–63)	41 (22–67)
Male/female	38/14	35/12
Sanders type II	26	22
Sanders type III	18	18
Sanders type VI	8	7

TABLE 2.—Radiographic Data at Final Follow-Up

	Preoperative		Postoperative		Follow-Up	
	Group A	Group B	Group A	Group B	Group A	Group B
Böhler angle	3.5 ± 12.7	4.2 ± 15.6	32.6 ± 9.3*	35.1 ± 8.4*	32.9 ± 5.6*	34.7 ± 15*
Gissane angle	119.7 ± 45.2	124.9 ± 11.3	122.1 ± 23	127.1 ± 19.4	121.3 ± 13.2	127.3. ± 16.5

$p = 0.0001$.
*The value is of statistical significance comparing with the preoperative value.

TABLE 3.—Average Scores Measured Using Different Scoring Systems at 1 yr Postoperative

	AOFA	FFI	CFSS
Group A	71.6 ± 12.5	21.4 ± 6.6	73.5 ± 8.3
Group B	72.3 ± 17.4	22.7 ± 5.2	75.1 ± 6.9
p	>0.05	>0.05	>0.05

definition of complications and evaluation of patients did not appear to be done by observers who were not involved in the care of the patients or blinded to treatment group, leading to the potential for detection bias. Issues such as soft tissue complications, the definition of infection, and the need for hardware removal are all subject to the issues of such bias. Therefore, I am most comfortable concluding that the open management of calcaneus fractures can be successfully accomplished using either metal or absorbable implants. There may be advantages to the bioabsorbable implants, which should be confirmed with additional higher quality randomized controlled trials.

M. F. Swiontkowski, MD

Twenty-one-Year Follow-up of Supination—External Rotation Type II—IV (OTA Type B) Ankle Fractures: A Retrospective Cohort Study

Donken CCMA, Verhofstad MHJ, Edwards MJ, et al (Radboud Univ Nijmegen Med Centre, The Netherlands; St Elisabeth Hosp, Tilburg, The Netherlands)
J Orthop Trauma 26:e108-e114, 2012

Objective.—To evaluate long-term results after protocoled treatment of supination—external rotation (SER) Type II—IV ankle injuries.
Design.—Retrospective cohort study.
Setting.—Level I trauma center.
Patients.—Two hundred seventy-six adult patients with an SER Type II—IV ankle fracture between January 1, 1985, and January 1, 1990. All patients were approached to participate in this study.
Intervention.—Fractures with tibiotalar congruity were treated nonoperative and unstable fractures with joint incongruity were treated operatively.
Mean Outcome Measurements.—1) a functional outcome questionnaire (Olerud score); 2) range of motion; 3) functional impairment (American

Medical Association guidelines); and 4) radiologic anatomic result (medial clear space widening; osteoarthritis; Cedell score).

Results.—After a median of 21 years in 54% (n = 148) of patients, follow-up was achieved. Seventy-six patients (51%) had a SER Type II injury, four patients (3%) a SER Type III injury, and 68 (46%) had sustained a SER Type IV. Excellent or good results were found in 92% (Olerud score), 97% (loaded dorsal range of motion), 92% (medial clear space widening), 97% (osteoarthritis), and 76% (Cedell score) of patients. Functional impairment expressed as percentage of whole person impairment varied between 0% and 16%. The various fracture types performed statistically equal on all outcome parameters. There was no difference between operative and nonoperative treatment. There was no correlation between the Olerud score and other parameters.

Conclusions.—The very long-term overall results of the stratified surgical treatment of SER Type II–IV ankle fractures is "excellent" or "good" in the majority of patients and therefore seems justified. Although additional soft tissue damage is unavoidable in case of operative treatment, it does not negatively affect outcome in the long term.

Level of Evidence.—Therapeutic Level IV. See Instructions for Authors for a complete description of levels of evidence (Fig 1, Table 3).

▶ It is a rare thing in the orthopedic literature for the results of an injury with more than 20 years of follow-up to be reported. This large cohort study gives us these results in more than 100 patients with supination external rotation ankle fractures.

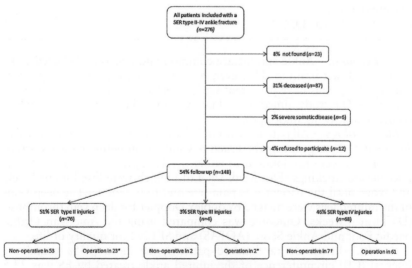

FIGURE 1.—Flowchart of patients at follow-up. (Reprinted from Donken CCMA, Verhofstad MHJ, Edwards MJ, et al. Twenty-one-year follow-up of supination—external rotation type II–IV (OTA type B) ankle fractures: a retrospective cohort study. *J Orthop Trauma.* 2012;26:e108-e114, with permission from Lippincott Williams & Wilkins.)

TABLE 3.—Percentage of Patients with 'Good' Or 'Excellent' Outcome in SER Type IV Injuries

	Olerud	ROM	OA	MCS	Cedell
Deltoid ligament rupture (n = 35)	94	85	82	100	82
Medial malleolar fracture (n = 28)	75	92	88	92	76
P	0.07	0.69	0.72	0.21	0.75
Posterior syndesmotic rupture (n = 34)	91	78	78	97	75
Posterior malleolar fracture (n = 34)	82	100	87	97	84
P	0.48	0.01	0.51	1.00	0.54

ROM, range of motion; OA, osteoarthritis; MCS, medial clear space; SER, supination–external rotation.

The vast majority of the original cohort was located (Fig 1). The results are generally good to excellent. We learn that the results of patients treated without surgery are as good as those treated with surgery. With this type of clinical research design, all this tells us is that the surgeons making the judgments regarding treatment were highly skilled because their predictions of who would benefit from surgery were highly accurate. This cohort study provided the orthopedic community with confidence that we can continue to inform our patients that they will, in more than 85% of cases, have good to excellent long-term ankle function.

M. F. Swiontkowski, MD

Elastic stockings or Tubigrip for ankle sprain: A randomised clinical trial
Sultan MJ, McKeown A, McLaughlin I, et al (Univ Hosp of South Manchester, Manchester, UK)
Injury 43:1079-1083, 2012

Background.—Ankle sprains are common and generally believed to be benign and self-limiting. However, a significant proportion of patients with ankle sprains have persistent symptoms for months or even years.

Aims.—The study aimed to evaluate whether elastic stockings improve recovery following ankle sprain.

Methodology.—All patients within 72 h of ankle sprain were identified in Accident & Emergency or the Fracture Clinic. Consenting patients, stratified for sex, were randomised to either: (i) Tubigrip or (ii) class II below knee elastic stockings (ESs, Medi UK Ltd.) which were fitted immediately and worn until the patient was pain-free and fully mobile. The deep veins of the injured legs were imaged by duplex Doppler for deep vein thrombosis (DVT) at 4 weeks. Outcome was compared using the American Orthopaedic Foot and Ankle Score (AOFAS) and SF12v2 for quality of life.

Results.—In the 36 randomised patients, the mean (95% confidence interval (CI)) circumference of the injured ankle treated by ES was 23.5 (23−24) cm initially and 22 (22−23) and 22 (21−22.5) cm at 4 and 8 weeks ($p < 0.001$) compared with 24 (23−25) cm initially and 24 (23−25) and 24 (23−24.5) cm using Tubigrip ($p < 0.001$). By 8 weeks, the mean AOFAS and SF12v2 scores were significantly improved by ES at 99

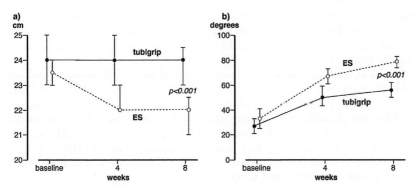

FIGURE 2.—(a) Mean (95,% CI) ankle circumference (cms) was significantly reduced by elastic stockings within four weeks and throughout the study. The range of ankle movements, (b), was also improved by ES at four and eight weeks. (Reprinted from Sultan MJ, McKeown A, McLaughlin I, et al. Elastic stockings or Tubigrip for ankle sprain: a randomised clinical trial. *Injury.* 2012;43:1079-1083, with permission from Elsevier.)

TABLE 3.—Time (Days) to Recovery (Mean 95% CI)

	ES (*n* = 18)	Tubigrip (*n* = 16)	ES v Tubigrip *p* Value
Using crutches	1.6 (1–3)	5.6 (2–10)	0.003
Taking analgesia	7.1 (5–10)	10.4 (6–18)	0.297
Return to work	5.2 (1–8)	10.1 (3–17)	0.11
Climb stairs unaided	9.5 (5–15)	12.7 (8–18)	0.242

(8.1) and 119 (118–121) compared with 88 (11) and 102 (99–107) with Tubigrip (*p* < 0.001). Of the 34 duplex images at 4 weeks, none had a DVT.

Conclusion.—Elastic compression improves recovery following ankle sprain (Fig 2, Table 3).

▶ Ankle sprains are very common and present to orthopedic surgeons as well as emergency department physicians, family physicians, and urgent care physician offices in large numbers. This well-done controlled trial demonstrates that elastic support stockings improve the rate of clinical and functional recovery. Their use should be incorporated into the routine management of these very common injuries.

M. F. Swiontkowski, MD

Outcomes of Operative Treatment of Unstable Ankle Fractures: A Comparison of Metallic and Biodegradable Implants

Noh JH, Roh YH, Yang BG, et al (Kangwon Natl Univ Hosp, Chuncheon-si, Gangwon-do, South Korea; Gachon Univ School of Medicine, Namdong-gu, Incheon, South Korea; Natl Police Hosp, Songpa-gu, Seoul, South Korea)
J Bone Joint Surg Am 94:e166.1-e166.7, 2012

Background.—Biodegradable implants for internal fixation of ankle fractures may overcome some disadvantages of metallic implants, such as imaging interference and the potential need for additional surgery to remove the implants. The purpose of this study was to evaluate the outcomes after fixation of ankle fractures with biodegradable implants compared with metallic implants.

Methods.—In this prospectively randomized study, 109 subjects with an ankle fracture underwent surgery with metallic (Group I) or biodegradable implants (Group II). Radiographic results were assessed by the criteria of the Klossner classification system and time to bone union. Clinical results were assessed with use of the American Orthopaedic Foot & Ankle Society (AOFAS) ankle-hindfoot scale, Short Musculoskeletal Function Assessment (SMFA) dysfunction index, and the SMFA bother index at three, six, and twelve months after surgery.

Results.—One hundred and two subjects completed the study. At a mean of 19.7 months, there were no differences in reduction quality between the groups. The mean operative time was 30.2 minutes in Group I and 56.4 minutes in Group II ($p < 0.001$). The mean time to bone union was 15.8 weeks in Group I and 17.6 weeks in Group II ($p = 0.002$). The mean AOFAS score was 87.5 points in Group I and 84.3 points in Group II at twelve months after surgery ($p = 0.004$). The mean SMFA dysfunction index was 8.7 points in Group I and 10.5 points in Group II at twelve months after surgery ($p = 0.060$). The mean SMFA bother index averaged 3.3 points in Group I and 4.6 points in Group II at twelve months after surgery ($p = 0.052$). No difference existed between the groups with regard to clinical outcomes for the subjects with an isolated lateral malleolar fracture.

Conclusions.—The outcomes after fixation of bimalleolar ankle fractures with biodegradable implants were inferior to those after fixation with metallic implants in terms of the score on the AOFAS scale and time to bone union. However, the difference in the final AOFAS score between the groups may not be clinically important. The outcomes associated with

TABLE 2.—Clinical Results*

	Group I (N = 53)	Group II (N = 47)	P Value
AOFAS score *(points)*			
3 mo	77.0 ± 6.2	75.0 ± 7.5	0.129
6 mo	85.4 ± 4.5	82.1 ± 7.5	0.009
12 mo	87.5 ± 3.8	84.3 ± 6.6	0.004
SMFA dysfunction index *(points)*			
Baseline	4.0 ± 1.8	4.2 ± 2.5	0.549
3 mo	23.2 ± 8.7	23.4 ± 9.8	0.800
6 mo	13.8 ± 5.6	17.0 ± 6.7	0.012
12 mo	8.7 ± 3.8	10.5 ± 5.3	0.060
SMFA bother index *(points)*			
Baseline	1.1 ± 2.1	1.8 ± 2.4	0.140
3 mo	24.6 ± 8.6	26.7 ± 10.6	0.475
6 mo	12.7 ± 4.8	15.6 ± 4.0	0.015
12 mo	3.3 ± 1.3	4.6 ± 1.5	0.052

AOFAS = American Orthopaedic Foot & Ankle Society, and SMFA = Short Musculoskeletal Function Assessment.
*The values are given as the mean score and the standard deviation. Two patients in Group II who had nonunion were excluded from the analysis.

the use of biodegradable implants for the fixation of isolated lateral malleolar fractures were comparable with those for metallic implants (Table 2).

▶ This well-done prospective randomized controlled trial answers the question of the relative impact of biodegradable implants compared with metal implants for internal fixation of ankle fractures. The development of biodegradable implants is predicated on a perceived lesser need to remove the implants, which is fairly common with metal implants. This study addresses the relatively early (1 year) outcomes for patients with lateral malleolar and bimalleolar fractures. We learn from this study that the times to union are longer for biodegradable implants, but this outcome measure is subject to detection bias. We also learn that the functional outcomes as judged by American Orthopedic Foot & Ankle Society score but not by the Short Musculoskeletal Function Assessment are inferior for the biodegradable implants. I think we can safely conclude that choosing biodegradable implants for ankle fixation are likely not worth the additional expense and that metal implants should likely remain the standard.

M. F. Swiontkowski, MD

Twenty-Two-Year Follow-up of Pronation External Rotation Type III–IV (OTA type C) Ankle Fractures: A Retrospective Cohort Study
Donken CCMA, Verhofstad MHJ, Edwards MJ, et al (Radboud Univ Nijmegen Med Centre, The Netherlands; Saint Elisabeth Hosp, Tilburg, The Netherlands)
J Orthop Trauma 26:e115-e122, 2012

Objective.—Long-term evaluation protocolled treatment of pronation external rotation (PER) type III–IV (OTA type C) ankle fractures.

Design.—Level III retrospective cohort study.

Setting.—Level I trauma center.

Patients.—A consecutive series of 98 patients with PER III–IV ankle fractures between 1985 and 1990.

Intervention.—Stable fractures with tibiotalar congruity were treated conservatively, whereas osteosynthesis was performed in unstable and displaced fractures to restore tibiotalar congruity.

Main Outcome Measurements.—Outcome parameters were (1) functional outcome questionnaire (Olerud score), (2) physical evaluation (loaded dorsal range of motion), (3) functional impairment (*AMA Guides*, 5th ed.), and (4) radiographic evaluation (Cedell score, medial clear space widening, and osteoarthritis).

Results.—After a median of 22 years, follow-up was achieved in 95% ($n = 60$) of living patients. Four patients had a true PER III injury, 5 patients had an unclear injury (between PER III and IV), and 51 patients (85%) sustained a PER IV injury. Excellent or good results were found in 90% of patients (Olerud score). Functional impairment, expressed as percentage of Whole Person Impairment, varied between 0% and 3%. Patients treated operatively and conservatively had statistically equivalent scores.

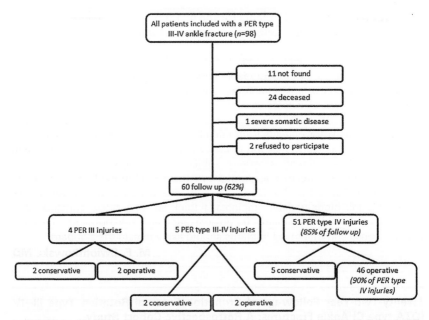

FIGURE 2.—Flowchart of patients at follow-up. (Reprinted from Donken CCMA, Verhofstad MHJ, Edwards MJ, et al. Twenty-two-year follow-up of pronation external rotation type III–IV (OTA type C) ankle fractures: a retrospective cohort study. *J Orthop Trauma*. 2012;26:e115-e122, with permission from Lippincott Williams & Wilkins.)

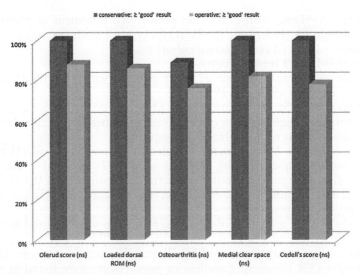

FIGURE 7.—Patients with excellent or good results; conservative treatment compared with operative treatment. (Reprinted from Donken CCMA, Verhofstad MHJ, Edwards MJ, et al. Twenty-two-year follow-up of pronation external rotation type III–IV (OTA type C) ankle fractures: a retrospective cohort study. *J Orthop Trauma*. 2012;26:e115-e122, with permission from Lippincott Williams & Wilkins.)

Conclusions.—The long-term result of surgical treatment of PER ankle fractures is "good" or "excellent" in the majority of patients.

Level of Evidence.—Therapeutic Level IV. See Instructions for Authors for a complete description of levels of evidence (Figs 2 and 7).

▶ This is a long-term (> 20-year) outcome cohort study on patients with pronation external rotation (PER) injuries that accompanies a much larger cohort study from the same institution and investigators reporting on supination external rotation (SER) injuries. As with the SER injuries, the long-term results are good to excellent in more than 90% of patients. The trend for better functional outcomes (not statistically significant) in patients treated nonoperatively is reflective of the judgment of the surgeons making treatment decisions for these patients. Almost certainly, the patients with PER injuries treated conservatively had minimally or nondisplace fractures. This article gives us confidence that we can continue to reassure our patients with these ankle fractures that they have a 90% chance of having a good to excellent long-term functional outcome.

M. F. Swiontkowski, MD

Femur

Spica Casting for Pediatric Femoral Fractures: A Prospective, Randomized Controlled Study of Single-Leg Versus Double-Leg Spica Casts

Leu D, Sargent MC, Ain MC, et al (The Johns Hopkins Univ/Johns Bayview Med Ctr, Baltimore, MD; et al)
J Bone Joint Surg Am 94:1259-1264, 2012

Background.—At many centers, double-leg spica casting is the treatment of choice for diaphyseal femoral fractures in children two to six years old. We hypothesized that such patients can be effectively treated with single-leg spica casting and that such treatment would result in easier care and better patient function during treatment.

Methods.—In a prospective, randomized controlled study, fifty-two patients two to six years old with a diaphyseal femoral fracture were randomly assigned to be treated immediately (after consent was obtained) with a single-leg (twenty-four patients) or double-leg (twenty-eight patients) spica cast. Serial radiographs were evaluated for maintenance of fracture reduction with respect to limb length, varus/valgus angulation, and procurvatum/recurvatum angulation. After cast removal, the performance version of the Activities Scale for Kids questionnaire and a custom-written survey were administered to the parents so that they could evaluate the ease of care and function of the children during treatment. Means were compared between treatment groups with use of Student t tests. P values of <0.05 were considered significant.

Results.—All limbs healed in satisfactory alignment. The children treated with a single-leg spica cast were more likely to fit into car seats ($p < 0.05$) and fit more comfortably into chairs ($p < 0.05$). Caregivers of patients

TABLE 1.—Comparison of Double-Leg and Single-Leg Spica Cast Groups

Parameter	Spica Cast Group*		P Value
	Double-Leg	Single-Leg	
Time in cast* *(days)*	44.15 (29 to 65) [27]	44.5 (−18 to 13) [23]	0.45
Shortening* *(mm)*	13.04 (0 to 26) [27]	13.64 (0 to 27) [23]	0.40
Varus (−)/valgus (+)* *(°)*	−1.46 (−18 to 13) [25]	−2.45 (−16 to 10) [23]	0.29
Procurvatum (+)/recurvatum (−)* *(°)*	6.46 (−3 to 35) [26]	6.74 (−10 to 17) [23]	0.28
Fits in previous car seat[†]	35 [23]	71 [21]	0.01[‡]
Comfort in chair* *(VAS score)*	6.26 (1 to 10) [23]	4.38 (1 to 10) [21]	0.032[‡]
Crawling[†]	57 [23]	52 [21]	0.33
Walking[†]	17 [23]	38 [21]	0.076
Independent movement[†]	7 [23]	6 [21]	0.44
Difficulty leaving residence* *(VAS score)*	6.74 (0 to 10) [23]	5.00 (0 to 10) [21]	0.066
Difficulty keeping child clean* *(VAS score)*	6.04 (2 to 10) [23]	6.05 (2 to 10) [21]	0.42
Difficulty keeping cast clean* *(VAS score)*	6.00 (0 to 10) [23]	6.10 (1 to 10) [21]	0.40
Cast needed trimming[†]	39 [23]	62 [21]	0.23
Time off work by caregiver[†]	79 [19]	52 [21]	0.052
Days off work by caregiver*	19 (0 to 59) [19]	10.38 (0 to 53) [21]	0.049[‡]
ASKp score*[§]	24.56 (8 to 58) [16]	26.15 (5 to 61) [21]	0.39

*The values are given as the mean (range) [total number of patients]. VAS = visual analog scale.
[†]The values are given as the percentage of patients [total number of patients].
[‡]A significant difference.
[§]ASKp denotes Activities Scale for Kids, performance version.

treated with a single-leg cast took less time off work ($p < 0.05$). There were no major complications.

Conclusions.—Treatment of pediatric femoral fractures with a single-leg spica cast is effective and safe, and postfracture patient care is facilitated.

Level of Evidence.—Therapeutic <u>Level I</u>. See Instructions for Authors for a complete description of levels of evidence (Table 1).

▶ This is a well-done randomized, controlled trial comparing single- to double-leg spica casting for children with femoral shaft fractures. The randomized design has resulted in the expected outcome—that the patients in each group were equivalent in terms of injury and other characteristics. The outcomes for fracture care were equivalent with substantive advantages to the single-leg cohort in car seat and general seating function. That parents found the single-leg cast to be more acceptable is no surprise. The orthopedic community desires evidence that the fracture outcomes are not compromised with the more adaptable single-leg cast and this article provides us with that reassurance.

M. F. Swiontkowski, MD

Comparison of Titanium Elastic Nail and Plate Fixation of Pediatric Subtrochanteric Femur Fractures
Li Y, Heyworth BE, Glotzbecker M, et al (Univ of Michigan, Ann Arbor; Children's Hosp Boston, MA)
J Pediatr Orthop 33:232-238, 2013

Background.—Studies have demonstrated a higher risk of complications when children with fractures in the proximal third of the femur and length-unstable fractures are treated with titanium elastic nails. Alternative treatment methods include open plating and submuscular plating. We are not aware of any published studies that directly compare titanium elastic nail and plate fixation of pediatric subtrochanteric femur fractures. The purpose of the present study was to retrospectively compare the outcomes and complications of titanium elastic nail and plate fixation of subtrochanteric femur fractures in children and young adolescents.

Methods.—A total of 54 children aged 5 to 12 years with subtrochanteric femur fractures treated with titanium elastic nails or plating at 2 institutions between 2003 and 2010 were identified. We retrospectively compared 25 children treated with titanium elastic nails to 29 children treated with either open plating or submuscular plating. Similar to previous studies, a fracture that was located within 10% of the total femur length below the lesser trochanter was classified as subtrochanteric. Outcomes were classified as excellent, satisfactory, or poor. A major complication was defined as any complication that led to unplanned surgery. Minor complications were defined as complications that resolved with nonoperative treatment or did not require any treatment.

Results.—Outcome scores were significantly better in the plating group ($P = 0.03$), but both groups demonstrated high rates of excellent and satisfactory results. The overall complication rate was significantly higher in the titanium elastic nails group (48%; 12 of 25) when compared with the plating group (14%; 4 of 29) ($P = 0.008$). Patients in the titanium elastic nails group were advanced to full weightbearing significantly earlier (6.6 vs. 9.9 wk) ($P = 0.005$). The major complication rate, length of hospitalization, and time to radiographic union were similar for the 2 groups.

Conclusions.—Our results indicate that plate fixation of pediatric subtrochanteric femur fractures is associated with better outcome scores and a lower overall complication rate when compared with titanium elastic nails.

Level of Evidence.—Therapeutic Level III (Tables 3 and 4).

▶ Femoral shaft fractures in children are fairly common but more proximal shaft fractures in the subtrochanteric region comprise less than 15% of the total femoral shaft fractures. This is a multicenter comparative cohort study that confirms that subcutaneous plating has better clinical and radiographic outcomes than flexible nailing (Tables 3 and 4). This is likely strongly related to the shorter working length of these nails in more proximal fractures with lower deforming force than midshaft fractures. Although this is not a prospective randomized controlled

TABLE 3.—Outcome Scores

	n (%)		
	Excellent Result	Satisfactory Result	Poor Result
Titanium elastic nails results in the present study*	13 (52)	10 (40)	2 (8)
Plating results in the present study*	25 (87)	3 (10)	1 (3)

*A patient's overall outcome was determined by the category with the worst result.

TABLE 4.—Complications

	Titanium Elastic Nails Group	Plating Group	P
Fracture malalignment	4	1	
Leg-length inequality	4	3	
Affected limb long	2	3	
Affected limb short	1	0	
Unknown	1	0	
Pain from prominent implants	3	0	
Knee stiffness	1	0	
Cellulitis at insertion site	1	0	
Saphenous nerve paresthesias	1	0	
Skin maceration from cast	1	0	
Total no. patients with complications [n (%)]	12* (48)	4 (14)	0.008

*Three patients had >1 complication.

trial and there is likely some selection and detection bias in play, the results seem strong enough to guide clinical decision making until better data are available.

M. F. Swiontkowski, MD

Nonisthmal femoral shaft nonunion as a risk factor for exchange nailing failure

Yang KH, Kim JR, Park J (Yonsei Univ, Seoul, Republic of Korea; Chonbuk Natl Univ, Jeonju, Republic of Korea)

J Trauma Acute Care Surg 72:E60-E64, 2012

Background.—Although nail exchange with a larger diameter nail after additional reaming is typically considered the gold standard for failed femoral nailing, some reports question the role of exchange nailing. The purpose of this study was to evaluate the risk factors affecting the outcome of exchange nailing for femoral shaft nonunion after initial nailing.

Methods.—Forty-one consecutive patients treated with exchange nailing between November 1996 and March 2010 for femoral shaft nonunion that was initially managed with an intramedullary nailing were retrospectively reviewed. Possible risk factors and outcome (bony union) of exchange nailing were evaluated.

Results.—Of the 41 femoral shaft nonunions treated with exchange nailing, 9 (22%) failed to achieve bony union. The union rate for isthmal nonunions was 87% (27 of 31 cases) and for nonisthmal nonunions was 50% (5 of 10 cases). Univariate and multivariate logistic regression analyses demonstrated that the anatomic site (isthmal vs. nonisthmal) was a significant risk factor for exchange nailing failure (univariate, $p = 0.021$; multivariate, $p = 0.016$).

Conclusions.—Although exchange nailing is an excellent choice for aseptic isthmal femoral shaft nonunion occurring after the initial nailing,

TABLE 2.—Univariate and Multivariate Logistic Regression Analyses to Identify the Risk Factors Affecting the Results of Exchange Nailing

Risk Factor	Univariate Analysis			Multivariate Analysis		
	Odds Ratio	95% Confidence Interval	P	Odds Ratio	95% Confidence Interval	p
Injury type (low vs. high)	0.23	0.03−2.00	0.180	NA	NA	NA
Fracture type (closed vs. open)	0.54	0.06−5.19	0.595	NA	NA	NA
Comminution grade (low vs. high)	2.76	0.39−19.81	0.312	NA	NA	NA
Initial nailing method (closed vs. open)	2.86	0.60−13.59	0.187	NA	NA	NA
Interlocking mode (dynamic vs. static)	1.37	0.24−7.88	0.725	NA	NA	NA
Nonunion type (hypertrophic vs. atrophic)	2.86	0.60−13.59	0.187	NA	NA	NA
Nonunion site (isthmal vs. nonisthmal)	**6.75**	**1.33−34.27**	**0.021**	**16.83**	**1.71−166.05**	**0.016**
Smoking (nonsmoker vs. smoker)	3.33	0.70−15.86	0.130	9.24	0.95−89.76	0.055
Severity (simple vs. recalcitrant)	0.45	0.05−4.20	0.481	NA	NA	NA
Over-reaming size (1 mm vs. at least 2 mm)	1.23	0.20−7.53	0.817	NA	NA	NA

NA, not applicable.
Significant results ($p < 0.05$) are marked in bold.

other treatment options such as augmentative plating should be considered for nonisthmal femoral shaft nonunions (Table 2).

▶ This cohort study of femoral nonunions emphasizes the location of the nonunion in regard to where it is in relation to the narrow portion of the femoral canal (the isthmus). Exchange nailing for isthmal nonunion is far more successful than in nonunions, where there is not a tight fit of the larger nail against the endosteal surface of the femur above and below the nonunion site. With a differential success rate of 87% for isthmal nonunions versus 50% for pre- or post-isthmal nonunions, the recommendation should be for surgeons to consider plate fixation in the pre- or post-isthmal femoral nonunion with a nail in place.

M. F. Swiontkowski, MD

Comparison of the 95-Degree Angled Blade Plate and the Locking Condylar Plate for the Treatment of Distal Femoral Fractures

Vallier HA, Immler W (Case Western Reserve Univ, Cleveland, OH)
J Orthop Trauma 26:327-333, 2012

Objectives.—In the distal femur, locked plating is efficacious when coronal fractures preclude the use of a conventional fixed-angle device. However, minimal comparative data exist for supracondylar fracture patterns, which could be treated with other devices. The purpose of this study was to compare the 95-degree angled blade plate (ABP) versus the

Locking Condylar Plate (LCP) by assessing complications and secondary procedures in fractures amenable to treatment with either implant.

Design.—Retrospective review.

Setting.—Level 1 trauma center.

Patients/Participants.—Seventy patients with 71 distal femoral fractures (OTA 33-A, 33-C1, 33-C2) amenable to either ABP or LCP with a mean age of 59.5 years (range, 20–92 years) were included. Seventeen fractures (24%) occurred adjacent to a previous knee arthroplasty (10 ABP and 7 LCP). The 2 groups were similar with respect to age, fracture pattern, and the presence of open fracture. Most injuries were the result of high-energy trauma, and 21% were open fractures.

Intervention.—Thirty-two fractures (45%) were treated with an ABP, and 39 (55%) were treated with the LCP.

Main Outcome Measures.—Complications, including infection, nonunion, and malunion, and secondary operations were determined.

Results.—After a mean of 26-month follow-up, 4 patients (6.0%) were treated for infections. Malunions occurred in 11% of LCP patients and in 1 ABP patient (3.4%, $P = 0.14$). All patients with malunions were older than 55 years. Seven patients (11%) were treated for nonunions. Six of the nonunions occurred after LCP (16% vs. 3.4%, $P = 0.11$) Complications were more frequent in LCP patients (35%) versus ABP patients (10%, $P = 0.001$). Complications were not related to fracture pattern, periprosthetic fracture, or open fracture. Mean age of patients with complications was 64 years (vs. 53 years, $P = 0.01$), and they were more likely to have lower energy mechanisms ($P = 0.017$). Overall, 18 patients (27%) underwent secondary procedures, including treatment of infection, nonunion, malunion, or prominent implant removal. Secondary procedures were more common after LCP (43%) versus ABP (6.9%, $P = 0.0008$) patients. Painful prominent implants were removed from 7 LCP patients (18%) and no ABP patients ($P = 0.01$).

Conclusions.—Distal femur fractures are often associated with prolonged healing and rehabilitation times, which increase substantially when complications occur. Internal fixation of these fractures may be performed successfully with ABP or LCP. In our review of fractures that could be treated with either implant, patients treated with locking plates had more complications and nonunions, requiring more secondary procedures to treat complications and to remove prominent implants. Furthermore, locking plates are substantially more expensive than conventional fixed-angle devices. Future investigation is needed in the form of a large randomized prospective study to clearly define clinical differences, functional outcomes, and costs of care.

Level of Evidence.—Therapeutic Level III. See Instructions for Authors for a complete description of levels of evidence (Tables 1 and 3).

▶ This is an interesting retrospective comparative cohort study comparing the use of 2 implants for the internal fixation of distal femur fractures. The 95° condylar blade plate is generally considered to be more difficult to use because

TABLE 1.—Demographic Information

	ABP (n = 32 Fractures)	LCP (n = 39 Fractures)	Total (n = 71 Fractures)	P
Male	7	20	27	0.008
Female	25	18	43	
Mean age (y)	60.6	58.6	55.5	0.79
Mechanism of injury				
Low energy (fall)	9	7	16	0.15
High energy:	23	31	54	0.23
MVC	10	14	24	0.34
MCA	1	7	8	0.02
Fall from height	9	6	15	0.09
GSW	2	2	4	0.42
Industrial	1	2	3	0.34
Open fracture	6	9	15	0.32
Closed fracture	26	30	56	
Fracture pattern*				
33-A (1-3)	21	20	41	0.16
33-A1	8	7	15	0.23
33-A2	6	5	11	0.25
33-A3	7	8	15	0.44
33-C (1-2)	11	19	30	
33-C1	3	8	11	0.10
33-C2	8	11	19	0.38
Periprosthetic fracture	10	7	17	0.10

Editor's Note: Please refer to original journal article for full references.
Thirty-two patients with 32 fractures were treated with an ABP, and 38 patients with 39 fractures were treated with a locking plate (LCP).
GSW, gunshot wound; MCA, motorcycle accident; MVC, motor vehicle collision.
*Fracture pattern as classified by the OTA.[25]

TABLE 3.—Characteristics of Patients Who Developed Complications Including Infection, Malunion, and Nonunion

	ABP (n = 3)	LCP (n = 13)	Total (n = 16)
Mean age (y)	60.3 (58−63)	64.7 (47−83)	63.9 (47−83)
Gender			
Female	3	11	14 (88%)
Male	0	2	2 (12%)
Mechanism			
Low energy	2	4	6 (38%)
High energy	1	9	10 (62%)
Fracture pattern			
33-A	1*	10*	11 (69%)
33-C	2*	3	5 (31%)
Open fracture	0	1	1 (6.3%)
Periprosthetic fracture	2	1	3 (19%)

*One patient in each of these groups had sustained a periprosthetic fracture.

the insertion of the blade has to be correct in all 3 planes, as it is a fixed angle implant. The fact of the matter is that the locking condylar buttress plate is also fixed angle. Although it can appear to be easier to insert, misapplication is very common, and this series proves that point. I think the findings of this cohort study could be interpreted as more experienced surgeons use the condylar blade plate with excellent results and the locking condylar buttress plate is not as easy to insert as it appears. Both implants require intimate knowledge of the principles of accurate insertion and a compulsive pursuit of accuracy in the operating room application.

M. F. Swiontkowski, MD

General Topics

Routine pin tract care in external fixation is unnecessary: A randomised, prospective, blinded controlled study

Camathias C, Valderrabano V, Oberli H (Univ Childrens Hosp Basel, Switzerland; Univ Hosp Basel, Switzerland; Natl Referral Hosp, Muntelier, Switzerland)
Injury 43:1969-1973, 2012

Introduction.—Pin site infections are seen in up to 40% of external fixators (ExFix) and are therefore the most common complication with this device. There is no consensus in the literature as to the appropriate regimen for pin tract care and infection prevention.

This study is the first intra-subject, randomised, prospective controlled trial comparing daily pin tract care to no pin tract care at all.

Method.—Consecutive patients series (56 patients, 16 female, age 4–68y, mean 24y, in total 204 pins) recruited in the National Referral Hospital in Honiara in the Solomon Islands over a 2 year period. Exclusion criteria were application of ExFix for less than two weeks or a non-standard ExFix.

Pin treatment was allocated into groups anatomically, proximal and distal. Randomisation was intra-subject and intra-group: 101 pins had daily pin site care and 103 had no treatment at all.

Endpoints.—Soft-tissue interface, stability of the pins, torsional stability as determined with a torque metre, osteolysis and pain. Assessment of pin sites blinded. Statistical analysis using the paired t test for parametric data and the Wilcoxon rank test for non-parametric data (Stat View).

Results.—No significant difference between the two groups. Soft-tissue interface 36% vs. 35% (granulation/secretion), stability 20 vs 25 pins with loosening. No significant osteolysis (7 vs. 6 pins). Torque: mean 0.75 Nm, max.: 3.05 Nm vs. 0.60 Nm, max.: 3.55 Nm, no significant difference. No differences in demographics (age, localisation, sex, time of fixation).

Conclusion.—This study shows that routine pin tract care is unnecessary in external fixation treatment of injuries (Figs 1 and 5).

▶ Debate regarding optimum pin care in patients with external fixation has been ongoing for the past 50 years. Few randomized trials have been conducted to address the issue. Opinions range from no specialized care, to peroxide, to saline/peroxide mixture or saline alone, dressings around the pin (or not), and the use of antibacterial topical applications. This is a very well-designed randomized control trial comparing no specialized treatment with active pin care. The

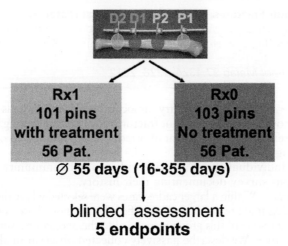

FIGURE 1.—Study design with randomisation and blinding. (Reprinted from the Injury, International Journal of the Care of the Injured. Camathias C, Valderrabano V, Oberli H. Routine pin tract care in external fixation is unnecessary: a randomised, prospective, blinded controlled study. *Injury.* 2012;43:1969-1973, Copyright 2012, with permission from Elsevier.)

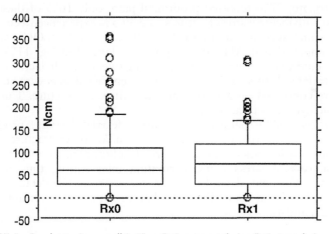

FIGURE 5.—Boxplot torsion overall in Ncm. Rx0: not treated pins, Rx1: treated pins. (Reprinted from the Injury, International Journal of the Care of the Injured. Camathias C, Valderrabano V, Oberli H. Routine pin tract care in external fixation is unnecessary: a randomised, prospective, blinded controlled study. *Injury.* 2012;43:1969-1973, Copyright 2012, with permission from Elsevier.)

design is appropriately complex (Fig 1) to account for all relevant variables. The outcomes of pin loosening to removal torque force all confirm that there is no advantage to active pin care over no specialized care.

This "noncare" should become the treatment standard for most situations in which external fixation is used.

M. F. Swiontkowski, MD

Atypical Femur Fractures: 81 Individual Personal Histories

Schneider JP, Hinshaw WB, Su C, et al (Arizona Community Physicians, Tucson; Harris Regional Hosp, Sylva, NC; IBM Global Services, Armonk, NY; et al)

J Clin Endocrinol Metab 97:4324-4328, 2012

Context.—An online voluntary association of individuals who had incurred one or more atypical femur fractures (AFFs) while taking bisphosphonates for prevention or treatment of osteoporosis provided an opportunity to collect long-term histories.

Setting.—Individuals from a nationwide general community completed an anonymous survey documenting their history.

Participants.—Within a larger cadre, cases were selected where the documentation, including fracture radiographs, verified the diagnosis based on published standards. Eighty-one of this group responded to the anonymous survey.

Interventions.—We describe passively collected observational data only.

Outcome Measures.—The incidence of a large number of potential variations was determined.

Results.—The mean duration of bisphosphonate treatment was 9.5 yr. Prevention was the initial indication in 68% of the subjects; 94% started on alendronate, 77% reported prodromal pain, only 16% of these were diagnosed with incident stress fractures, and 39.5% experienced a contralateral AFF from less than 1 month to 49 months after the first. Of 71 subjects with a completed first AFF, 38% reported delayed healing, 11% had a complete contralateral AFF, and 22% underwent prophylactic rodding for a contralateral stress AFF. Forty-four percent of subjects with complete AFFs were continued on a bisphosphonate after the fracture. Thirty-five percent incurred a metatarsal fracture.

Conclusions.—AFF patients experienced delayed healing, prodromal pain, and persisting risk of a contralateral and/or other fracture. Femur pain evaluation in patients on long-term bisphosphonates may facilitate early diagnosis of stress AFFs, permitting intervention, thus reducing completed and/or contralateral or other fracture risk. The details of these histories will assist in counseling regarding prognosis after an initial AFF (Tables 1, 2, and 4).

▶ In our collective ongoing attempt to gain greater insight into the risks of atypical femur fractures after bisphosphonate use, this group of investigators takes an interesting and unique approach using web-based social media. This is a convenience sample of responders to an invitation to participate in a survey. As with any convenience sample, the respondents may be different from the overall population of patients with atypical femur fractures. Important take-home messages from these data are the duration of therapy at more than 9 years and the incidence of bilateral fractures. The duration would support the current recommendation of a 1- to 2-year drug holiday after 5 to 7 years on therapy. The data do not confirm whether this strategy will decrease the incidence of these fractures, however. The fact that nearly 40% of patients sustain a contralateral fracture

TABLE 1.—Patient Demographics

Gender	78 Women, 3 Men
Median age (n = 71) at initially diagnosed complete fracture	64 yr (range, 43.5–82)
Median age (n = 10) at initially diagnosed stress fracture	68 yr (range, 57–89)
Median age (n = 81) at the time of survey closure mid-2011	67 yr (range, 53–92)
Ever a smoker	2.5% (2/81)
Regular prednisone (or equivalent) use	7.4% (6/81)
Estrogen replacement therapy	47% (37/78)
Reported physical activity level before fracture	
Low	3.7%
Average	34.6%
Somewhat greater than average	30.7%
Much greater than average	21.0%

TABLE 2.—BP Use

Duration of BP use before initially diagnosed complete AFF (n = 71)	9.15 yr (range, 1.5–15)
Duration of BP use before initially diagnosed stress AFF (n = 10)	9.10 yr (range, 6–12)
BP initially prescribed for prevention based on a diagnosis of osteopenia	68% (53/78)
Alendronate (Fosamax) initially prescribed	94% (76/81)
Risedronate (Actonel) initially prescribed	5% (4/81)
Zoledronic acid initially prescribed for bone loss, not metastatic disease	1
Respondents prescribed 2 BPs	27
Respondents prescribed 3 BPs	3
Initial alendronate dose prescribed for prevention was 10 mg/d or 70 mg/wk	66% (50/76))
Continued on BP after initially diagnosed complete AFF	44% (31/71)
Still on BP at time of contralateral stress fracture or AFF	34% (11/32)
Continued BP after bilateral complete AFF	2

TABLE 4.—Atypical Fracture Outcome

Delayed union of first complete fracture (see *Results*)	38% (27/71)
Portion with delayed union requiring additional surgery to promote union	63% (17/27)
Portion of initial complete fractures followed by a complete contralateral fracture	13% (9/71)
Portion of initial complete fractures having contralateral prophylactic rodding	25% (18/71)
Portion of all 81 patients who underwent surgery on both femurs	33% (27/81)
Portion of 10 initial unilateral stress fractures subsequently having bilateral stress fractures	50% (5/10)
Initial rodded stress fracture followed by rodding of a contralateral stress fracture	40% (4/10)
Portion of all initially diagnosed fractures who stopped BP by that time or within 3 months and later incurred a second femoral fracture	35.5% (22/62)
Portion of all initially diagnosed fractures who did not stop BP and later incurred a second femoral fracture	52.6% (10/19)
Metatarsal fracture occurred during or after BP treatment	34.6% (28/81)
Stress or complete fracture of a bone in the pelvis (n = 2)	2.5%
Osteonecrosis of the jaw (n = 3)	3.7%

should encourage us to follow these patients closely and to consider advanced imaging such as bone scans or magnetic resonance imaging with any contralateral symptoms. Additionally, that 77% reported prodromal pain should raise awareness among all physicians to evaluate patients on bisphosphonate therapy with imaging at the earliest sign of thigh or hip pain. Finally, the high rate of delayed healing adds further data to the growing body of literature on treatment of these fractures. Treatment of teriparatide should be considered at the earliest indication of delayed healing.

M. F. Swiontkowski, MD

The Effects of Clopidogrel (Plavix) and Other Oral Anticoagulants on Early Hip Fracture Surgery

Collinge CA, Kelly KC, Little B, et al (Harris Methodist Fort Worth Hosp/John Peter Smith Orthopedic Surgery Residency, TX; Dallas Veterans Affairs Med Ctr, TX; Tarleton State Univ, Stephenville, TX; et al)
J Orthop Trauma 26:568-573, 2012

Objective.—Risk for bleeding complications during and after early hip fracture surgery for patients taking clopidogrel and other anticoagulants have not been defined. The purpose of this study is to assess the perioperative bleeding risks and clinical outcome after early hip fracture surgery performed on patients taking clopidogrel (Plavix) and other oral anticoagulants.

Design.—Study design is a retrospective cohort analysis using data extracted from hospital records and state death records.

Setting.—Regional medical center (level II trauma).

Methods.—Data for 1118 patients ≥60 years of age who had surgical treatment for a hip fracture between 2004 and 2008 were reviewed. Eighty-two patients undergoing late surgery (>3 days after admission) were excluded. Patients taking clopidogrel were compared against those not taking clopidogrel. In addition, patients taking clopidogrel only were compared against cohorts of patients taking both clopidogrel and aspirin, aspirin only, warfarin only, or no anticoagulant.

Results.—Seventy-four of 1036 patients (7%) were taking clopidogrel, although control groups included 253 patients on aspirin alone, 90 patients on warfarin, and 619 taking no anticoagulants. No significant differences were noted between patients taking clopidogrel and those not taking clopidogrel in estimated blood loss, transfusion requirement, final blood count, hematoma evacuation, hospital length of stay (LOS), or mortality while in hospital or at 1 year. A higher American Society of Anesthesiologists score was seen in the clopidogrel and warfarin groups ($P = 0.05$ each), increased LOS in the clopidogrel group ($P = 0.05$), and higher rate of deep vein thrombosis seen in those patients taking warfarin ($P = 0.05$). Clopidogrel only versus aspirin versus both aspirin and clopidogrel, versus no anticoagulant versus warfarin showed no significant differences in estimated blood loss, transfusion requirement, final blood count, bleeding or perioperative complications, or mortality.

Conclusions.—Patients undergoing early hip fracture surgery who are taking clopidogrel, aspirin, or warfarin (with regulated international normalized ratio) are not at substantially increased risk for bleeding, bleeding complications, or mortality. Comorbidities and American Society of Anesthesiologists scores were significantly higher in the clopidogrel

TABLE 1.—Baseline Patient and Injury Characteristics

	Clopidogrel (n=74)	No Anticoagulant (n=619)	P	Aspirin Only (n=253)	P	Warfarin (n=90)	P
Average age (yrs)	78.9 ± 8.1	80.8 ± 8.8	0.20	81.2 ± 8.7	0.20	81.4 ± 7.7	0.99
% Female	68.9	72.1%	0.67	70%	0.98	70	0.98
ASA*	3.4 ± 0.6	3.1 ± 0.6	0.05	3.2 ± 0.6	0.05	3.4 ± 0.5	0.99
Admission Hgb*	12.1 ± 1.9	12.2 ± 2.5	0.80	12.1 ± 1.7	0.93	12.3 ± 1.7	0.33
Fracture type (%)							
Neck	36 (48.4%)	303 (48.9%)	0.93	119 (47%)	—	48 (53.3)	—
Inter/pertrochanteric	34 (44.6%)	275 (44.3%)		119 (47%)	0.94	37 (40.0)	0.83
Subtrochanteric	4 (5.4%)	41 (6.6%)	—	15 (5.9%)	—	5 (5.6)	—
Repair %	54.1	60.1	0.38	61.3	0.33	48.9	0.66
Replacement %	45.9	39.9	—	38.7	—	51.1	—
Average time to operating room (days)*[a]	1.66 + 1.0	1.55 + 0.9	0.39	1.52 + 1.0	0.33	1.88 + 1.0	0.22
Average procedure time (min)[a]*	63.5 ± 30.9	59.2 ± 37.0	0.90	57.6 ± 28.2	0.90	71.6 ± 41.4	0.30

Repair defined as sliding hip screw or intramedullary nail; replacement defined as hemiarthroplasty or total joint replacement.
Bonferroni correction for multiple comparisons.
Hgb, hemoglobin.
*Results reported as mean ± standard deviation.

TABLE 2.—Clinical Outcomes, Bleeding, and Mortality Data

	Clopidogrel* (n = 74)	No Anticoagulants (n = 619)	P	Aspirin Only (n = 253)	P	Warfarin (n = 90)	P
Average EBL (cc)	165.6 ± 135	138.6 ± 125.9	0.63	144.3 ± 133.6	0.50	184.2 ± 206	0.86
Hematoma requiring evacuation (%)	2 (2.7%)	13 (1.5%)	0.93	3 (1.2%)	0.69	1 (1.1%)	0.86
DVT (%)	0	10 (1.1%)	0.56	1 (0.4%)	0.51	7 (7.8%)	0.05
Pulmonary embolus (%)	0	2	0.49	0	0.99	0	0.99
Average units of blood transfused	1.7 ± 1.9 (0–8)	1.5 ± 2.1 (0–37)	0.90	1.4 ± 1.7	0.50	1.6 ± 2.9	0.90
Required blood transfusion (%)	62.2%	54.5%	0.26	55.3%	0.36	55.6%	0.49
Average final hospital Hgb	10.1 ± 1.1	10.2 + 1.2	0.39	10.0 ± 1.1	0.36	10.2 ± 1.2	0.90
Average postoperative LOS	6.4 ± 4.1 (2–20)	5.5 ± 3.6 (0–50)	0.05	5.2 ± 2.6	0.05	6.6 ± 4.2 (2–23)	0.50
In-hospital mortality (%)	1 (1.4)	12 (1.4%)	0.92	4 (1.6%)	0.69	1 (1.1%)	0.57
Mortality <30 days (%)	8 (10.8%)	35 (4.0%)	0.14	11 (4.3%)	0.07	7 (7.8)	0.69
Mortality <1 year (%)	21 (28.4%)	162 (18.6%)	0.79	50 (19.8%)	0.16	18 (20.0)	0.29

Bonferroni correction for multiple comparisons.
*Comparison/reference group.

TABLE 4.—Clinical Outcomes, Bleeding, and Mortality Data: Clopidogrel Subgroup Analysis

	Clopidogrel Only (n = 40)	No Anticoagulants (n = 619)	P	Clopidogrel and Aspirin (n = 34)	P
EBL (cc)	147.1 ± 92.8	135.9 ± 122.6	0.54	190 ± 172.9	0.58
Hematoma requiring evacuation (%)	0	10 (1.6%)	0.89	1 (2.9%)	0.78
DVT (%)	0	9 (1.5%)	0.95	0	0.99
Pulmonary embolus (%)	0	2 (0.3%)	0.26	0	0.99
Units of blood transfused	1.4 ± 1.7	1.5 ± 2.3	0.50	2.0 ± 2.1	0.74
Required blood transfusion (%)	55.0	55.3	0.89	69.7	0.17
Final hospital Hgb	10.1 ± 1.2	10.2 ± 1.2	0.52	10.1 ± 1.0	0.99
Postoperative LOS	6.0 ± 3.4	5.6 ± 4.0	0.61	6.6 ± 4.8	0.75
In hospital mortality (%)	0 (0.0%)	8 (1.3%)	0.98	1 (2.9%)	0.78
Mortality <30 days (%)	3 (17.5%)	39 (6.3%)	0.23	1 (2.9%)	0.13
Mortality <1 year (%)	10 (25.0%)	117 (18.9%)	0.46	7 (23.6%)	0.82

group, which may have resulted in the increased postoperative LOS in this group (Tables 1, 2, and 4).

▶ The use of clopidogrel and aspirin is widespread in patients with ischemic heart disease, particularly in whom stents have been inserted. The clinical situation of timing for patients with hip fracture who are on these medications is very common. This is a very well-conducted, retrospective cohort study where appropriate statistical analyses have been conducted. The outcomes of interest were in terms of transfusion, deep vein thrombosis, death, and estimated blood loss. Patients on warfarin and those with clopidogrel alone as well as clopidogrel plus aspirin were analyzed separately. The conclusion that these medications should not produce a decision to delay surgery seems well founded.

M. F. Swiontkowski, MD

PCR-hybridization after sonication improves diagnosis of implant-related infection

Esteban J, Alonso-Rodriguez N, del-Prado G, et al (IIS-Fundacion Jimenez Diaz, Madrid, Spain; et al)
Acta Orthop 83:299-304, 2012

Purpose.—We wanted to improve the diagnosis of implant-related infection using molecular biological techniques after sonication.

Methods.—We studied 258 retrieved implant components (185 prosthetic implants and 73 osteosynthesis implants) from 126 patients. 47

TABLE 3.—Comparison of Results From PCR and Culture

		PCR		Culture	
	Total no. of Samples	+	−	+	−
Clinical infection					
Yes	109	78	31	67	42
No	149	27	122	10	139
Culture					
Positive	77	59	18		
Negative	181	46	135		

TABLE 4.—Results Obtained From Arthroplasty and Fracture Patients in this Series

		Culture		PCR	
Patients With Retrieved Implants	Total no. of Cases	+	−	+	−
All arthroplasty patients under study	75	29	46	40	35
All fracture (nailing and/or osteosynthesis) patients under study	51	16	35	16	35
All patients	126	45	81	56	70

patients had a clinical diagnosis of infection (108 components) and 79 patients did not (150 components). The fluids from sonication of retrieved implants were tested in culture and were also analyzed using a modified commercial PCR kit for detection of Gram-positive and Gram-negative bacteria (GenoType BC; Hain Lifescience) after extraction of the DNA.

Results.—38 of 47 patients with a clinical diagnosis of infection were also diagnosed as being infected using culture and/or PCR (35 by culture alone). Also, 24 patients of the 79 cases with no clinical diagnosis of infection were identified microbiologically as being infected (4 by culture, 16 by PCR, and 4 by both culture and PCR). Comparing culture and PCR, positive culture results were obtained in 28 of the 79 patients and positive PCR results were obtained in 35. There were 21 discordant results in patients who were originally clinically diagnosed as being infected and 28 discordant results in patients who had no clinical diagnosis of infection.

Interpretation.—For prosthetic joint infections and relative to culture, molecular detection can increase (by one tenth) the number of patients diagnosed as having an infection. Positive results from patients who have no clinical diagnosis of infection must be interpreted carefully (Tables 3-5).

▶ Infection following internal fixation of fractures can be difficult to diagnose. Furthermore, differentiation of colonization from infection-producing symptoms or clinical problems can be even more difficult. Molecular biologic techniques are being more widely used in academic centers to diagnose implant-related infection, particularly related to joint replacement. This well-done cohort study confirms that investment in these systems may not be all that helpful in identifying prosthetic-related infection as it relates to internal fixation and, therefore, unlikely to be used in most community settings. Nevertheless, research should continue in attempts to improve the diagnostic techniques, particularly surrounding the issue

TABLE 5.—Results Obtained From Patients With or Without Clinical Diagnosis of Infection in Our Series

Patients With Retrieved Implants	Total no. of Cases	Culture +	Culture −	PCR +	PCR −
Arthroplasty cases with clinical infection	31	24	7	26	5
Arthroplasty cases without clinical infection	44	5	39	14	30
Fracture cases with clinical infection	16	12	4	8	8
Fracture cases without clinical infection	35	4	31	8	27
Patients with clinical diagnosis of infection	47	36	11	34	13
Patients without clinical diagnosis of infection	79	9	70	22	57

in which nonunion of fracture may be in part related to difficult-to-diagnose infection or colonization of the implant.

M. F. Swiontkowski, MD

Early Initiation of Bisphosphonate Does Not Affect Healing and Outcomes of Volar Plate Fixation of Osteoporotic Distal Radial Fractures
Gong HS, Song CH, Lee YH, et al (Seoul Natl Univ Bundang Hosp, Seongnam, South Korea)
J Bone Joint Surg Am 94:1729-1736, 2012

Background.—Bisphosphonates can adversely affect fracture-healing because they inhibit osteoclastic bone resorption. It is unclear whether bisphosphonates can be initiated safely for patients who have sustained an acute distal radial fracture. The purpose of this randomized study was to determine whether the early use of bisphosphonate affects healing and outcomes of osteoporotic distal radial fractures treated with volar locking plate fixation.

Methods.—Fifty women older than fifty years of age who had undergone volar locking plate fixation of a distal radial fracture and had been diagnosed with osteoporosis were randomized to Group I (n = 24, initiation of bisphosphonate treatment at two weeks after the operation) or Group II (n = 26, initiation of bisphosphonate treatment at three months). Patients were assessed for radiographic union and other radiographic parameters (radial inclination, radial length, and volar tilt) at two, six, ten, sixteen, and twenty-four weeks, and for clinical outcomes that included Disabilities of the Arm, Shoulder and Hand (DASH) scores, wrist motion, and grip strength at twenty-four weeks. The two groups were compared with regard to the time to radiographic union, the radiographic parameters, and the clinical outcomes.

Results.—No significant differences were observed between the two groups with respect to radiographic or clinical outcomes after volar locking plate fixation. All patients obtained fracture union, and the mean times to radiographic union in Groups I and II were similar (6.7 and 6.8 weeks, respectively; $p = 0.65$). Furthermore, the time to radiographic union was not related to osteoporosis severity or fracture type.

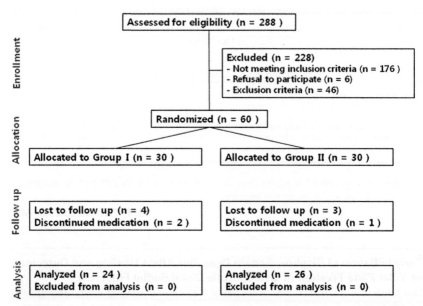

FIGURE 1.—A CONSORT flow diagram for enrollment and analysis. Group I had initiation of bisphosphonate medication at two weeks postoperatively, and Group II had initiation of bisphosphonate medication at three months postoperatively. (Reprinted from Gong HS, Song CH, Lee YH, et al. Early initiation of bisphosphonate does not affect healing and outcomes of volar plate fixation of osteoporotic distal radial fractures. *J Bone Joint Surg Am.* 2012;94:1729-1736, with permission from The Journal of Bone and Joint Surgery, Incorporated.)

TABLE 1.—Radiographic and Clinical Outcomes at Twenty-four Weeks Postoperatively

	Group I (Started Bisphosphonates at 2 Weeks)* (N = 24)	Group II (Started Bisphosphonates at 3 Months)* (N = 26)	P Value
Time to radiographic healing	6.7 ± 1.5	6.8 ± 1.6	0.650
Proportion with healing at 6 weeks	20/24	20/26	0.814
Radiographic parameters			
Radial inclination *(deg)*	20 ± 2	19 ± 2	0.211
Radial length *(mm)*	10 ± 2	10 ± 2	0.883
Volar tilt *(deg)*	5 ± 4	6 ± 3	0.365
DASH scores *(points)*	17 ± 14 (range, 0-46)	15 ± 14 (range, 0-45)	0.610
Wrist ranges of motion *(deg)*			
Flexion	50 ± 10	51 ± 14	0.784
Extension	64 ± 10	66 ± 10	0.532
Supination	74 ± 13	77 ± 9	0.316
Pronation	66 ± 12	65 ± 12	0.937
Grip strength *(kg)*	13.6 ± 5.3	13.8 ± 5.4	0.885

*The values are given as the mean and standard deviation, except for the proportion with healing at six weeks.

Conclusions.—In patients with an osteoporotic distal radial fracture treated with volar locking plate fixation, the early initiation of bisphosphonate treatment did not affect fracture-healing or clinical outcomes.

Level of Evidence.—Therapeutic Level I. See Instructions for Authors for a complete description of levels of evidence (Fig 1, Table 1).

▶ This relatively well-done randomized clinical trial examines early versus delayed institution of bisphosphonate therapy for patients undergoing volar locking plate fixation of distal radius fractures. It is a relatively small number of patients, but with these results it is apparent that if there is an impact of bisphosphonate therapy on clinical or functional outcomes in these patients, it must be very small indeed. A fragility fracture is the biggest predictor of the next fracture, and the orthopedic community needs to take the lead in the diagnosis and appropriate care of patients with confirmed osteoporosis. With another study of similar design in patients with intertrochanteric fractures treated with internal fixation, we can safely conclude that early treatment of patients with fragility fractures does not negatively impact clinical or functional outcomes.

M. F. Swiontkowski, MD

Hip Fracture

Incidence of subsequent hip fractures is significantly increased within the first month after distal radius fracture in patients older than 60 years
Chen C-W, Huang T-L, Su L-T, et al (China Med Univ Hosp, Taichung, Taiwan)
J Trauma Acute Care Surg 74:317-321, 2013

Background.—Distal radius fracture is recognized as an osteoporosis-related fracture in aged population. If another osteoporosis-related fracture occurs in a short period, it represents a prolonged hospitalization and a considerable economic burden to the society. We evaluated the relationship between distal radius fracture and subsequent hip fracture within 1 year, especially in the critical time and age.

Methods.—We identified newly diagnosed distal radius fracture patients in 2000 to 2006 as an exposed cohort (N = 9,986). A comparison cohort (N = 81,227) was randomly selected from patients without distal radius fracture in the same year of exposed cohort. The subjects were followed up for 1 year since the recruited date. We compared the sociodemographic factors between two cohorts. Furthermore, the time interval following the previous distal radial fracture and the incidence of subsequent hip fracture was studied in detail.

Results.—The incidence of hip fracture within 1 year increased with age in both cohorts. The risk was 5.67 times (84.6 vs. 14.9 per 10,000 person-years) greater in the distal radial fracture cohort than in the comparison cohort. The multivariate Cox proportional hazard regression analyses showed the hazard ratios of hip fracture in relation to distal radial fracture was 3.45 (95% confidence interval = 2.59—4.61). The highest incidence was within the first month after distal radial fracture, 17-fold higher than the comparison cohort (17.9 vs. 1.05 per 10,000). Among comorbidities,

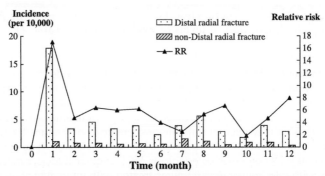

FIGURE 2.—Incidence rates of hip fracture in cohorts with and without distal radius fracture and relative risk by follow-up month. (Reprinted from Chen C-W, Huang T-L, Su L-T, et al. Incidence of subsequent hip fractures is significantly increased within the first month after distal radius fracture in patients older than 60 years. *J Trauma Acute Care Surg*. 2013;74:317-321, with permission from Lippincott Williams & Wilkins.)

TABLE 1.—Incidence of Hip Fracture Measured by Sociodemographic Factor and Baseline Comorbidity in Cohorts With and Without Distal Radius Fracture

| | Distal Radius Fracture | | | | | | | |
| | − | | | | + | | | |
Variable	Total (N)	Case* (n)	Person Year	Rate†	Total (N)	Case* (n)	Person Year	Rate†	Rate Ratio
All	81,227	121	81,163	14.9	9,986	84	9,933	84.6	5.67
Sex									
Female	40,539	64	40,505	15.8	6,224	65	6,185	105.1	6.65
Male	40,688	57	40,658	14.0	3,762	19	3,748	50.7	3.62
Age (yr)									
30−39	25,603	7	25,599	2.7	1,514	4	1,511	26.5	9.68
40−49	23,562	10	23,556	4.2	1,975	8	1,969	40.6	9.57
50−59	14,858	12	14,853	8.1	2,357	8	2,351	34.0	4.21
≥60	17,204	92	17,155	53.6	4,140	64	4,103	156.0	2.91
Occupation									
White collar	37,380	33	37,361	8.8	3,484	22	3,471	63.4	7.18
Blue collar	29,537	46	29,514	15.6	4,556	38	4,529	83.9	5.38
Others	14,310	42	14,288	29.4	1,946	24	1,933	124.2	4.22
Urbanization									
Low	2,748	9	2,743	32.8	448	3	446	67.3	2.05
Moderate	22,991	37	22,971	16.1	3,337	33	3,316	99.5	6.18
High	55,488	75	55,449	13.5	6,201	48	6,171	77.8	5.75
Income (USD)									
<500	26,958	73	26,919	27.1	4,051	45	4,026	111.8	4.12
500−999	36,051	43	36,028	11.9	4,617	36	4,591	78.4	6.57
≥1,000	18,218	5	18,215	2.7	1,318	3	1,316	22.8	8.30

+, distal radius fracture cohort; −, nondistal radius fracture cohort.
*Subsequent hip fracture case number.
†Per 10,000 person years.

age >60 years was also a significant factor associated with hip fracture (hazard ratio = 8.67, 95% confidence interval = 4.51−16.7).

Conclusions.—Patients with distal radius fracture and age >60 years will significantly increase the incidence of subsequent hip fracture, especially within the first month.

Level of Evidence.—Prognostic/epidemiologic study, level II (Fig 2, Table 1).

▶ This is an important demographic analysis that confirms the clinical association between distal radius fracture and subsequent hip fracture. A review of these data should prompt orthopedic surgeons treating distal radius fracture patients to assure that they obtain proper bone health evaluations to include vitamin D level measurement and a double-energy X-ray absorptiometry scan. Who performs these assessments and subsequent evaluation and treatment is not important; it is the role in patient education and referral for these assessments that is the critical role that the orthopedic surgeon is best positioned to fulfill.

M. F. Swiontkowski, MD

Catastrophic Failure After Open Reduction Internal Fixation of Femoral Neck Fractures With a Novel Locking Plate Implant
Berkes MB, Little MTM, Lazaro LE, et al (Hosp for Special Surgery, NY)
J Orthop Trauma 26:e170-e176, 2012

Objectives.—To determine if the use of a novel proximal femoral locking plate could reduce the incidence of femoral neck shortening and improve clinical outcomes after open reduction internal fixation (ORIF) for femoral neck fractures as compared with historical controls.

Design.—Single surgeon, retrospective case—control study.

Setting.—Academic level I trauma center.

Patients/Participants.—Twenty-one femoral neck fractures treated with the posterolateral femoral locking plate (Synthes, Inc, Paoli, PA) were eligible for inclusion. Eighteen met inclusion/exclusion criteria with a mean follow-up of 16 months.

Intervention.—ORIF of femoral neck fracture with the posterolateral femoral locking plate. This consists of a side plate with multiple locking screws directed into the femoral head at converging/diverging angles and a single shaft screw. Intraoperative compression was achieved with partially threaded screws before locking screw insertion.

Main Outcome Measurements.—Maintenance of reduction was assessed by comparing immediate postoperative and final follow-up radiographs. Clinical outcome was assessed with Harris Hip Scores after 1 year. Complications and secondary operations were noted.

Results.—Seven (36.8%) of 18 patients experienced catastrophic failure. Five of these patients required total hip replacement, whereas the remaining 2 died before further treatment. The remaining 11 patients (61.1%) achieved bony union; the average displacement of the center of the head did not differ when compared with historical controls (0.78 mm inferiorly, 1.62 mm medially, and 2.4 degrees of increased varus vs. 0.86 mm, 1.23 mm, and 0.6 degree). Complications in this group include 1 instance of screw fracture, 2 total hip replacements, and a peri-implant subtrochanteric femur fracture.

The average patient age and proportion of displaced fractures did not differ between the historical control and experimental groups. Fracture displacement was strongly associated with catastrophic failure in the experimental group only. Average Harris Hip Scores was significantly worse compared with that of historical controls (67.9 vs. 84.7, $P = 0.05$).

Conclusions.—ORIF of femoral neck fractures using a locking plate construct yielded unacceptably poor outcomes in this patient population. We hypothesize that the stiffness of this construct prevents any fracture site micromotion, placing the mechanical burden on the implant, which can result in failure at the bone—screw interface or fatigue failure of the implant itself (Fig 5).

▶ Over the past 5 to 7 years, locked plate technology has captured the attention of the orthopedic trauma community. Plates have been designed for every metaphyseal and diaphyseal fracture application including the proximal femur. This cohort study elucidates a major failure of design and/or application of one such locking plate for femoral neck fractures. The patient cohort in which these plates were used was younger with higher energy injuries as one would suspect. The 37% failure rate should direct the orthopedic community away from further

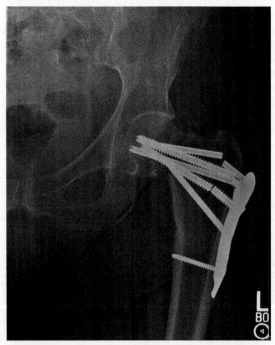

FIGURE 5.—A postoperative AP radiograph of the hip demonstrating screw failure and varus collapse. Note failure of all 5.0- and 7.3-mm locking screws with subsequent varus displacement. (Reprinted from Berkes MB, Little MTM, Lazaro LE, et al. Catastrophic failure after open reduction internal fixation of femoral neck fractures with a novel locking plate implant. *J Orthop Trauma*. 2012;26:e170-e176, with permission from Lippincott Williams & Wilkins.)

routine use of this implant (Fig 5). Although the retrospective cohort design introduces issues of selection and detection bias, the data are so convincing that further study with randomized designs is probably not warranted.

M. F. Swiontkowski, MD

Does early administration of bisphosphonate affect fracture healing in patients with intertrochanteric fractures?

Kim T-Y, Ha Y-C, Kang B-J, et al (Chung-Ang Univ College of Medicine, Seoul, Korea)
J Bone Joint Surg Br 94-B:956-960, 2012

This prospective multicentre study was undertaken to determine whether the timing of the post-operative administration of bisphosphonate affects

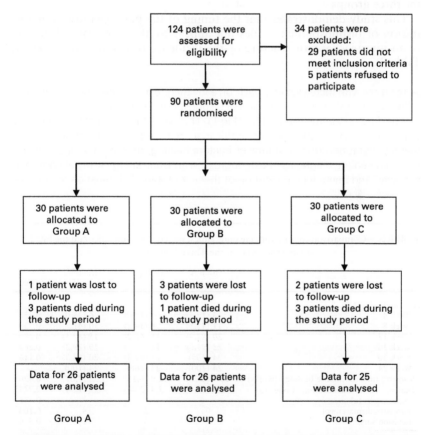

FIGURE 1.—Flow diagram of patient involvement in the study. (Reprinted from Kim T-Y, Ha Y-C, Kang B-J, et al. Does early administration of bisphosphonate affect fracture healing in patients with intertrochanteric fractures? *J Bone Joint Surg Br.* 2012;94-B:956-960, with permission from British Editorial Society of Bone and Joint Surgery.)

fracture healing and the rate of complication following an intertrochanteric fracture. Between August 2008 and December 2009, 90 patients with an intertrochanteric fracture who underwent internal fixation were randomised to three groups according to the timing of the commencement of risedronate treatment after surgery: Group A (from one week after surgery), Group B (from one month after surgery), and Group C (from three months after surgery). The radiological time to fracture healing was assessed as the primary endpoint, and the incidence of complications, including excessive displacement or any complication requiring revision surgery, as the secondary endpoint. The mean time to fracture healing post-operatively in groups A, B and C was 10.7 weeks (SD 4.4), 12.9 weeks (SD 6.2) and 12.3 weeks (SD 7.1), respectively ($p = 0.420$). At 24 weeks after surgery, all fractures had united, except six that had a loss of fixation. Functional outcomes at one year after surgery according to the Koval classification ($p = 0.948$) and the incidence of complications ($p = 0.386$) were similar in the three groups.

This study demonstrates that the timing of the post-operative administration of bisphosphonates does not appear to affect the rate of healing of an intertrochanteric fracture or the incidence of complications (Fig 1, Table 2).

▶ In an era with increased emphasis on early diagnosis and treatment of patients with fragility fractures, the question of bisphosphonate therapy's impact on fracture healing is extremely important (Fig 1). This well-done clinical trial addresses that issue. In a way, the findings of this trial, that the timing of bisphosphonate therapy institution does not impact fracture healing, makes it easier to recommend immediate diagnosis of osteoporosis with Dual-energy x-ray absorptiometry scan and immediate institution of therapy (Table 2). It must be recognized

TABLE 2.—Comparisons of Fracture Healing Times, Functional Outcomes and the Incidence of Complications in the Three Study Groups

	Group A (n = 26)	Group B (n = 26)	Group C (n = 25)	p-Value[†]
Fracture healing* (n, %)				
Week 4	3 (12.5)	3 (13.0)	6 (25.0)	0.428
Week 8	11 (45.8)	8 (34.8)	10 (41.7)	0.739
Week 12	20 (83.3)	15 (65.2)	15 (62.5)	0.230
Week 16	22 (91.7)	17 (73.9)	19 (79.2)	0.269
Week 20	24 (100)	21 (91.3)	20 (83.3)	0.116
Week 24	24 (100)	23 (100)	24 (100)	-
Mean (SD) time to fracture healing* (weeks)	10.7 (4.36)	12.9 (6.15)	12.3 (7.07)	0.420[‡]
Mean (SD) Koval classification at one year	2.4 (1.66)	2.4 (2.06)	2.2 (1.54)	0.948[‡]
Complications (n)				0.386
Excessive displacement	0	2	4	0.103
Revision surgery	2	3	1	0.550

*Excluding patients requiring revision surgeries.
[†]Pearson's chi-squared test, unless otherwise stated.
[‡]Analysis of variance (ANOVA).

that this trial was conducted in patients with intertrochanteric fractures, and there may be differential effects on other fractures, although this would seem to be unlikely.

M. F. Swiontkowski, MD

Comparative Effectiveness of Regional *versus* General Anesthesia for Hip Fracture Surgery in Adults
Neuman MD, Silber JH, Elkassabany NM, et al (Univ of Pennsylvania, Philadelphia; Univ of Pennsylvania School of Medicine, Philadelphia; et al)
Anesthesiology 117:72-92, 2012

Background.—Hip fracture is a common, morbid, and costly event among older adults. Data are inconclusive as to whether epidural or spinal (regional) anesthesia improves outcomes after hip fracture surgery.

Methods.—The authors examined a retrospective cohort of patients undergoing surgery for hip fracture in 126 hospitals in New York in 2007 and 2008. They tested the association of a record indicating receipt of regional *versus* general anesthesia with a primary outcome of inpatient mortality and with secondary outcomes of pulmonary and cardiovascular complications using hospital fixed-effects logistic regressions. Subgroup analyses tested the association of anesthesia type and outcomes according to fracture anatomy.

Results.—Of 18,158 patients, 5,254 (29%) received regional anesthesia. In-hospital mortality occurred in 435 (2.4%). Unadjusted rates of mortality and cardiovascular complications did not differ by anesthesia type. Patients receiving regional anesthesia experienced fewer pulmonary complications (359 [6.8%] *vs.* 1,040 [8.1%], $P < 0.005$). Regional anesthesia was associated with a lower adjusted odds of mortality (odds ratio: 0.710, 95% CI 0.541, 0.932, $P = 0.014$) and pulmonary complications (odds ratio: 0.752, 95% CI 0.637, 0.887, $P < 0.0001$) relative to general anesthesia. In subgroup analyses, regional anesthesia was associated with improved survival and fewer pulmonary complications among patients with intertrochanteric fractures but not among patients with femoral neck fractures.

Conclusions.—Regional anesthesia is associated with a lower odds of inpatient mortality and pulmonary complications among all hip fracture patients compared with general anesthesia; this finding may be driven by a trend toward improved outcomes with regional anesthesia among patients with intertrochanteric fractures (Table 3).

▶ This is a large cohort study using an administrative data set that focuses on the critical outcomes following hip fracture surgery as they relate to the type of anesthesia utilized. Without randomization we cannot be completely confident of the findings, as patients treated using general anesthesia may well be very different than those who received regional anesthesia; the review of important factors

TABLE 3.—Comparison of Unadjusted In-Hospital Outcomes by Anesthesia Type within 126 Hospitals in New York State, 2007–2008

	General Anesthesia	Regional Anesthesia	P Value
Discharges (%)	12,904 (71.1)	5,254 (28.9)	—
Mortality (%)	325 (2.5)	110 (2.1)	0.090
Cardiac complications	—	—	—
Congestive heart failure (%)	230 (1.8)	93 (1.8)	0.955
Acute myocardial infarction (%)	266 (2.1)	97 (1.9)	0.348
Cardiac arrest (%)	410 (3.2)	142 (2.7)	0.091
Any cardiac complication (%)	688 (5.3)	250 (4.8)	0.113
Pulmonary complications	—	—	—
Aspiration (%)	333 (2.6)	133 (2.5)	0.849
Infectious pneumonia (%)	359 (2.8)	153 (2.9)	0.631
Respiratory failure (%)	641 (5.0)	180 (3.4)	<0.0001
Any pulmonary complication (%)	1,040 (8.1)	359 (6.8)	0.005

does not identify important differences. One condition that comes to mind is patients who are on Clopridel for significant cardiovascular issues, as they are generally not felt to be eligible for regional anesthesia. Regardless, it does appear that patients receiving regional anesthesia have a lower risk of significant pulmonary morbidity and mortality, and regional anesthesia should probably be the first proposal to patients who are undergoing hip fracture surgery.

M. F. Swiontkowski, MD

TRIGEN INTERTAN Intramedullary Nail Versus Sliding Hip Screw: A Prospective, Randomized Multicenter Study on Pain, Function, and Complications in 684 Patients with an Intertrochanteric or Subtrochanteric Fracture and One Year of Follow-up

Matre K, Vinje T, Havelin LI, et al (Haukeland Univ Hosp, Bergen, Norway; et al)
J Bone Joint Surg Am 95:200-208, 2013

Background.—Both intramedullary nails and sliding hip screws are used with good results in the treatment of intertrochanteric and subtrochanteric fractures. The aim of our study was to assess whether use of the TRIGEN INTERTAN nail, as compared with a sliding hip screw, resulted in less postoperative pain, improved functional mobility, and reduced surgical complication rates for patients with an intertrochanteric or subtrochanteric fracture.

Methods.—In a prospective, randomized multicenter study, 684 elderly patients were treated with the INTERTAN nail or with a sliding hip screw with or without a trochanteric stabilizing plate. The patients were assessed during their hospital stay and at three and twelve months postoperatively. A visual analogue scale (VAS) pain score was recorded at all time points, and functional mobility was assessed with use of the timed Up & Go test.

The Harris hip score (HHS) was used to assess hip function more specifically. Quality of life was measured with the EuroQol-5D (EQ-5D). Radiographic findings as well as intraoperative and postoperative complications were recorded and analyzed.

Results.—Patients treated with an INTERTAN nail had slightly less pain at the time of early postoperative mobilization (VAS score, 48 versus 52; $p = 0.042$), although this did not influence the length of the hospital stay and there was no difference at three or twelve months. Regardless of the fracture and implant type, functional mobility, hip function, patient satisfaction, and quality-of-life assessments were comparable between the groups at three and twelve months. The numbers of patients with surgical complications were similar for the two groups (twenty-nine in the sliding-hip-screw group and thirty-two in the INTERTAN group, $p = 0.67$).

Conclusions.—INTERTAN nails and sliding hip screws are similar in terms of pain, function, and reoperation rates twelve months after treatment of intertrochanteric and subtrochanteric fractures (Tables 2 and 3).

▶ This is a well-done randomized controlled trial (RCT) comparing an intramedullary nail (IMN) with sliding hip screw in intertrochanteric and subtrochanteric fractures. As with most RCTs and meta-analyses on this topic, the results are comparable with higher technical complications with the IMN. There is ample evidence in the literature, including this study, that should cause us to continue the selection of the sliding hip screw for most intertrochanteric hip fractures and the IMN for most (and nearly all) subtrochanteric hip fractures. IMN technique is more difficult and has a higher rate of complications. It requires compulsivity in patient positioning, intraoperative imaging, and placement of the starting point

TABLE 2.—Primary Outcomes

	INTERTAN	Sliding Hip Screw	Mean Difference (95% Confidence Interval)	P Value*
Mean VAS score for pain				
Postop.				
At rest	22 (n = 283)	21 (n = 289)	1.1 (−2.3-4.5)	0.54[†]
At mobilization	48 (n = 269)	52 (n = 284)	−3.7 (−7.4-0.04)	**0.042[†]**
3 mo	25 (n = 226)	25 (n = 206)	−0.5 (−4.6-3.6)	0.82
12 mo	17 (n = 185)	17 (n = 192)	0.05 (−4.0-4.1)	0.98
Timed Up & Go test				
Postop. *(no. [%] of patients)*				
Total no. assessed	306/341	295/343		0.14
Unable to perform test	167 (55%)	163 (55%)		0.87
Test performed, not passed[‡]	7 (2%)	6 (2%)		0.83
Test performed and passed[‡]	132 (43%)	126 (43%)		0.92
Mean score *(sec)*				
Postop.	74 (n = 132)	69 (n = 126)	5.1 (−3.5-14.3)	0.20[†]
3 mo	29 (n = 177)	29 (n = 164)	0.04 (−4.3-4.4)	0.99
12 mo	27 (n = 154)	25 (n = 160)	1.3 (−3.6-6.2)	0.60

*Significant p value is in bold.
[†]Adjusted p values; adjustments were made because of differences in the time distribution of patient examinations. The unadjusted p value for pain at mobilization was 0.053.
[‡]A timed Up & Go test of more than three minutes and thirty seconds was considered to be a test not passed.

TABLE 3.—Intraoperative, Early, and Late Postoperative Complications and Reoperations in the Two Treatment Groups

	INTERTAN* (N = 341)	Sliding Hip Screw* (N = 343)	P Value[†]
Intraop. complications			
Technical or implant-related (n = 643)[‡]	62/328 (18.9%)	21/315 (6.7%)	**<0.001**
Requiring surgical intervention[§]	4	2	0.41
Other in-hospital complications			
General medical	104	110	0.79
Early postop. death	8	14	0.20
Postop. surgical complications	32 (9.4%)	29 (8.5%)	0.67
(including those with nonop. treatment)[#]			
Major	26 (7.6%)	27 (7.9%)	0.90
Minor	7 (2.1%)	2 (0.6%)	0.09
Reoperation in 1st 12 mo	28 (8.2%)	27 (7.9%)	0.87
Indications for reoperations			
Major reoperations**	23 (6.7%)	28 (8.2%)	0.48
Cutout	6 (1.8%)	9 (2.6%)	
Infection	2 (0.6%)	3 (0.9%)	
Fracture around implant	5 (1.5%)	1 (0.3%)	
Mechanical failure/nonunion	3 (0.9%)	10 (2.9%)	
Poor reduction/implant position	4 (1.2%)	3 (0.9%)	
Other	3 (0.9%)	2 (0.6%)	
Minor reoperations	5 (1.5%)	1 (0.3%)	0.10
Removal of drain		1	
Adding distal locking screw	3		
Removal of distal locking screw	1		
Removal of separate lag screw	1		
1-yr mortality[††]	24.6%	25.4%	0.83

*The values are given as the number of patients with the percentage in parentheses unless otherwise indicated.
[†]Pearson chi-square test. The significant p value is in bold.
[‡]Technical or implant-related problems were mainly minor problems without any crucial influence on the surgical procedure or the outcome of the operation. Exceptions are listed in the row below.
[§]One femoral fracture after nailing was treated with a long INTERTAN nail as planned. One long nail was converted to a short nail because of distal anterior cortex penetration. Two planned long nails were converted to a short nail because of a short femur in one case and a narrow femur in the other. One intraoperative fissure with a sliding hip screw was treated with a longer plate. Another intraoperative fracture/fissure with a sliding hip screw was not detected initially and was treated with a reoperation eleven days later.
[#]More than one complication per patient is possible. Seven patients in the INTERTAN group and two patients in the sliding-hip-screw group with a cutout left surgically untreated are included.
**More than one reason per patient possible.
[††]Kaplan-Meier survival analyses.

after an excellent reduction of the fracture. Each has its role, but sliding screws should remain the workhorse for most of the intertrochanteric hip fractures.

M. F. Swiontkowski, MD

More re-operations after uncemented than cemented hemiarthroplasty used in the treatment of displaced fractures of the femoral neck: An observational study of 11 116 hemiarthroplasties from a national register
Gjertsen J-E, Lie SA, Vinje T, et al (Norwegian Arthroplasty Register, Norway)
J Bone Joint Surg Br 94-B:1113-1119, 2012

Using data from the Norwegian Hip Fracture Register, 8639 cemented and 2477 uncemented primary hemiarthroplasties for displaced fractures of the femoral neck in patients aged >70 years were included in a prospective observational study. A total of 218 re-operations were performed after cemented and 128 after uncemented procedures. Survival of the hemiarthroplasties was calculated using the Kaplan-Meier method and hazard rate ratios (HRR) for revision were calculated using Cox regression analyses. At five years the implant survival was 97% (95% confidence interval (CI) 97 to 97) for cemented and 91% (95% CI 87 to 94) for uncemented hemiarthroplasties. Uncemented hemiarthroplasties had a 2.1 times increased risk of revision compared with cemented prostheses (95% confidence interval 1.7 to 2.6, $p < 0.001$). The increased risk was mainly caused by revisions for peri-prosthetic fracture (HRR = 17), aseptic loosening (HRR = 17), haematoma formation (HRR = 5.3), superficial infection (HRR = 4.6) and dislocation (HRR = 1.8). More intra-operative complications, including intra-operative death, were reported for the cemented hemiarthroplasties. However, in a time-dependent analysis, the HRR for re-operation in both groups increased as follow-up increased.

This study showed that the risk for revision was higher for uncemented than for cemented hemiarthroplasties (Fig 1, Tables 1 and 2).

▶ This hip fracture study is very worthy of note and should impact treatment decision making worldwide. The use of uncemented prostheses should be the treatment of choice for older patients with displaced femoral neck fractures where arthroplasty is the best decision for the patient. With a differential implant

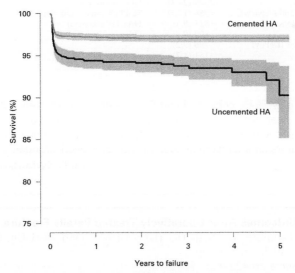

FIGURE 1.—Adjusted survival with 95% confidence intervals for patients with cemented and uncemented hemiarthroplasty (HA) with all re-operations as the endpoint. (Reprinted from Gjertsen J-E, Lie SA, Vinje T, et al. More re-operations after uncemented than cemented hemiarthroplasty used in the treatment of displaced fractures of the femoral neck: an observational study of 11 116 hemiarthroplasties from a national register. *J Bone Joint Surg Br.* 2012;94-B:1113-1119, with permission from British Editorial Society of Bone and Joint Surgery.)

TABLE 1.—Baseline Characteristics of Patients

	Cemented Hemiarthroplasty (n = 8639)	Uncemented Hemiarthroplasty (n = 2477)	p-Value
Mean age at fracture (yrs) (range)	83.5 (70 to 104)	83.8 (70 to 103)	0.067*
Female (n, %)	6450 (74.7)	1825 (73.7)	0.322†
ASA‡ class (n, %)			0.394†
1	345 (4.0)	85 (3.4)	
2	2912 (33.7)	872 (35.2)	
3	4727 (54.7)	1346 (54.3)	
4	515 (6.0)	142 (5.7)	
5	4 (0.0)	2 (0.1)	
Data missing	136 (1.6)	30 (1.2)	
Cognitive impairment (n, %)			<0.001†
Yes	2173 (25.2)	705 (28.5)	
Uncertain	962 (11.1)	273 (11.0)	
No	5281 (61.1)	1457 (58.8)	
Data missing	223 (2.6)	42 (1.7)	

*independent t-test
†Pearson chi-squared test
‡ASA, American Society of Anesthesiologists

TABLE 2.—Type of Implants

Cemented Hemiarthroplasty (n = 8639)		Uncemented Hemiarthroplasty (n = 2477)	
Name	Number (%)	Name	Number (%)
Exeter/V40 (Stryker)	2907 (33.6)	Corail (DePuy)	1869 (75.5)
Charnley (DePuy)	2085 (24.1)	Filler (Biotechni)	361 (14.6)
Spectron (Smith and Nephew)	1066 (12.3)	SL-PLUS (Smith and Nephew)	158 (6.4)
Lubinus SP II (LINK)	825 (9.5)	HACTIV (Biomed)	37 (1.5)
Titan (DePuy)	809 (9.4)	Other	52 (2.1)
Charnley Modular (DePuy)	796 (9.2)		
Other	151 (1.7)		

survival rate of 97% for cemented and 91% for uncemented stems, this recommendation is clear. When one considers that these are registry data, where experimental design and bias in treatment decision making do not come into play, the impact on our treatment recommendation should be even stronger.

M. F. Swiontkowski, MD

Knee

Functional Outcomes After Operatively Treated Patella Fractures

Lebrun CT, Langford JR, Sagi HC (Univ of Maryland Med Ctr, Baltimore; Florida Orthopaedic Inst, Tampa)
J Orthop Trauma 26:422-426, 2012

Objectives.—To evaluate the midterm functional outcomes of patients with isolated operatively treated patella fractures.

Design.—Prospective cohort and retrospective clinical and radiographic assessment.

Setting.—A Level I and Level II trauma center.

Patients/Participants.—Two hundred forty-one patients underwent operative intervention for a displaced patella fracture between 1991 and 2007. After appropriate exclusions, 110 patients met criteria. A total of 40 (36%) patients with isolated, unilateral, operatively treated patella fractures with minimum 1-year follow-up agreed to participate in this study and return for functional testing. Mean follow-up was 6.5 years (range, 1.25–17 years).

Intervention.—Enrolled patients were treated with one of the following methods: standard tension band with Kirschner wires, tension band through 2 cannulated screws, longitudinal anterior banding with cerclage, or partial patellectomy.

Main Outcome Measurements.—All enrolled patients were evaluated with the SF-36 and an injury-specific questionnaire (Knee Injury and Osteoarthritis Outcome Scores) and asked to self-report symptomatic hardware. Patients were also evaluated by physical examination assessing range of motion and Biodex bilateral quadriceps isometric and isokinetic comparisons.

Results.—The mean normalized SF-36 physical composite score and the mean normalized Knee Injury and Osteoarthritis Outcome Scores subscale scores (pain, 71.7; symptoms, 66.3; activities of daily living, 75.1; sport/recreation, 45.2; quality of life, 49.6) were statistically different ($P < 0.05$) from reference population norms. Removal of symptomatic fixation was required in 52% of the patients treated with osteosynthesis, whereas 38% of those with retained fixation self-reported implant-related pain at least some of the time. Eight patients (20%) had an extensor lag greater than 5°. A restricted range of flexion of greater than 5° was noted in 15 patients (38%) and restricted range of extension of greater than 5° was noted in 6 patients (15%). Biodex dynamometric testing revealed a mean isometric extension deficit of 26% between the uninvolved and involved sides for peak torque. Extension power was also tested with an angular velocity of 90°/sec and 180°/sec and mean deficits of 31% and 29% were noted, respectively, when compared with the contralateral extremity.

Conclusions.—At a mean of 6.5 years after operative treatment for patella fractures, significant symptomatic complaints and functional deficits persist based on validated outcome measures as well as objective physical evaluations. This study fills a void in the literature regarding the functional outcomes of these patients. It also underscores the complexity associated with treating this common fracture and should help guide surgeons to better counsel patients on the expected long-term function after operative treatment of patella fractures (Tables 1 and 3).

▶ This is a large retrospective cohort study defining the long-term outcomes of patellar fracture operative management. The results are generally poor, likely related to significant quadriceps atrophy and patellofemoral arthritis. The authors take pains to evaluate whether the responding patients are different from the nonresponders in terms of their fracture and operative management decisions

TABLE 1.—SF-36 Outcome Scores

SF-36 Outcome Scores	Mean	Range	95% Confidence Interval
Physical component score	40.9	15.7–58.5	37.8–44
Mental component score	52.3	22.8–68.1	49.5–55.1

Operative Treatment	Mean MCS	Mean PCS
Tension band with Kirschner wires (N = 15)	54	42
Tension band through cannulated screws (N = 10)	53	46
Longitudinal anterior banding with cerclage (N = 2)	55	38
Partial patellectomy (N = 13)	45	40

Data displayed are summation of the entire study population.
MCS, mental component score; PCS, physical component score. Data displayed as means for the different operative treatments.

TABLE 3.—Characteristics of Respondent and Nonrespondent Groups

	Respondent Group (N = 40)	Nonrespondent Group (N = 110)	Significant Difference
Age	52	50	NS ($P = 0.63$)
Sex	48% men	52% men	NS ($P = 0.713$)
Fracture classification			
OTA 34-C1	30%	32%	NS ($P = 1.00$)
OTA 34-C2	15%	17%	NS ($P = 0.809$)
OTA 34-C3	55%	51%	NS ($P = 0.714$)
Gustilo and Anderson classification			
Closed	73%	77%	NS ($P = 0.671$)
Type I open	20%	15%	NS ($P = 0.621$)
Type II open	5%	6%	NS ($P = 1.00$)
Type III open	3%	2%	NS ($P = 0.565$)

NS, not significant. Two-tailed P values are reported. A t test was used for continuous data. Fisher exact test used for categorical data.

and they are not (Table 3). However, it is conceivable that the responding patients are those with greater functional deficits. Regardless, these results are concerning. It seems that the biggest gains in terms of improving patient functional outcomes are likely not related to operative techniques, but rather improved methods for regaining quadricep strength and early full range of motion.

M. F. Swiontkowski, MD

Pelvic and Acetabular Fracture

Embolization of Pelvic Arterial Injury is a Risk Factor for Deep Infection After Acetabular Fracture Surgery

Manson TT, Perdue PW, Pollak AN, et al (Univ of Maryland, Baltimore)
J Orthop Trauma 27:11-15, 2013

Objective.—To determine whether embolization of pelvic arterial injuries before open reduction and internal fixation (ORIF) of acetabular fractures is associated with an increased rate of deep surgical site infection.

Methods.—Retrospective review of patients who underwent ORIF of acetabular fractures at our institution from 1995 through 2007 (n = 1440). We compared patients with acetabular fractures who underwent angiography and embolization of a pelvic artery (n = 12) with those who underwent angiography but did not undergo embolization (n = 14). Primary outcome was presence of infection requiring return to the operating room.

Result.—Seven (58%) of the 12 patients who underwent embolization developed deep surgical site infection compared with only 2 (14%) of the patients who underwent angiography but did not require pelvic vessel embolization ($P < 0.05$, Fisher exact test).

Conclusions.—The combination of an acetabular fracture that requires ORIF and a pelvic arterial injury that requires angiographic embolization is rare. However, the 58% infection rate of the patients who underwent embolization before ORIF is an order of magnitude higher than typical historical controls (2%–5%) and significantly higher than that of the control group of patients who underwent angiography without embolization (14%). In addition, a disproportionate number of the patients who developed infection had their entire internal iliac artery embolized. Surgeons should be aware that embolization of a pelvic arterial injury is associated with a high rate of infection after subsequent ORIF of an acetabular fracture. Embolization of the entire iliac artery should be avoided whenever possible (Table 3).

▶ This small retrospective comparative cohort study documents the increased risk of deep infection after acetabular fracture surgery that occurs related to prior angiographic embolization for control of hemorrhage. Of course, there are the standard issues of detection and selection bias as well as local treatment effects, but this magnitude of risk would seem to far exceed the power of these factors to eliminate all the differences in the 2 treatment groups. This finding should impact the threshold for proceeding with angiographic embolization for hemorrhage control

TABLE 3.—Demographic Data for Patients With Acetabular Fractures Who Had Undergone Angiography, Comparing Those Who Did and Those Who Did Not Undergo Embolization

	Embolization (n = 12)	No Embolization (n = 14)	P
ISS	36.5	24.6	<0.05*
Intensive care unit stay, d	23.5	11.6	<0.05*
Hospital length of stay, d	29.6	18.4	0.06*
Age, yr	37.7	33.7	NS*
Body mass index, kg/m²	26.2	27.5	NS*
Glasgow Coma Scale score	13.2	12.5	NS*
Initial systolic blood pressure, mmHg	127.3	120.6	NS*
Initial heart rate, bpm	113.9	105.6	NS*
Complex acetabular fracture pattern, %	83.3	64.3	NS†

NS, not significant.
*Student *t* test.
†Fisher exact test.

in younger patients where acetabular open reduction and internal fixation is required.

M. F. Swiontkowski, MD

Two to Twenty-Year Survivorship of the Hip in 810 Patients with Operatively Treated Acetabular Fractures

Tannast M, Najibi S, Matta JM (Hip and Pelvis Inst, Santa Monica, CA)
J Bone Joint Surg Am 94:1559-1567, 2012

Background.—The aims of the study were (1) to determine the cumulative two to twenty-year survivorship of the hip after open reduction and internal fixation of displaced acetabular fractures, (2) to identify factors predicting conversion to total hip arthroplasty or hip arthrodesis, and (3) to create a predictive model that calculates an individual's probability of early need for total hip arthroplasty or hip arthrodesis.

Methods.—Eight hundred and sixteen acetabular fractures treated with open reduction and internal fixation by one surgeon over a twenty-six-year period were analyzed. Cumulative two to twenty-year Kaplan-Meier

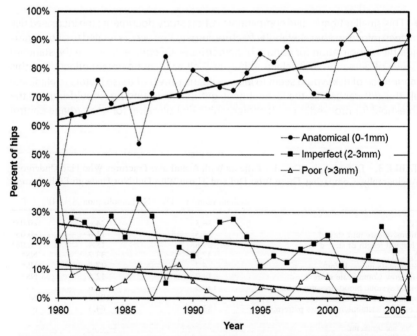

FIGURE 1.—Time dependence of the utilization of the accuracy of reduction (Fig 1B). (Reprinted from Tannast M, Najibi S, Matta JM. Two to twenty-year survivorship of the hip in 810 patients with operatively treated acetabular fractures. *J Bone Joint Surg Am.* 2012;94:1559-1567, with permission from The Journal of Bone and Joint Surgery, Incorporated.)

survivorship analyses of the hip, including best and worst-case scenarios, were performed with total hip arthroplasty or hip arthrodesis as the end point. Univariate and multivariate Cox regression analyses were performed to identify negative predictors, which were then used to construct a nomogram for predicting an individual's probability of needing an early total hip arthroplasty.

Results.—The cumulative twenty-year survivorship of the 816 hips available for follow-up was 79% at twenty years. The best and worst-case scenarios corresponded to cumulative twenty-year survivorship of 86% and 52%, respectively. Significant independent negative predictors were nonanatomical fracture reduction, an age of more than forty years, anterior

TABLE 3.—Survivorship According to Fracture Type and Other Characteristics

	Survivorship (95% Confidence Interval)* (%)				Median Time to Failure[†]
	Two Years	Five Years	Ten Years	Twenty Years	
Entire series (n = 816)	91 (90-92)	88 (87-90)	85 (84-87)	79 (76-81)	1.5
Simple fracture type (n = 241)	91 (89-93)	86 (84-89)	84 (81-87)	73 (68-79)	1.3
Anterior wall (n = 12)	91 (82-100)[‡]	68 (53-84)[‡]	68 (53-84)[‡]	34 (9-59)[‡]	2.3
Anterior column (n = 80)	95 (92-97)	92 (88-95)	87 (83-91)	77 (70-85)	3.0
Posterior wall (n = 107)	88 (84-91)	82 (78-86)	81 (77-85)	76 (71-82)	1.2
Posterior column (n = 14)	100	100	100	100	—
Transverse (n = 28)	89 (83-95)	89 (83-95)	89 (83-95)	89 (83-95)	0.3
Associated fracture type (n = 575)	92 (91-93)	89 (88-91)	86 (84-87)	80 (78-83)	1.6
Posterior column, posterior wall (n = 26)	85 (78-92)	85 (78-92)	85 (78-92)	85 (78-92)	0.5
Transverse, posterior wall (n = 143)	89 (86-91)	85 (82-88)	81 (78-85)	74 (68-80)	1.5
T-shaped (n = 96)	89 (85-92)	85 (81-89)	77 (72-81)	74 (68-79)	1.6
Anterior column, posterior hemitransverse (n = 76)	92 (89-95)	92 (89-95)	88 (84-92)	75 (65-84)	1.3
Both columns (n = 234)	96 (94-97)[§]	93 (91-95)[§]	91 (89-93)[§]	87 (83-90)[§]	2.2
Initial displacement					
≥20 mm (n = 226)	86 (84-89)[‡]	84 (81-86)[‡]	78 (75-81)[‡]	68 (63-73)[‡]	1.3
<20 mm (n = 590)	93 (92-95)[§]	90 (89-91)[§]	88 (86-89)[§]	83 (81-85)[§]	1.9
Treatment delay					
<21 days (n = 730)	93 (92-94)[§]	89 (88-91)[§]	86 (85-88)[§]	79 (77-82)[§]	2.0
≥21 days (n = 86)	82 (78-86)[‡]	80 (75-84)[‡]	74 (69-79)[‡]	74 (69-79)[‡]	0.9
Previous surgery					
Yes (n = 5)	60 (38-82)[‡]	30 (6-54)[‡]	—	—	0.8
No (n = 811)	92 (91-93)[§]	89 (87-90)[§]	85 (84-87)	79 (77-81)	1.6
Age					
<40 yr (n = 386)	96 (95-97)[§]	95 (94-96)[§]	92 (91-94)[§]	87 (84-89)[§]	2.3
40-65 yr (n = 318)	88 (86-90)[‡]	83 (81-86)[‡]	81 (79-83)[‡]	74 (71-77)[‡]	1.3
>65 yr (n = 112)	83 (79-87)[‡]	79 (75-83)[‡]	70 (65-76)[‡]	51 (38-64)[‡]	0.8
>75 yr (n = 42)	80 (73-87)[‡]	74 (66-83)[‡]	65 (54-76)[‡]	—	0.6
Approach					
Ilioinguinal (n = 323)	94 (94-96)[§]	92 (91-94)[§]	90 (88-92)[§]	84 (81-87)[§]	2.0
Kocher-Langenbeck (n = 352)	90 (88-91)	86 (84-88)	84 (82-86)	80 (77-83)	1.2
Extended iliofemoral (n = 129)	90 (87-93)[‡]	86 (83-90)[‡]	79 (75-83)[‡]	67 (61-73)[‡]	2.2
Ilioinguinal and Kocher-Langenbeck (n = 12)	92 (84-100)	83 (73-94)	73 (59-86)	—	3.5

*Based on Kaplan-Meier cumulative survivorship analysis.
[†]Calculated for failures only.
[‡]Significantly lower compared with hips without the specific criterion.
[§]Significantly higher compared with hips without the specific criterion.

hip dislocation, postoperative incongruence of the acetabular roof, involvement of the posterior acetabular wall, acetabular impaction, a femoral head cartilage lesion, initial displacement of the articular surface of ≥20 mm, and utilization of the extended iliofemoral approach.

Conclusions.—Open reduction and internal fixation of displaced acetabular fractures was able to successfully prevent the need for subsequent total hip arthroplasty within twenty years in 79% of the patients. The results represent benchmark comparative data for any future and past studies on the outcome of surgical fixation of acetabular fractures (Fig 1B, Table 3).

▶ This very large cohort study represents the career focus of the senior author, Dr Matta, on providing surgical reduction of displaced acetabular fractures. There are multiple take-home messages. The first is that experience matters as the surgeon's results in terms of reduction improve over time. Whether or not the same results can be obtained for surgeons with lower volumes is subject to question. Patient referral to high-volume surgeons seems appropriate given this experience. The second is that surgical approaches have changed over time with the increased experience. This evolution is toward less soft-tissue disrupting approaches. Finally, good clinical results in nearly 80% of patients at 20 years are possible with this standard setting clinical experience. Patients should not have these data reported to them as the expected outcomes because they likely represent the best case scenario that doubtfully can be reproduced with lesser experience.

M. F. Swiontkowski, MD

Radiographic Changes of Implant Failure After Plating for Pubic Symphysis Diastasis: An Underappreciated Reality?

Collinge C, Archdeacon MT, Dulaney-Cripe E, et al (Harris Methodist Fort Worth Hosp and John Peter Smith Orthopaedic Surgery Residency Program, TX; Univ of Cincinnati Academic Med Ctr, OH; Wright State Univ, Dayton, OH; et al)
Clin Orthop Relat Res 470:2148-2153, 2012

Background.—Implant failure after symphyseal disruption and plating reportedly occurs in 0% to 21% of patients but the actual occurrence may be much more frequent and the characteristics of this failure have not been well described.

Questions/Purposes.—We therefore determined the incidence and characterized radiographic implant failures in patients undergoing symphyseal plating after disruption of the pubic symphysis.

Methods.—We retrospectively reviewed 165 adult patients with Orthopaedic Trauma Association (OTA) 61-B (Tile B) or OTA 61-C (Tile C) pelvic injuries treated with symphyseal plating at two regional Level I and one Level II trauma centers. Immediate postoperative and latest followup anteroposterior radiographs were reviewed for implant loosening or breakage

TABLE 2.—Radiographic Data

Variable	Data
Mean pubic diastasis on injury AP radiograph	37 mm (range, 9—118 mm)
Mean pubic space on immediate postoperative radiograph	*4.9 mm (range, 2—10 mm)
Mean pubic space on final followup radiograph	†8.4 mm (range, 3—23 mm)
Patients with fixation failure and pubic space widening of 2—9 mm	77 (59%)
Patients with fixation failure and pubic space widening of ≥ 10 mm	7 (5.5%)
Changes in plate-screw construct associated with symphyseal widening	
Screws loosened only	67 (71%)
Broken screws only	5 (5%)
Combination of loosened and broken screws	16 (17%)
Plate breakage	7 (7%)
Patients reoperated for failed fixation	1 (1%)

*Statistically different from the injury radiograph ($p < 0.05$).
†Statistically different from the immediate postoperative radiograph ($p < 0.05$).

and for recurrent diastasis of the pubic symphysis. The minimum followup was 6 months (average, 12.2 months; range, 6—65 months).

Results.—Failure of fixation, including screw loosening or breakage of the symphyseal fixation, occurred in 95 of the 127 patients (75%), which resulted in widening of the pubic symphyseal space in 84 of those cases (88%) when compared with the immediate postoperative radiograph. The mean width of the pubic space measured 4.9 mm (range, 2—10 mm) on immediate postoperative radiographs; however, on the last radiographs, the mean was 8.4 mm (range, 3—21 mm), representing a 71% increase. In seven patients (6%), the symphysis widened 10 mm or more; however, only one of these patients required revision surgery.

Conclusions.—Failure of fixation with recurrent widening of the pubic space can be expected after plating of the pubic symphysis for traumatic diastasis. Although widening may represent a benign condition as motion is restored to the pubic symphysis, patients should be counseled regarding a high risk of radiographic failure but a small likelihood of revision surgery.

Level of Evidence.—Level IV, case series. See Guidelines for Authors for a complete description of levels of evidence (Table 2).

▶ This large cohort study from 3 experienced pelvic fracture surgery centers confirms that hardware loosening or breakage after open reduction with internal fixation of symphyseal disruption is the rule rather than the exception, with 75% of patients experiencing this outcome. Widening of the symphysis when compared with the original postoperative reduction is even more common. Despite these alarming statistics, actual revision of anterior pelvic fixation is relatively uncommon. These findings are not surprising given the normal motion at the symphysis; it only makes sense that more motion than is physiologic at this site would occur after disruption of the critical support soft tissues. Given these findings, perhaps we should reconsider the early approach of 2-hole plate fixation that allows this type of motion without catastrophic failure.

M. F. Swiontkowski, MD

Failure of Locked Design-Specific Plate Fixation of the Pubic Symphysis: A Report of Six Cases

Moed BR, Grimshaw CS, Segina DN (Saint Louis Univ School of Medicine, MO; Holmes Regional Trauma Ctr, Melbourne, FL)

J Orthop Trauma 26:e71-e75, 2012

Objectives.—Physiological pelvic motion has been known to lead to eventual loosening of screws, screw breakage, and plate breakage in conventional plate fixation of the disrupted pubic symphysis. Locked plating has been shown to have advantages for fracture fixation, especially in osteoporotic bone. Although design-specific locked symphyseal plates are now available, to our knowledge, their clinical use has not been evaluated and there exists a general concern that common modes of failure of the locked plate construct (such as pullout of the entire plate and screws) could result in complete and abrupt loss of fixation. The purpose of this study was to describe fixation failure of this implant in the acute clinical setting.

Design.—Retrospective analysis of multicenter case series.

Setting.—Multiple trauma centers.

Patients.—Six cases with failed fixation, all stainless steel locked symphyseal plates and screws manufactured by Synthes (Paoli, PA) and specifically designed for the pubic symphysis, were obtained from requests for information sent to orthopaedic surgeons at 10 trauma centers. A four-hole plate with all screws locked was used in 5 cases. A six-hole plate with 4 screws locked (two in each pubic body) was used in one.

Intervention.—Fixation for disruption of the pubic symphysis using an implant specifically designed for this purpose.

Main Outcome Measurements.—Radiographic appearance of implant failure.

Results.—Magnitude of failure ranged from implant loosening (3 cases), resulting in 10-mm to 12-mm gapping of the symphyseal reduction, to early failure (range, 1−12 weeks), resulting in complete loss of reduction (3

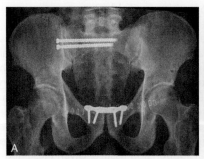
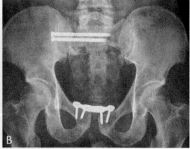

FIGURE 2.—Anteroposterior radiographs of Case 5 (Table 1 in the original article) showing (A) the immediate postoperative film and (B) when the patient returned for follow-up 10 weeks after surgery. (Reprinted from Moed BR, Grimshaw CS, Segina DN. Failure of Locked Design-Specific Plate Fixation of the Pubic Symphysis: a Report of Six Cases. *J Orthop Trauma.* 2012;26:e71-e75, with permission from Lippincott Williams & Wilkins.)

TABLE 1.—Case Data

Case No.	Age (Years)	Sex	Mechanism of Injury	Associated Injuries	OTA Type 61-	Time From Injury to Fixation (Hours)	Plate Type	Number of Locked Screws in Plate	Time From Fixation to Failure (Weeks)	Posterior Fixation Used	Mode of Failure
1	45	M	All terrain vehicle accident	Yes	C1.2	36	Six-hole symphyseal locking	4	3	Yes	Unscrewing of locked screws and pullout from bone
2	54	M	Fall off a horse	No	C1.3	46	Four-hole symphyseal locking	4	1	Yes	Loosening of symphyseal hardware*
3	64	M	Motorcycle accident	Yes	C1.3	96	Four-hole symphyseal locking	4	12	Yes	Loosening of symphyseal hardware*
4	44	M	Motorcycle accident	Yes	B1.1	96	Four-hole symphyseal locking	4	12	No	Loosening of symphyseal hardware*
5	42	M	Fall from a height	No	C1.3	24	Four-hole symphyseal locking	4	Sometime before 10†	Yes	Construct pullout from bone
6	40	M	Fall from a height	No	B1.1	24	Four-hole symphyseal locking	4	Sometime before 12†	No	Broken screws at screw/plate interface

OTA, Orthopaedic Trauma Association; M, male
*Minor failure with loosening of the screw–bone interface and approximately 10 mm of gapping of the pubic symphyseal reduction.
†No follow-up between hospital discharge and examination showing failure.

cases). Failure mechanism included construct pullout, breakage of screws at the screw/plate interface, and loosening of the locked screws from the plate and/or bone. Backing out of the locking screws resulting from inaccurate insertion technique was also observed.

Conclusions.—Failure mechanisms of locked design-specific plate fixation of the pubic symphysis include those seen with conventional uniplanar fixation as well as those common to locked plate technology. Specific indications for the use of these implants remain to be determined (Fig 2, Table 1).

▶ Locked implant technology has spread to every fracture in which internal fixation is considered appropriate and involves every trauma implant manufacturer. The complications regarding the use of locked implants are large in number but relatively poorly defined in the literature. This small cohort study details complications related to locked symphyseal fixation and no doubt represents a small number of complications related to the use of these devices. It is likely that use of nonlocked technology in symphyseal disruption is advisable because the joint has some small amount of motion even in the uninjured pelvis.

M. F. Swiontkowski, MD

Radial Head and Neck Fractures

Comparison of Early Mobilization Protocols in Radial Head Fractures
Paschos NK, Mitsionis GI, Vasiliadis HS, et al (Univ of Ioannina, Greece)
J Orthop Trauma 27:134-139, 2013

Objectives.—We compared 2 different protocols of early mobilization with a protocol of delayed mobilization in patients with simple radial head fractures (B2.1 type of Orthopaedic Trauma Association Classification). An attempt to correlate certain characteristics of the radial head fractures with outcome was made.

Design.—Prospective randomized comparative study.

Setting.—Level 1 trauma center.

Patients/Participants.—One hundred eighty consecutive patients were randomly allocated into 3 different protocols.

Intervention.—In the first group, immediate mobilization of the elbow joint was applied. In the second, a sling was used for 2 days and then active mobilization was introduced. The third protocol represented the control group where immobilization in a cast for 7 days before the mobilization was applied.

Main Outcome Measurements.—Broberg and Morrey score, The American Shoulder and Elbow Surgeons-Elbow score, visual analogue scale, and grip and pinch strength were evaluated.

Results.—The 2 protocols introducing early mobilization resulted in better outcome compared with immobilization. The first protocol resulted in worse pain in the first 3 days. Range of motion, strength, and functional outcome was better in patients allocated to the second protocol. These differences were more evident in displaced fractures. A fragment

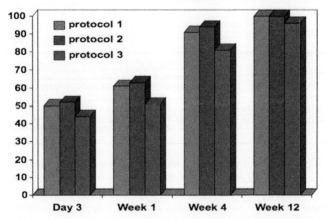

FIGURE 3.—Progress of the clinical score in nondisplaced fractures (21-B2.1.1). (Reprinted from Paschos NK, Mitsionis GI, Vasiliadis HS, et al. Comparison of early mobilization protocols in radial head fractures. *J Orthop Trauma.* 2013;27:134-139, with permission from Lippincott Williams & Wilkins.)

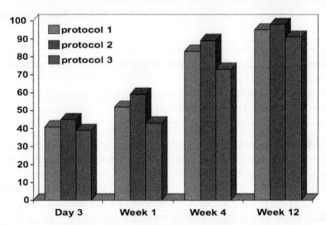

FIGURE 4.—Progress of the clinical score in displaced fractures (21-B2.1.2). (Reprinted from Paschos NK, Mitsionis GI, Vasiliadis HS, et al. Comparison of early mobilization protocols in radial head fractures. *J Orthop Trauma.* 2013;27:134-139, with permission from Lippincott Williams & Wilkins.)

displacement of more than 4 mm and an angulation of more than 30 degrees proved to impair outcome.

Conclusions.—Early mobilization of simple radial head fractures seemed to be a safe and an effective treatment option. It seems that a delay of 48 hours before early mobilization could be advantageous. Individualization of treatment in accordance to the characteristics of fracture could be a decisive factor for outcome.

Level of Evidence.—Therapeutic Level I. See Instructions for Authors for a complete description of levels of evidence. (Figs 3 and 4, Table 1).

▶ Partial articular radial head fractures (OTA/AO B2.1 or Mason 2) are fairly common injuries. It has been standard treatment for at least 30 years to avoid

TABLE 1.—Patient Demographics and Excellent/Good Score

	Protocol A	Protocol B	Protocol C	Total
Male/female	28/32	27/33	26/34	81/99
Age, yrs	37.9	35.3	36.7	36.8
Dominant hand/nondominant	31/29	32/28	30/30	93/87
Nondisplaced/displaced	40/20	38/22	38/22	116/64
Good and excellent score/total in nondisplaced	39/40	37/38	34/38	110/116
Good and excellent score/total in displaced	14/20	21/22	15/22	50/64
Good and excellent score/total	53/60	58/60	49/60	160/180

immobilization for more than 10 to 14 days to achieve optimum motion and function. This randomized comparative study addresses the question of how fast to have the patient start working on elbow range of motion. It appears that earlier is better than a week of immobilization and that 2 days of immobilization in a sling may be the optimum way to treat patients with these injuries for both displaced and nondisplaced fractures (Figs 3 and 4). This protocol should be adopted by those who treat patients with this injury (Table 1).

M. F. Swiontkowski, MD

Short- to mid-term results of metallic press-fit radial head arthroplasty in unstable injuries of the elbow

Flinkkilä T, Kaisto T, Sirniö K, et al (Oulu Univ Hosp, Finland)
J Bone Joint Surg Br 94-B:805-810, 2012

We assessed the short- to mid-term survival of metallic press-fit radial head prostheses in patients with radial head fractures and acute traumatic instability of the elbow.

The medical records of 42 patients (16 males, 26 females) with a mean age of 56 years (23 to 85) with acute unstable elbow injuries, including a fracture of the radial head requiring metallic replacement of the radial head, were reviewed retrospectively. Survival of the prosthesis was assessed from the radiographs of 37 patients after a mean follow-up of 50 months (12 to 107). The functional results of 31 patients were assessed using range-of-movement, Mayo elbow performance score (MEPS), Disabilities of the Arm, Shoulder and Hand (DASH) score and the RAND 36-item health survey.

At the most recent follow-up 25 prostheses were still well fixed, nine had been removed because of loosening, and three remained implanted but were loose. The mean time from implantation to loosening was 11 months (2 to 24). Radiolucent lines that developed around the prosthesis before removal were mild in three patients, moderate in one and severe in five. Range of movement parameters and mass grip strength were significantly lower in the affected elbow than in the unaffected side. The mean MEPS score was 86 (40 to 100) and the mean DASH score was 23 (0 to 81). According to RAND-36 scores, patients had more pain and lower physical function scores than normal population values.

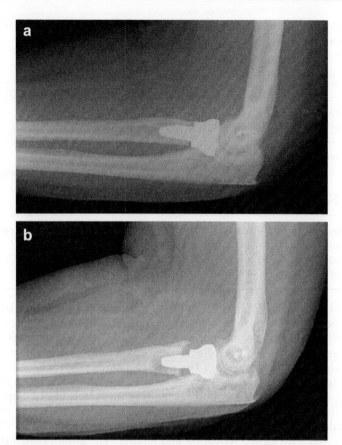

FIGURE 1.—Radiographs of a 64-year-old woman who underwent replacement of the radial head after a 'terrible triad' injury, a) three weeks post-operatively, and b) at 27 months post-operatively, showing severe osteolysis and a loose prosthesis, which was subsequently removed as a result of pain and crepitus. (Reprinted from Flinkkilä T, Kaisto T, Sirniö K, et al. Short- to mid-term results of metallic press-fit radial head arthroplasty in unstable injuries of the elbow. *J Bone Joint Surg Br.* 2012;94-B:805-810, with permission from British Editorial Society of Bone and Joint Surgery.)

TABLE 1.—Range-of-Movement Measurements in the Affected and Unaffected Elbows

Mean Range of Movement (°) (Range)	Affected	Unaffected	*p*-Value*
Flexion arc	117 (75 to 155)	150 (140 to 160)	< 0.01
Flexion	136 (90 to 160)	149 (140 to 155)	< 0.01
Extension	20 (−10 to 40)	0 (−10 to 5)	< 0.01
Forearm rotation arc	148 (45 to 180)	150 (140 to 160)	< 0.01
Pronation	75 (20 to 90)	88 (80 to 90)	< 0.01
Supination	73 (0 to 90)	84 (70 to 90)	< 0.01

*Paired *t*-test.

Loosening of press-fit radial head prostheses is common, occurs early, often leads to severe osteolysis of the proximal radius, and commonly requires removal of the prosthesis (Fig 1, Table 1).

▶ This is a carefully conducted outcome study of patients treated with press fit radial head prostheses for significant radial head fractures associated with elbow instability. The results are concerning, with early failure occurring in one third requiring early removal. The functional outcomes from these severe injuries were far from acceptable (Table 1). Continued research into surgical techniques to improve the outcomes after these injuries is justified.

M. F. Swiontkowski, MD

Tibia Fractures

Open Reduction and Intramedullary Nail Fixation of Closed Tibial Fractures
Bishop JA, Dikos GD, Mickelson D, et al (Stanford Univ School of Medicine, Redwood City, CA; Ortholndy, Indianapolis, IN; Univ of Washington, Seattle)
Orthopedics 35:e1631-e1634, 2012

Some tibial shaft fractures cannot be accurately reduced using closed or percutaneous techniques during an intramedullary nailing procedure. Under these circumstances, a formal open reduction can be performed. Direct exposure of the fracture facilitates accurate reduction but does violate the soft tissue envelope. The purpose of this study was to evaluate the safety and efficacy of open reduction prior to intramedullary nailing.

Using the trauma database at a Level I trauma center, 11 uncomplicated closed displaced tibia fractures treated with formal open reduction prior to intramedullary nailing were identified and matched with a cohort of 21 fractures treated with closed reduction and nailing. The authors attempted to match 2 controls to each patient to improve the power of the study. Clinical and radiographic outcomes were compared. All fractures ultimately healed within 5° of anatomic alignment. No infections or nonunions occurred in the open reduction group, and 1 deep infection and 1 nonunion occurred in the closed reduction group. No significant differences existed between the study groups.

Although closed reduction and intramedullary nailing remains the treatment of choice for most significantly displaced tibial shaft fractures, open reduction with respectful handling of the soft tissue envelope can be safe and effective and should be considered when less invasive techniques are unsuccessful (Tables 1 and 2).

▶ Closed reduction and interlocking nail fixation can be technically difficult on occasion. This is generally related to the fracture pattern or soft tissue interposition, which prevents realignment of the fracture surfaces with manipulation. A general rule of thumb is that if you cannot reduce the fracture adequately with manual force, and placing percutaneous manipulation pins in both fragments does not allow realignment, then a limited-incision open reduction is a wise

TABLE 1.—Baseline Demographic Characteristics of Cases and Controls Demonstrating No Significant Difference Between Groups

Variable	Open Reduction(n = 11)	Closed Reduction(n = 21)	P
Mean age(range), y	38.2 (16-56)	37.6 (15-53)	.90
No. of men	8	15	.938
No. of smokers	5	10	.981
No. of diabetes mellitus	0	0	N/A

Abbreviation: N/A, not applicable.

TABLE 2.—Outcomes of Surgical of Surgical Treatment in Case and Control Groups

		No.		
Variable	Open Reduction (n = 11)		Closed Reduction (n = 21)	P
Infection			1	.478
Nonunion	0		1	.444
Malunion	0		0	N/A

Abbreviation: N/A, not applicable.

choice. This is a matched cohort series from a busy level-one center that confirms that these limited incisions do not place the patient at additional risk. The rule of thumb should continue. Stated another way, 15 to 20 inches of struggling should prompt the small incision to remove barriers to reduction and allow direct reduction techniques.

M. F. Swiontkowski, MD

Functional Impact of Tibial Malrotation Following Intramedullary Nailing of Tibial Shaft Fractures

Theriault B, Turgeon AF, Pelet S (CHA-Hôpital de l'Enfant-Jésus, Québec, Canada)
J Bone Joint Surg Am 94:2033-2039, 2012

Background.—Tibial malrotation is a complication that is seen in approximately 30% of patients following locked intramedullary nailing. In this cohort study, we evaluated the hypothesis that tibial malrotation would lead to impaired functional outcomes.

Methods.—Patients with a unilateral tibial shaft fracture who were managed with intramedullary nailing between 2003 and 2007 were identified with use of ICD-10 (International Classification of Diseases, 10th Revision) codes. After institutional review board approval and written informed consent had been obtained, specific assessment of eligible patients was achieved with use of computed tomography, functional measures (Lower Extremity Functional Scale, Olerud-Molander Score, six-minute walk test), and physical examination. Measures were compared between patients

TABLE 1.—Functional Outcomes in the Groups with and without Malrotation*

Variable	Tibial Rotation ≥10° (N = 29)	Tibial Rotation <10° (N = 41)	P Value
LEFS *(points)*	70.8 ± 8.6	72.6 ± 8.7	0.41
Olerud-Molander *(points)*	76.6 ± 20.0	83.2 ± 19.0	0.18
Six-minute walk test *(m)*	566.0 ± 76.8	583.6 ± 86.3	0.38

*The values are given as the mean and the standard deviation.

with and without tibial malrotation (defined as tibial rotation of ≥10°) on imaging studies.

Results.—Of the 288 patients who were identified, 100 were eligible for the study and seventy consented to participate. The mean duration of follow-up (and standard deviation) for these seventy patients was 58 ± 11 months. Twenty-nine patients (41%) had tibial malrotation. Lower Extremity Functional Scale scores were similar between the groups with and without malrotation (mean, 70.8 ± 8.6 points compared with 72.6 ± 8.7 points; $p = 0.41$). The results for the other functional tests were also similar.

Conclusions.—Despite high rates of tibial malrotation following locked intramedullary nailing of isolated tibial diaphyseal fractures, this finding does not have a significant intermediate-term functional impact (Table 1).

► Tibial malrotation following closed intramedullary interlocking nailing is very common, involving 20% to 30% of patients. This is because the reduction is done closed without direct visualization of the fracture site. Most often the rotation is external but can be internal. This cohort study demonstrates that on a population basis, this malrotation does not necessarily impact the patient's functional outcome. This information will directly benefit clinicians who must discuss asymmetric rotation noted by themselves or their patients in terms of its implication on patient function. It will be very helpful in the decision-making surrounding early return to the operating room to correct the deformity. This can be very difficult to perform and is rarely successful without removal of the nail and further overreaming before reinsertion of the nail.

M. F. Swiontkowski, MD

A Comparison of Two Approaches for the Closed Treatment of Low-Energy Tibial Fractures in Children
Silva M, Eagan MJ, Wong MA, et al (Los Angeles Orthopaedic Hosp, CA; Univ of California, Los Angeles)
J Bone Joint Surg Am 94:1853-1860, 2012

Background.—Many orthopaedic surgeons treat tibial shaft fractures in children with a period of non-weight-bearing after application of a long leg cast, presumably to prevent fracture angulation and shortening. We hypothesized that allowing children to immediately bear weight as tolerated in a cast with the knee in 10° of flexion would lessen disability, without increasing the risk of unacceptable shortening or angulation.

Methods.—We divided eighty-one children, between the ages of four and fourteen years, with a low-energy, closed tibial shaft fracture into two groups. One group (forty children) received a long leg cast with the knee flexed 60° and were asked not to bear weight. The second group (forty-one children) received a long leg cast with the knee flexed 10° and were encouraged to bear weight as tolerated. All patients were switched to short leg walking casts at four weeks. We compared time to healing, overall alignment, shortening, and physical disability as determined by the Activities Scale for Kids-Performance (ASK-P) questionnaire.

Results.—The mean time to fracture union was 10.8 weeks in both groups ($p = 0.47$). At the time of healing, mean coronal alignment was within 1.3° in both groups, mean sagittal alignment was within 1°, and mean shortening was <0.5 mm, with no significant differences. The ASK-P scores showed that both groups had overall improvement in physical

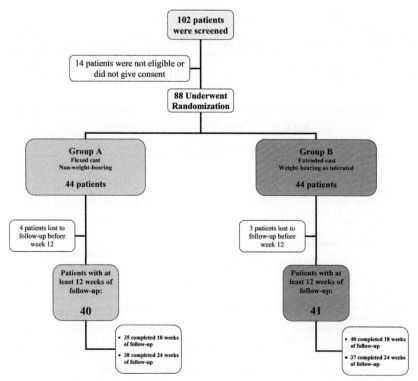

FIGURE 1.—Patient distribution in this study. (Reprinted from Silva M, Eagan MJ, Wong MA, et al. A comparison of two approaches for the closed treatment of low-energy tibial fractures in children. *J Bone Joint Surg Am.* 2012;94:1853-1860, with permission from The Journal of Bone and Joint Surgery, Incorporated.)

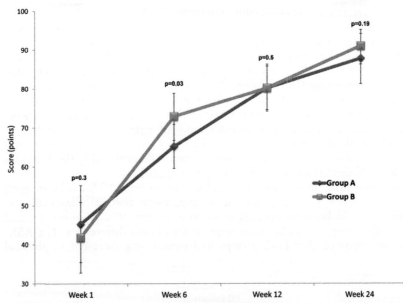

FIGURE 2.—The mean total scores (and 95% confidence intervals) on the Activities Scale for Kids-Performance (ASK-P) questionnaire. The patients in Group B showed greater functional improvement than those in Group A at six weeks after the fracture ($p = 0.03$). (Reprinted from Silva M, Eagan MJ, Wong MA, et al. A comparison of two approaches for the closed treatment of low-energy tibial fractures in children. *J Bone Joint Surg Am.* 2012;94:1853-1860, with permission from The Journal of Bone and Joint Surgery, Incorporated.)

TABLE 1.—Fracture Alignment and Shortening

	Group A* (N = 40)	Group B* (N = 41)	P Value
Prereduction radiographs			
Coronal plane angulation (varus or valgus)	$1.3° \pm 2.65°$ (0° to 14.4°)	$2.21° \pm 2.64°$ (0° to 13.0°)	0.13
Sagittal plane angulation (procurvatum or recurvatum)	$0.7° \pm 1.0°$ (0° to 4.0°)	$1.8° \pm 2.84°$ (0° to 12.2°)	0.02
Shortening (*mm*)	0.5 ± 0.97 (0 to 3.6)	1.4 ± 2.42 (0 to 9.2)	0.02
Postreduction radiographs			
Coronal plane angulation (varus or valgus)	$1.2° \pm 1.7°$ (−0 to 5.7°)	$1.64° \pm 2.0°$ (0° to 9.5°)	0.26
Sagittal plane angulation (procurvatum or recurvatum)	$1.1° \pm 1.6°$ (0° to 5.2°)	$1.3° \pm 2.4°$ (0° to 10.2°)	0.62
Shortening (*mm*)	0.6 ± 1.0 (0 to 3.0)	1.2 ± 2.78 (0 to 14.1)	0.22
Radiographs at the time of union			
Coronal plane angulation (varus or valgus)	$1.26° \pm 1.9°$ (0° to 5.7°)	$1.2° \pm 1.7°$ (0° to 5.0°)	0.93
Sagittal plane angulation (procurvatum or recurvatum)	$1.0° \pm 1.7°$ (0° to 6.0°)	$0.6° \pm 1.3°$ (0° to 5.0°)	0.2
Shortening (*mm*)	0.1 ± 0.5 (0 to 3.0)	0.5 ± 2.2 (0 to 12.2)	0.2

*The data are given as the mean and the standard deviation, with the range in parentheses.

functioning over time. However, at six weeks, the children who were allowed to bear weight as tolerated had better overall scores ($p = 0.03$) and better standing skills ($p = 0.01$) than those who were initially instructed to be non-weight-bearing.

Conclusions.—Children with low-energy tibial shaft fractures can be successfully managed by immobilizing the knee in 10° of flexion and encouraging early weight-bearing, without affecting the time to union or increasing the risk of angulation and shortening at the fracture site (Figs 1 and 2, Table 1).

▶ This is a well-done controlled trial comparing 2 methods of managing low-energy tibia fractures in children. The outcome measurements are important to both treating physicians and patients and parents: tibial alignment and function. We can safely conclude that weight bearing as tolerated with slight knee flexion is a safe way to manage children with these common fractures. There is no doubt based on the trial design (Fig 1) and the outcomes (Fig 2, Table 1) that this is an equivalent method to the traditional non—weight-bearing strategy.

M. F. Swiontkowski, MD

Upper Extremity: Pediatrics

Postoperative Radiographs After Pinning of Supracondylar Humerus Fractures: Are They Necessary?

Karamitopoulos MS, Dean E, Littleton AG, et al (Alfred I. duPont Hosp for Children, Wilmington, DE)
J Pediatr Orthop 32:672-674, 2012

Background.—The purpose of this study was to evaluate the necessity of early postoperative radiographs after pinning of supracondylar humerus fractures by determining both the percentage of patients who displayed change in fracture fixation and whether these changes affected their outcome.

Methods.—A series of 643 consecutive patients who underwent operative management of Gartland type II and III fractures at our institution between January 2002 and December 2010 were reviewed. Demographic data were obtained through chart review, including age, sex, extremity, fracture type, and mechanism. Intraoperative fluoroscopic images were compared with postoperative radiographs to identify changes in fracture alignment and pin placement.

Results.—A total of 643 patients (320 females, 323 males) with a mean age of 6.1 years (range, 1.1 to 16.0) were reviewed. Fifty-seven percent of fractures were classified as type II and 43% were type III. The overall complication rate was 8.8% (57/643). Pin backout or fracture translation was seen in 32 patients (4.9%) at the first postoperative visit. All of these patients sustained type III fractures. One of these patients required further operative management. Patients with changes in pin or fracture alignment did not demonstrate a statistically significant difference in time to first postoperative visit ($P = 0.23$), days to pin removal ($P = 0.07$), or average follow-up time ($P = 0.10$). Fracture severity did not correlate with change in alignment ($P = 0.952$). No postoperative neurological complications were observed in patients with alignment changes.

Conclusions.—Mild alignment changes and pin migration observed in postoperative radiographs after pinning of supracondylar humerus fractures have little effect on clinical management parameters or long-term sequelae. Radiographs can therefore be deferred until the time of pin removal provided adequate intraoperative stability was obtained.

Level of Evidence.—Level IV.

▶ In this era of examining all extraneous sources of waste, the question of the impact of postoperative radiographs is pertinent. In children with this very common fracture, there is the additional issue of radiation exposure. We would not want to expose children to additional radiation if there are no clinical decisions impacted by the radiograph. Although a retrospective analysis, this study makes the point that we do not change what we do based on these radiographs in the case of pinning of supracondylar humerus fractures. Therefore, unless there is a marked change in the clinical situation such as new trauma, the postoperative radiographs are unnecessary. I agree with their analysis of the data and with their conclusions. We need more studies like this to decrease the number of unnecessary imaging studies.

M. F. Swiontkowski, MD

Re-displacement of stable distal both-bone forearm fractures in children: A randomised controlled multicentre trial

Colaris JW, Allema JH, Biter LU, et al (Erasmus Med Ctr, Rotterdam, The Netherlands; Haga Ziekenhuis, Den Haag, The Netherlands; Sint Franciscus Ziekenhuis, Rotterdam, The Netherlands; et al)

Injury 44:498-503, 2013

Introduction.—Displaced metaphyseal both-bone fractures of the distal forearm are generally reduced and stabilised by an above-elbow cast (AEC) with or without additional pinning. The purpose of this study was to find out if re-displacement of a reduced stable metaphyseal both-bone fracture of the distal forearm in a child could be prevented by stabilisation with Kirschner wires.

Methods.—Consecutive children aged < 16 years with a displaced metaphyseal both-bone fracture of the distal forearm ($n = 128$) that was stable after reduction were randomised to AEC with or without percutaneous fixation with Kirschner wires. The primary outcome was re-displacement of the fracture.

Results.—A total of 67 children were allocated to fracture reduction and AEC and 61 to reduction of the fracture, fixation with Kirschner wires and AEC. The follow-up rate was 96% with a mean follow-up of 7.1 months.

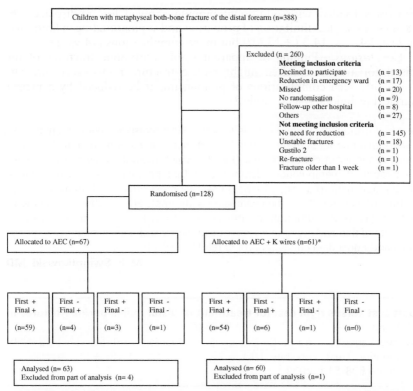

FIGURE 2.—Flowchart of enrolment in the study. (Reprinted from the Injury, International Journal of the Care of the Injured. Colaris JW, Allema JH, Biter LU, et al. Re-displacement of stable distal both-bone forearm fractures in children: A randomised controlled multicentre trial. *Injury.* 2013;44:498-503, Copyright 2013, with permission from Elsevier.)

TABLE 2.—Data on the Outcomes

	AEC n = 67	K Wires + AEC n = 61
Re-displacement (%)*	44.8	8.2
Days in cast	33.4 (±8.8)	32.2 (±6.1)
Days until first clinical examination	68.4 (±25.4)	69.7 (±28.5)
Days until final clinical examination	216.3 (±49.1)	215.5 (±47.2)
Referral to physiotherapy (%)	54.5	35.6
Number of visits to physiotherapy	3.9 (±7.3)	2.6 (±6.1)
Limitation of wrist flexion—extension of the fractured arm, degrees	4.4 (±6.2)	3.8 (±7.4)
Limitation of elbow flexion—extension of the fractured arm, degrees	0.5 (±2.0)	0.2 (±2.1)
VAS cosmetics fractured arm by parents	8.5 (±1.8)	8.0 (±2.2)
VAS cosmetics fractured arm by orthopaedic surgeon	8.9 (±1.2)	8.4 (±1.3)
Total ABILHAND score at final clinical examination	41.5 (±1.6)	41.9 (±0.4)

Values are presented as mean (±standard deviation) unless stated otherwise. AEC: above elbow cast; K wires: Kirschner wires; VAS: visual analogue scale.
*Significant difference ($p < 0.0001$).

Fractures treated with additional pinning showed less re-displacement (8% vs. 45%), less limitation of pronation and supination (mean limitation 6.9 ($\pm$9.4)° vs. 14.3 ($\pm$13.6)°) but more complications (14 vs. 1).

Conclusions.—Pinning of apparent stable both-bone fractures of the distal forearm in children might reduce fracture re-displacement. The frequently seen complications of pinning might be reduced by a proper surgical technique (Fig 2, Table 2).

▶ Most orthopedic surgeons have experienced a redisplacement of a metaphyseal both-bone forearm fracture in a child that required a reduction. This well-done randomized controlled trial (Fig 2), which included only those fractures that required manipulation, demonstrates that percutaneous K-wire fixation as a supplement to an above-elbow cast will most often result in maintenance of the original reduction when compared with simple above-elbow cast immobilization (Table 2). Although this practice will likely be slow to be adopted, the strength of this evidence should move us toward this change in treatment strategy until additional data either confirm or refute these findings.

M. F. Swiontkowski, MD

Soft cast versus rigid cast for treatment of distal radius buckle fractures in children

Witney-Lagen C, Smith C, Walsh G (Calderdale and Huddersfield NHS Foundation Trust, Yorkshire, UK)
Injury 44:508-513, 2013

Introduction.—Buckle fractures are extremely common and their optimum management is still under debate. This study aimed to ascertain whether buckle fractures of the distal radius can be safely and effectively treated in soft cast with only a single orthopaedic outpatient clinic appointment.

Methods.—A total of 232 children with buckle fractures of the distal radius were included in the study. 111 children with 112 distal radius fractures were treated in full rigid cast and 121 children with 123 fractures were treated with soft cast. The rigid cast children attended outpatient clinic for removal of cast at 3 weeks. Soft casts were removed by parents unwinding the cast at home after 3 weeks. Follow-up was conducted prospectively by telephone questionnaire at an average of 6 weeks post-injury.

Results.—Outcome data were available for 117 children treated in soft cast and for 102 children treated in rigid cast. The most common mechanism of injury was a fall sustained from standing or running, followed by falls from bikes and then trampoline accidents. Overall, both groups recovered well. Overall satisfaction with the outcome of treatment was 97.4% in soft cast and 95.2% in rigid cast. Casts were reported as comfortable by 95.7% in soft cast and 93.3% in rigid cast. Cast changes were required for 6.8% of soft casts and 11.5% of rigid casts. The most frequent cause for changing rigid casts was getting the cast wet. None of the improved scores seen in the soft cast group were statistically significant. No re-fractures

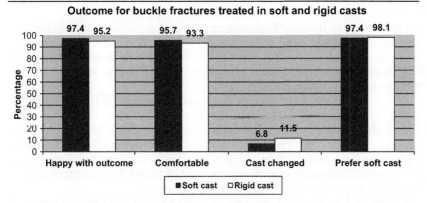

FIGURE.—Outcome for buckle fractures treated in soft and rigid casts. (Reprinted from the Injury, International Journal of the Care of the Injured. Witney-Lagen C, Smith C, Walsh G. Soft cast versus rigid cast for treatment of distal radius buckle fractures in children. *Injury.* 2013;44:508-513, Copyright 2013, with permission from Elsevier.)

were seen in either group. Nearly all (94.9%) children in soft cast did bathe, shower or swim in their cast. Parents of both groups preferred treatment with soft cast (*p* < 0.001). Reasons given for preferring the soft cast included the ability to get the cast wet, avoidance of the plaster saw and not having to take time off work to attend a follow-up visit for cast removal.

Conclusion.—Buckle fractures of the distal radius can be safely and effectively treated in soft cast with only a single orthopaedic outpatient clinic appointment (Fig).

▶ The orthopedic community has long been guilty of overtreating distal radial buckle fractures in children. This sequential outcome study comparing the outcomes and ease of treatment for rigid cast immobilization demonstrates that a limited period of immobilization in a soft cast provides basically identical results to rigid cast immobilization for lower cost and less exposure to radiation from radiographs with greater parental satisfaction (Fig). Short-term immobilization in a soft cast should be standard treatment with the exception of children at high risk for reinjury in the period immediately after immobilization.

M. F. Swiontkowski, MD

Below-elbow cast for metaphyseal both-bone fractures of the distal forearm in children: A randomised multicentre study

Colaris JW, Biter LU, Allema JH, et al (Erasmus Med Ctr, Rotterdam, The Netherlands; Sint Franciscus Hosp, Rotterdam, The Netherlands; HAGA Hosp, The Hague, The Netherlands; et al)
Injury 43:1107-1111, 2012

Introduction.—Minimally displaced metaphyseal both-bone fractures of the distal forearm in children are often treated with an above-elbow cast (AEC). Treatment with a below-elbow cast (BEC) could give more comfort, but might lead to fracture displacement reducing pronation and supination. Because this has not been systematically investigated, we set up a randomised multicentre study. The purpose of this study was to find out whether BEC causes equal limitation of pronation and supination but with higher comfort level, compared with AEC.

Patients and Methods.—In four hospitals, consecutive children aged < 16 (mean 7.1) years with a minimally displaced metaphyseal both-bone fracture of the distal forearm were randomised to 4 weeks BEC ($n = 35$) or 4 weeks AEC ($n = 31$). Primary outcome was limitation of pronation and supination 6 months after initial trauma. The secondary outcomes were cast comfort, limitation of flexion/extension of wrist/elbow, complications, cosmetics, complaints, and radiological assessment.

Results.—A group of 35 children received BEC and 31 children received AEC. All children attended for the final examination at a mean follow-up of 7.0 months (range 5.0–11.6 months). Limitation of pronation and supination 6 months after initial trauma showed no significant difference between the two groups [4.4° (±5.8) for BEC and 5.8° (±9.8) for AEC]. Children treated with BEC had significantly higher cast comfort on a visual analogue scale [5.6 (±2.7) vs. 8.4 (±1.4)] and needed significantly less help with dressing (8.2 days vs. 15.1 days). Six complications occurred in the BEC group and 14 in the AEC group. Other secondary outcomes were similar between the two groups.

Conclusions.—Children with minimally displaced metaphyseal both-bone fractures of the distal forearm should be treated with a below-elbow cast (Tables 3 and 5).

▶ Although small in terms of the numbers of subjects randomized, this carefully conducted randomized, controlled trial provides us with the answer that below-

TABLE 3.—Limitation of Pronation and Supination of Fractured Arm

	BEC	AEC
Two months after the fracture		
None	15	10
1–10°	10	8
11–20°	3	6
21–30°	3	2
>31°	3	3
Total	34	29
Mean limitation/SD (°)	9.1 (±12.2)*	10.7 (±12.2)*
Six months after the fracture		
None	17	18
1–10°	14	7
11–20°	4	3
21–30°	0	2
>31°	0	1
Total	35	31
Mean limitation in degrees (SD)	4.4 (±5.8)*	5.8 (±9.8)*

BEC: below-elbow cast; AEC: above-elbow cast; SD = standard deviation.
Data are presented as numbers (unless otherwise indicated).
Three children missed the two-month examination.
*No significant difference in mean limitation of pronation and supination between both groups.

TABLE 5.—Data on Radiological Outcomes

| | Below-Elbow Cast | | | Above-Elbow Cast | | |
	Trauma	Removal of Cast	Final Clinical Examination	Trauma	Removal of Cast	Final Clinical Examination
AP ulna	6.5 (±4.1)[2]	5.5 (±4.2)	3.3 (±2.6)[2]	6.7 (±4.3)[2]	6.6 (±4.0)	4.4 (±3.1)[2]
AP radius	3.5 (±2.8)	4.0 (±3.8)	2.3 (+2.7)	4.2 (±3.3)[2]	4.3 (⊥4.2)	2.8 (±2.6)[2]
Lateral ulna	6.9 (±4.8)[2]	4.3 (±3.3)	3.3 (±2.6)[2]	7.9 (±5.4)[12]	5.8 (±4.7)[1]	4.0 (±3.2)[2]
Lateral radius	9.0 (±4.9)[12]	11.4 (±6.9)[1]	4.8 (±3.4)[2]	8.7 (±5.0)[12]	12.2 (±5.8)[1]	6.3 (±5.0)[2]

Radioulnar angulations: anteroposterior (AP) ulna, AP radius; and sagittal angulations (lateral ulna, lateral radius) presented in degrees as mean (±standard deviation).
No significant differences between below-elbow cast and above-elbow cast groups.
Significant differences (*p*-value < 0.05) were found between [1]trauma radiographs and radiographs removal of cast and [2]radiographs final examination.

elbow casting is adequate to maintain alignment for pediatric both-bone forearm fractures involving the metaphysis. Readers must be careful to limit these findings to those fractures, length stable, in the metaphysis. The radiographic and functional outcome data were no different, which allows us to use the less encumbering form of immobilization to the benefit of patients and their parents alike.

M. F. Swiontkowski, MD

Natural History of Unreduced Gartland Type-II Supracondylar Fractures of the Humerus in Children: A Two to Thirteen-Year Follow-up Study

Moraleda L, Valencia M, Barco R, et al (Hospital Universitario La Paz, Madrid, Spain)
J Bone Joint Surg Am 95:28-34, 2013

Background.—The preferred treatment of type-II supracondylar humeral fractures remains controversial. The purpose of this study was to evaluate the long-term clinical and radiographic outcome of type-II supracondylar humeral fractures in children treated with immobilization in a splint without reduction.

Methods.—The medical records of forty-six consecutive patients who sustained a supracondylar Gartland type-II fracture of the humerus treated with immobilization in a splint were reviewed. Age at the time of fracture, sex, side involved, dominant extremity, duration of immobilization, and complications were recorded. Radiographic assessment included the Baumann angle, carrying angle, and lateral humerocapitellar angle. Patients returned for clinical evaluation, and the Mayo Elbow Performance Score and the criteria of Flynn et al. were recorded. Patients completed the Quick-DASH, an abbreviated form of the Disabilities of the Arm, Shoulder and Hand questionnaire, to measure disability.

Results.—The average age (and standard deviation) at the time of fracture was 5.5 ± 2.6 years. The average duration of follow-up was 6.6 ± 2.8 years. The initial lateral humerocapitellar angle was a mean of

TABLE 1.—Range of Motion and Alignment

	Injured Side* (deg)	Uninjured Side* (deg)	P Value
Flexion	137.9 ± 9.1	144.8 ± 7.1	<0.001[†]
Extension	13.2 ± 5.9	7.4 ± 5.1	<0.001[†]
Total flexion-extension	153.8 ± 9.5	152.2 ± 8.1	0.083
Pronation	80.7 ± 4.6	81.7 ± 3.6	0.06
Supination	82.9 ± 3.5	83.2 ± 2.9	0.42
Carrying angle	+9 ± 8.1	+12.1 ± 4.9	0.003[†]

*The values are given as the mean and the standard deviation.
[†]Significant.

TABLE 2.—Clinical Results in Forty-six Patients

Parameter*	Result
Pain (no. of patients)	7 (15.2%)
Instability (no. of patients)	3 (6.5%)
QuickDASH[†]	10 ± 15.3
QuickDASH-Sports[†]	4.7 ± 12.2
MEPS[†]	95.6 ± 10.5
Flynn criteria (no. of patients)	
Excellent	26 (56.5%)
Good	11 (23.9%)
Fair	3 (6.5%)
Poor	6 (13%)
Clinical instability	3 (6.5%)

*DASH = Disabilities of the Arm, Shoulder and Hand questionnaire, and MEPS = Mayo Elbow Performance Score.
[†]The values are given as the mean and the standard deviation.

12.8° ± 9.8°, the mean Baumann angle was 12° ± 5.7°, and the mean radiographic carrying angle was 9° ± 11.3°. There were significant differences between injured and uninjured elbows at the time of follow-up with regard to flexion (mean, 137.9° ± 9.1° for injured and 144.8° ± 7.1° for uninjured elbows; $p < 0.001$), extension (mean, 13.2° ± 5.9° for injured and 7.4° ± 5.1° for uninjured elbows; $p < 0.001$), clinical carrying angle (mean, 9° ± 8.1° for injured and 12.1° ± 4.9° for uninjured elbows; $p = 0.003$), radiographic carrying angle (mean, 8.9° ± 8.1° for injured and 14.2° ± 5.5° for uninjured elbows; $p < 0.001$), and lateral humerocapitellar angle (mean, 30.5° ± 11° for injured and 41.9° ± 9.9° for uninjured elbows; $p < 0.001$). The mean score was 10 ± 15.3 points for the QuickDASH questionnaire, 4.7 ± 12.2 points for the QuickDASH-sports questionnaire, and 95.6 ± 10.5 for the Mayo Elbow Performance Score. According to the Flynn criteria, results were satisfactory in 80.4% of the patients.

Conclusions.—Patients with a type-II supracondylar fracture of the humerus treated conservatively had a mild cubitus varus deformity and a mild increase in elbow extension, although functional results were excellent in the majority of patients (Tables 1-3).

▶ Clinical decision making regarding type 2 supracondylar humerus fractures in children remains a bit of a dilemma. To reduce and pin the fracture by flexing the

TABLE 3.—Radiographic Results

	Injured Side*	Uninjured Side*	P Value
Lateral humerocapitellar angle (*deg*)	30.5 ± 11	41.9 ± 9.9	<0.001[†]
Baumann angle (*deg*)	12.8 ± 7.5	17.1 ± 7.3	0.007[†]
Carrying angle (*deg*)	8.9 ± 8.1	14.2 ± 5.5	<0.001[†]

*The values are given as the mean and the standard deviation.
[†]Significant.

elbow seems straightforward but is not without risk of negatively impacting the outcome. This retrospective report gives us the parameters of what we can discuss with parents regarding the option of conservative care with immobilization. We can now weigh the decision to intervene with reduction pinning vs immobilization in situ with a strong understanding of the minor degree of hyperextension and varus deformity that is likely to occur.

M. F. Swiontkowski, MD

The Efficacy of Intra-Articular Injections for Pain Control Following the Closed Reduction and Percutaneous Pinning of Pediatric Supracondylar Humeral Fractures: A Randomized Controlled Trial

Georgopoulos G, Carry P, Pan Z, et al (Children's Hosp Colorado, Aurora)
J Bone Joint Surg Am 94:1633-1642, 2012

Background.—The purpose of this single-blinded, randomized, controlled trial was to compare the analgesic efficacy of intra-articular injections of bupivacaine or ropivacaine with that of no injection for postoperative pain control after the operative treatment of supracondylar humeral fractures in a pediatric population.

Methods.—Subjects (n = 124) were randomized to treatment with 0.25% bupivacaine (Group B) (n = 42), 0.20% ropivacaine (Group R) (n = 39), or no injection (Group C) (n = 43). The opioid doses and the times of administration as well as child-reported pain severity (Faces Pain Scale-Revised) and parent-reported pain severity (Total Quality Pain Management survey) were recorded.

Results.—The proportion of subjects who required morphine and/or fentanyl injections was significantly ($p = 0.004$) lower in Group B (10%) as compared with Group R (36%) and Group C (44%). On the basis of the log-rank test, the opioid-free survival rates were significantly greater in Group B as compared to Groups C and R. Total opioid consumption (morphine equivalent mg/kg) in the first seventy-two hours postoperatively was significantly less in Group B as compared with Group C (mean difference, 0.225; [95% confidence interval (CI), 0.0152 to 0.435]; $p = 0.036$). Parent-reported pain scores were also significantly lower in Group B as compared with both Group C (mean difference, 1.81 [95% CI, 0.38 to

3.25]; $p = 0.014$) and Group R (mean difference, 1.66; 95% CI, 0.20 to 3.12; $p = 0.027$). There were no significant differences across the three groups in terms of self-reported pain. Differences between Groups R and C were not significant for any of the outcome variables.

Conclusions.—The intra-articular injection of 0.25% bupivacaine significantly improves postoperative pain control following the closed reduction and percutaneous pinning of supracondylar humeral fractures in pediatric patients.

Level of Evidence.—Therapeutic Level I. See Instructions for Authors for a complete description of levels of evidence (Figs 1 and 2, Table 1).

▶ This very well done randomized clinical trial confirms that postfixation aspiration of intraarticular hematoma and injection of ropivacaine is safe and effective in improving postoperative pain in children undergoing percutaneous reduction and fixation of supracondylar humerus fractures. The differences are clinically meaningful. Let us hope that it does not take 10 years for this practice to be widely

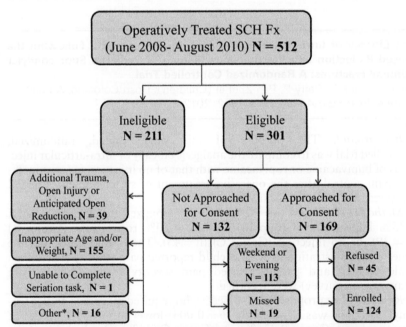

*Other category includes following reasons: operating surgeon was not a co-investigator (n = 3), study materials were not available in subjects' primary language (n = 10), revision pinning (n=1), legal guardian was not present for consent (n = 1) and injury occurred > 7 days prior to surgery (n = 1).

FIGURE 1.—Summary of enrollment. SCH Fx = supracondylar humeral fracture. (Reprinted from Georgopoulos G, Carry P, Pan Z, et al. The efficacy of intra-articular injections for pain control following the closed reduction and percutaneous pinning of pediatric supracondylar humeral fractures: a randomized controlled trial. *J Bone Joint Surg Am.* 2012;94:1633-1642, with permission from The Journal of Bone and Joint Surgery, Incorporated.)

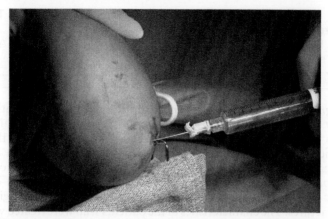

FIGURE 2.—Intra-articular injection of local anesthesia was given once the joint had been successfully aspirated. The intra-articular injections were performed with a 20-gauge needle through either an olecranon fossa or lateral approach. (Reprinted from Georgopoulos G, Carry P, Pan Z, et al. The efficacy of intra-articular injections for pain control following the closed reduction and percutaneous pinning of pediatric supracondylar humeral fractures: a randomized controlled trial. *J Bone Joint Surg Am.* 2012;94:1633-1642, with permission from The Journal of Bone and Joint Surgery, Incorporated.)

TABLE 1.—Demographic Data and Clinical Characteristics

	Control (N = 43)	Ropivacaine (N = 39)	Bupivacaine (N = 42)	P Value
Age* *(yr)*	6.92 ± 1.99	6.73 ± 2.21	6.86 yr ± 1.74	0.6719
Sex *(percentage of patients)*				0.9614
M	58.1%	53.8%	57.1%	
F	41.9%	46.2%	42.9%	
Fracture type *(percentage of patients)*				0.3705
Flexion	0.0%	0.0%	2.4%	
II	62.8%	46.2%	54.8%	
III	37.2%	53.8%	42.9%	
Time from initial injury to surgery *(percentage of patients)*				0.8315
<24 hr	83.72%	76.92%	78.57%	
24 to 48 hr	9.30%	10.26%	14.29%	
>48 hr	6.98%	12.82%	7.14%	
No. of pins* *(percentage of patients)*	2.40 ± 0.54	2.49 ± 0.56	2.63 ± 0.58	0.1483
Pin configuration *(percentage of patients)*				0.8346
Lateral or medial only	93.02%	94.87%	90.24%	
Lateral and medial	6.98%	5.13%	9.76%	
Preop. pain score* *(points)*	2.72 ± 2.75	2.84 ± 2.85	2.93 ± 3.03	0.9523
Preop. opioids* *(morphine equivalent mg/kg)*	0.02 ± 0.04	0.02 ± 0.04	0.04 ± 0.06	0.3130
Operative time* *(min)*	29.16 ± 10.07	30.85 ± 12.28	28.19 ± 8.68	0.6969
Intraop. opioids* *(morphine equivalent mg/kg)*	0.13 ± 0.07	0.15 ± 0.09	0.13 ± 0.07	0.5024

*The values are given as the mean and the standard deviation.

accepted in the orthopedic community and that dissemination of this information is prompt and effective.

M. F. Swiontkowski, MD

Type II Supracondylar Humerus Fractures: Can Some Be Treated Nonoperatively?

Spencer HT, Dorey FJ, Zionts LE, et al (Univ of California, Los Angeles; Children's Hosp Los Angeles, CA; et al)
J Pediatr Orthop 32:675-681, 2012

Background.—The range of injury severity that can be seen within the category of type II supracondylar humerus fractures (SCHFs) raises the question whether some could be treated nonoperatively. However, the clinical difficulty in using this approach lies in determining which type II SCHFs can be managed successfully without a surgical intervention.

Methods.—We reviewed clinical and radiographic information on 259 pediatric type II SCHFs that were enrolled in a prospective registry of elbow fractures. The characteristics of the patients who were treated without surgery were compared with those of patients who were treated surgically. Treatment outcomes, as assessed by the final clinical and radiographic alignment, range of motion of the elbow, and complications, were compared between the groups to define clinical and radiographic features that related to success or failure of nonoperative management.

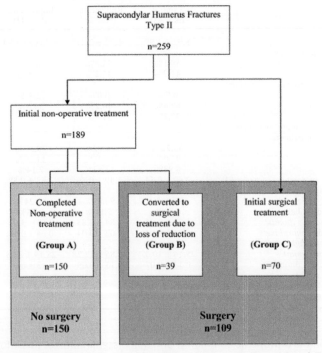

FIGURE 1.—Study population. (Reprinted from Spencer HT, Dorey FJ, Zionts LE, et al. Type II supracondylar humerus fractures: can some be treated nonoperatively? *J Pediatr Orthop.* 2012;32:675-681, with permission from Lippincott Williams & Wilkins.)

Results.—During the course of treatment, 39 fractures were found to have unsatisfactory alignment with nonoperative management and were taken for surgery. Ultimately, 150 fractures (57.9%) were treated nonoperatively, and 109 fractures (42.1%) were treated surgically. At final follow-up, outcome measures of change in carrying angle, range of motion, and complications did not show clinically significant differences between treatment groups. Fractures without rotational deformity or coronal angulation and with a shaft-condylar angle of >15 degrees were more likely to be associated with successful nonsurgical treatment. A scoring system was developed using these features to stratify the severity of the injury. Patients with isolated extension deformity, but none of the other features, were more likely to complete successful nonoperative management.

Conclusions.—This study suggests that some of the less severe pediatric type II SCHFs can be successfully treated without surgery if close follow-up is achieved. Fractures with initial rotational deformity, coronal malalignment, and significant extension of the distal fragment are likely to fail a nonoperative approach. An algorithm using the initial radiographic characteristics can aid in distinguishing groups (Figs 1 and 4, Table 5).

▶ The question of when a type 2 distal humerus fracture needs pin stabilization after reduction is relevant and one that all surgeons who treat these fractures struggle with. This is a very well-done retrospective analysis of decision factors that impact outcome. The blinded analysis of the x-rays is particularly important

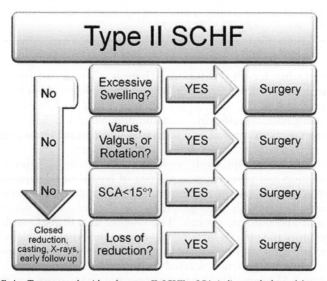

FIGURE 4.—Treatment algorithm for type II SCHFs. SCA indicates shaft-condylar angle; SCHF, supracondylar humerus fracture. (Reprinted from Spencer HT, Dorey FJ, Zionts LE, et al. Type II supracondylar humerus fractures: can some be treated nonoperatively? *J Pediatr Orthop.* 2012;32:675-681, with permission from Lippincott Williams & Wilkins.)

TABLE 5.—Multivariate Logistic Regression Analysis for Initial Treatment Groups Among the 259 Fractures Being Analyzed for Initial Treatment Decision

Initial Radiographic Features	n	Odds Ratio	SE	95% Confidence Interval	P
Rotational deformity	23	6.67	3.90	2.12-20.96	0.001
Varus malalignment	40	2.52	1.09	1.08-5.89	0.033
Valgus malalignment	27	3.10	1.50	1.20-8.03	0.020
Shaft-condylar angle < 15 degrees	49	2.96	1.19	1.35-6.52	0.007
Shaft-condylar angle < 30 degrees	140	3.48	1.36	1.62-7.49	0.001

in increasing the validity of the conclusions. Although an element of varus, valgus, or rotational malalignment prompts the question of whether these are actually type 3 fractures of low severity, the conclusions of this investigation are pragmatic and useful. The treatment diagram (Fig 4) is particularly useful and will serve as a clinical decision-making tool in the future. The most important take-home fact is that fractures with more than 15° of extension, whether accompanied by malalignment in any other plane, should be strongly considered for pin fixation after reduction. Those with less extension than that at the fracture site can be treated with reduction and splint/casting.

M. F. Swiontkowski, MD

Postoperative Pain Control After Supracondylar Humerus Fracture Fixation
Swanson CE, Chang K, Schleyer E, et al (Drexel Univ College of Medicine, Philadelphia, PA)
J Pediatr Orthop 32:452-455, 2012

Background.—Postoperative pain control in pediatric patients has become a priority for all institutions. There is a paucity of literature on pain control after orthopedic procedures in the pediatric population. The purpose of this study is to compare the efficacy of acetaminophen with narcotic analgesics, specifically, acetaminophen/codeine and morphine, for pain management after closed reduction and percutaneous pinning of displaced supracondylar humerus fractures in children.

Methods.—We retrospectively evaluated 217 patients who received closed reduction and percutaneous pinning of type II or III supracondylar humerus fractures at our institution from 2003 to 2009. Hospital charts were reviewed to obtain demographic data. Patients were divided into narcotic and non-narcotic groups. The Oucher and FLACC scales were used to quantify the effectiveness of the pain control that was delivered.

Results.—A total of 174 patients were treated with non-narcotic pain medications and 43 patients received narcotics. The average age of these patients was 5.45 years. The mean postoperative pain score for the non-narcotic group was 1.9, whereas the mean postoperative pain score for the

TABLE 1.—Medication Dosing Regimen

Analgesics	Dose
Acetaminophen	10-15 mg/kg Q4-6 h
Morphine	0.05-0.1 mg/kg Q3-4 h
Codeine	0.5-1.0 mg/kg Q4-6 h
Percocet	1-2 tabs 325 mg/5mg Q4-6 h

TABLE 2.—Pain Scores by Fracture Type

	Acetaminophen (Mean Pain Score)	Narcotic (Mean Pain Score)	
Gartland type II	1.9 (n = 77)	1.2 (n = 13)	$P = 0.20$
Gartland type III	1.9 (n = 90)	2.5 (n = 27)	$P = 0.15$
	$P = 0.99$	$P = 0.038$	

TABLE 3.—Pain Scores by Age

	Acetaminophen (Mean Pain Score)	Narcotic (Mean Pain Score)	
Below 6 yo	1.5 (n = 123)	1.9 (n = 48)	$P = 0.21$
Above 6 yo	2.3 (n = 80)	2.7 (n = 86)	$P = 0.13$
	$P = 0.0089$	$P = 0.0081$	

narcotic group was 2.2. This difference was not statistically significant. To account for the difference of age in patients and severity of fracture type, we created an age-matched cohort of patients with only type III supracondylar fractures. The average age of this group was 6.22 years. The mean pain score for the acetaminophen subgroup was 2.1 compared with a mean pain score of 2.4 for the narcotic subgroup. This difference was not statistically significant. Severe nausea or vomiting attributed to either class of medication was not observed. In addition, no patients developed a compartment syndrome.

Conclusions.—Acetaminophen is as effective as narcotic analgesics for providing pain control after supracondylar fracture surgery in children and is historically associated with fewer side effects. It is our recommendation to use acetaminophen alone for postoperative pain control in these patients.

Level of Evidence.—III (Tables 1-3).

▶ Pain control following operative management of supracondylar humeral fractures in children is an important issue. We want to minimize pain while still allowing the patient to be alert and cooperative for serial examinations to avoid missing compartmental syndrome. Although this is not a randomized trial, which would be ideal, the findings are worthy of note. Acetaminophen alone seems to be adequate for postoperative pain management in children with these injuries. This study should be followed by a randomized trial to finally confirm this effect.

M. F. Swiontkowski, MD

Upper Extremity

Predictors of Diagnosis of Ulnar Neuropathy After Surgically Treated Distal Humerus Fractures

Wiggers JK, Brouwer KM, Helmerhorst GTT, et al (Massachusetts General Hosp, Boston)
J Hand Surg 37A:1168-1172, 2012

Purpose.—Ulnar nerve dysfunction is a common sequela of surgical treatment of distal humerus fractures. This study addresses the null hypothesis that different types of distal humerus injuries have comparable rates of diagnosis of ulnar neuropathy.

Methods.—We assessed diagnosis of ulnar neuropathy in 107 consecutive adults who had a surgically treated fracture of the distal humerus followed up at least 6 months after injury. Diagnosis of ulnar neuropathy was defined as documentation of sensory and motor dysfunction of the ulnar nerve in the medical record. Fractures were categorized as either columnar fractures or fractures of the capitellum and trochlea. The explanatory (independent) variables included age, sex, fracture type, AO type, associated wound, associated elbow dislocation, mechanism of trauma, ipsilateral skeletal injury, olecranon osteotomy, implant over or below the medial epicondyle, infection, time from injury to surgery, the number of surgeries within 4 weeks and 6 months of injury, the total number of surgeries, and whether the nerve was transposed.

Results.—Postoperative ulnar neuropathy was diagnosed in 17 of 107 patients (16%), including 16 of 59 columnar fractures (21%). The only risk factor for ulnar neuropathy was columnar fracture.

Conclusions.—Patients with columnar fractures might be at higher risk for the development of postoperative ulnar neuropathy than patients with capitellum and trochlea fractures, regardless of whether the ulnar nerve was transposed.

Type of Study/Level of Evidence.—Prognostic IV.

▶ This retrospective analysis of patients with distal humerus fractures identifies C type distal humerus fractures as being the highest risk for ulnar nerve policy regardless of whether or not the nerve is transposed. This is likely due to the higher energy imparted to the distal humerus in the mechanism of injury as well as the need for greater degrees of surgical dissection to stabilize the fracture. The information is interesting but really of limited clinical use except to discuss the issue with patients prior to operative intervention, particularly where a clear exam of ulnar nerve function is not possible.

M. F. Swiontkowski, MD

Management of First-Time Dislocations of the Shoulder in Patients Older Than 40 Years: The Prevalence of Iatrogenic Fracture

Atoun E, Narvani A, Even T, et al (Royal Berkshire Hosp, Reading, UK)
J Orthop Trauma 27:190-193, 2013

Objective.—To evaluate the prevalence of iatrogenic humeral neck fracture after attempted closed reduction in patients older than 40 years who present with a first-time anterior dislocation.

Design.—Retrospective cohort study, evidence-based medicine level IV.

Patients.—Ninety-two patients older than 40 years (mean 66.6 years of age) with a first-time anterior dislocation of the shoulder.

Intervention.—Closed reductions by the emergency medicine physicians under conscious sedation, in the emergency department.

Main Outcome Measurements.—Prevalence of iatrogenic fracture on postreduction radiographs.

Results.—Nineteen (20.7%) patients were diagnosed with a concomitant greater tuberosity fracture on initial radiograph. In the postreduction radiographs, 5 patients (5.4%) were identified with a postreduction humeral neck fracture, and all of them had a greater tuberosity fracture on initial radiographs. A highly significant association ($P < 0.0001$) was observed between the finding of a greater tuberosity fracture on the initial radiographs and the occurrence of iatrogenic humeral neck fracture after close reduction.

Discussion.—Previous case reports have described an iatrogenic humeral neck fracture with reduction attempt of shoulder dislocation. In our retrospective study, 21% of the cohort of patients older than 40 years had a concomitant greater tuberosity fracture; 26% of them had an iatrogenic humeral neck fracture after reduction attempt under sedation in the emergency room. These patients ended up with poor outcome.

Conclusions.—Patients older than 40 years, presenting with a first-time anterior shoulder dislocation with an associated fracture of the greater tuberosity have a significant rate of iatrogenic humeral neck fracture during closed reduction under sedation (Table).

▶ This retrospective review paints us a cautionary tale regarding attempting closed reduction of patients over the age of 40 with anterior shoulder dislocation. Radiographic interpretation with a glenohumeral dislocation can be difficult. However, a tuberosity fracture is often seen with the most irregular x-ray beam orientation. This fracture should prompt the treating physician to use fluoroscopy for the attempted reduction and to insist on maximal muscle relaxation for the reduction maneuver.

M. F. Swiontkowski, MD

TABLE.—Patients Data - Procedures and Complications

	Sex	Age	Initial Injury	First Surgery	Complication	Second Surgery	Complication	Third Surgery
1	F	57	ADGTF	ORIF retrograde wire	AVN	CSRA	Brachial plexus injury	
2	M	46	ADGTF	ORIF retrograde wire	AVN stiffness	AR		
3	F	40	ADGTF	ORIF locking plate	Brachial artery and plexus injury, nonunion	HA	Cuff failure	RSA
4	M	48	ADGTF	HA	Tuberosities nonunion	Revision HA		
5	F	86	ADGTF	HA	Anterior dislocation	Refused		

ADGTF, Anterior Dislocation with fracture of Greater tuberosity; AR, arthroscopic release; AVN, Avascular necrosis; CSRA, Copeland surface replacement arthroplasty; F, female; HA Hemiarthroplasty; M, male; ORIF, open reduction and internal fixation; RSA, reverse shoulder arthroplasty.

External fixation versus open reduction with plate fixation for distal radius fractures: A meta-analysis of randomised controlled trials
Esposito J, Schemitsch EH, Saccone M, et al (Univ of Toronto, Ontario, Canada)
Injury 44:409-416, 2013

Background.—Both external fixation and open reduction with internal fixation (ORIF) using plates have been recommended for treatment of distal radius fractures. We conducted a systematic review and meta-analysis of randomised controlled trials comparing external fixation to ORIF.

Methods.—MEDLINE, EMBASE, and COCHRANE databases were searched from inception to January 2011 for all trials involving use of external fixation and ORIF for distal radius fractures. Eligibility for inclusion in the review was: use of random allocation of treatments; treatment arm receiving external fixation; and treatment arm receiving ORIF with plate fixation. Eligible studies were obtained and read in full by two co-authors who then

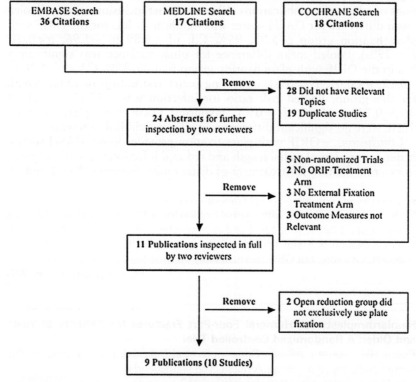

FIGURE 1.—Flow diagram of RCTs comparing open reduction internal fixation to external fixation for management of distal radius fractures. (Reprinted from the Injury, International Journal of the Care of the Injured. Esposito J, Schemitsch EH, Saccone M, et al. External fixation versus open reduction with plate fixation for distal radius fractures: a meta-analysis of randomised controlled trials. *Injury.* 2013;44:409-416, Copyright 2013, with permission from International Society for Adult Congenital Heart Disease.)

	Open Reduction with Plate			External Fixation				Mean Difference	Mean Difference
Study or Subgroup	Mean	SD	Total	Mean	SD	Total	Weight	IV, Random, 95% CI	IV, Random, 95% CI
Abramo et al, 2009	8.7	8.9	26	14	13	24	21.2%	-5.30 [-11.53, 0.93]	
Egol et al, 2008	13	30.9	44	17.2	33.7	44	7.2%	-4.20 [-17.71, 9.31]	
Rozental et al, 2009	4	8	23	9	18	22	15.3%	-5.00 [-13.20, 3.20]	
Wei et al, 2009 (RCP)	18	12	12	18	14	22	13.6%	0.00 [-8.96, 8.96]	
Wei et al, 2009 (VP)	4	5	12	18	14	22	20.2%	-14.00 [-20.50, -7.50]	
Wilcke et al, 2011	7	9.9	33	11	13.4	30	22.5%	-4.00 [-9.87, 1.87]	
Total (95% CI)			150			164	100.0%	-5.92 [-9.89, -1.96]	

Heterogeneity: Tau² = 9.23; Chi² = 8.16, df = 5 (P = 0.15); I² = 39%
Test for overall effect: Z = 2.93 (P = 0.003)

-20   -10   0   10   20
Favours ORIF   Favours Ex-fix

FIGURE 2.—Table and forest plot illustrating the meta-analysis of the Disabilities of Arm, Shoulder and Hand (DASH) score. RCP = radial column plate, VP = volar plate. (Reprinted from the Injury, International Journal of the Care of the Injured. Esposito J, Schemitsch EH, Saccone M, et al. External fixation versus open reduction with plate fixation for distal radius fractures: a meta-analysis of randomised controlled trials. *Injury.* 2013;44:409-416, Copyright 2013, with permission from International Society for Adult Congenital Heart Disease.)

independently applied the Checklist to Evaluate a Report of a Nonpharmacological Trial. Pooled mean differences were calculated for the following continuous outcomes: wrist range of motion; radiographic parameters; grip strength; and Disabilities of the Arm, Shoulder, and Hand (DASH) score. Pooled risk ratios were calculated for rates of complications and reoperation.

Results.—The literature search strategy identified 52 potential publications of which nine publications (10 studies) met inclusion criteria. Pooled mean difference for DASH scores was significantly less for the ORIF with plate fixation group (−5.92, 95% C.I. of −9.89 to −1.96, $p < 0.01$, $I^2 = 39\%$). Pooled mean difference for ulnar variance was significantly less in the ORIF with plate fixation group (−0.70, 95% C.I. of −1.20 to −0.19, $p < 0.01$, $I^2 = 0\%$), indicating better restoration of radial length for this group. Pooled risk ratio for infection was 0.37 (95% C.I. of 0.19−0.73, $p < 0.01$, $I^2 = 0\%$), favouring ORIF with plate fixation. There were no significant differences in all other clinical outcomes.

Conclusions.—ORIF with plate fixation provides lower DASH scores, better restoration of radial length and reduced infection rates as compared to external fixation for treatment of distal radius fractures (Figs 1 and 2).

▶ This is a well-conducted (Fig 1) randomized controlled trial comparing external fixation to open reduction with internal fixation for distal radius fractures. The data clearly support better functional and radiographic outcomes for ORIF (Fig 2). External fixation will still have a role for patients with significant soft tissue concomitant injury, but ORIF has justifiably become the treatment of choice.

M. F. Swiontkowski, MD

Hemiarthroplasty for Humeral Four-Part Fractures for Patients 65 Years and Older: A Randomized Controlled Trial
Boons HW, Goosen JH, van Grinsven S, et al (Elkerliek Hosp, Helmond, The Netherlands; Rijnstate Hosp, Arnhem, The Netherlands)
Clin Orthop Relat Res 470:3483-3491, 2012

Background.—Four-part fractures of the proximal humerus account for 3% of all humeral fractures and are regarded as the most difficult fractures to treat in the elderly. Various authors recommend nonoperative treatment or hemiarthroplasty, but the literature is unclear regarding which provides better quality of life and function.

Questions/Purposes.—We therefore performed a randomized controlled trial to compare (1) function, (2) strength, and (3) pain and disability in patients 65 years and older with four-part humeral fractures treated either nonoperatively or with hemiarthroplasty.

Methods.—We randomly allocated 50 patients to one of the two approaches. There were no differences in patient demographics between

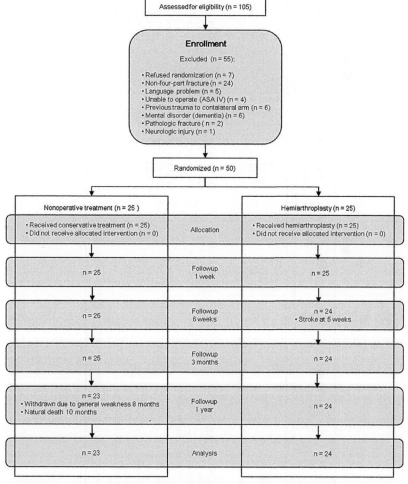

FIGURE 2.—A flow diagram shows the selection process of the patients through the study. (With kind permission from Springer Science+Business Media: Boons HW, Goosen JH, van Grinsven S, et al. Hemiarthroplasty for humeral four-part fractures for patients 65 years and older: a randomized controlled trial. *Clin Orthop Relat Res.* 2012;470:3483-3491.)

TABLE 2.—Differences in Effect between the Two Groups During the First Year of Followup

Variable	3-month Followup			12-month Followup		
	Nonoperative Treatment	Hemiarthroplasty	P Value	Nonoperative Treatment	Hemiarthroplasty	P Value
VAS pain	37 (21.3)	19 (18.0)	0.002	25 (1–93)*	23 (1–65)*	0.725
VAS disability	42 (25.6)	50 (20.6)	0.282	31 (24.7)	46 (25.7)	0.051
SST	48 (20.2)	41 (18.4)	0.209	23 (0–92)*	25 (8–100)*	0.592
Abductor strength (N)% contralateral shoulder	30 (0–98)*	20 (0–35)*	0.015	42 (28.5)	24 (12.5)	0.008
				71	54	0.051
ROM						
Forward flexion (°)	88 (45–130)	68 (45–105)	0.00	94 (45–165)	98 (45–165)	0.86
Abduction (°)	78 (30–130)	61 (45–75)	1	87 (30–130)	77 (45–165)	0.36
External rotation (°)	14 (5–20)	13 (5–20)	0.02	19 (15–25)	17 (10–25)	0.10
Internal rotation (lumbar level)	L5	L5	0.66	L3	L3	
CMS	54 (14.1)	48 (13.4)	0.125	60 (17.6)	64 (15.8)	0.413
Total pain (15)	9 (2.7)	11 (3.3)		10 (3.6)	13 (2.6)	
Activity (20)	11 (4.5)	9.3 (4.1)		12 (4.9)	13 (5.4)	
Mobility (40)	15 (4.8)	12 (4.5)		18 (6.9)	20 (8.3)	
Strength (25)	18 (5.0)	15 (5.7)		19 (4.7)	18 (4.7)	
Percentage contralateral shoulder				62	65	0.479

*Median value (range), all others are mean (SD); SST = Simple Shoulder Test; CMS = Constant-Murley score.

the two groups. The Constant- Murley score was the primary outcome measure. Secondary outcome measures were the Simple Shoulder Test, abduction strength test as measured by a myometer, and VAS scores for pain and disability. All patients were assessed at 12 months.

Results.—We found no between-group differences in Constant-Murley and Simple Shoulder Test scores at 3- and 12-months followup. Abduction strength was better at 3 and 12 months in the nonoperatively treated group although the nonoperatively treated patients experienced more pain at 3 months; this difference could not be detected after 12 months.

Conclusions.—We observed no clear benefits in treating patients 65 years or older with four-part fractures of the proximal humerus with either hemi-arthroplasty or nonoperative treatment.

Level of Evidence.—Level I, therapeutic study. See Instructions for Authors for a complete description of levels of evidence (Fig 2, Table 2).

▶ Arthroplasty for severely displaced or comminuted proximal humerus fractures in the elderly does not produce predictable favorable pain or functional outcomes. Recent cohort studies have documented poor range of motion with mid-range chronic pain in a large percentage of patients treated by experienced surgeons. This long overdue controlled trial addresses the question as to whether superior results could be obtained with nonoperative treatment. The answer is equivalent results but not superior results. The trial is well conducted, and the reporting is detailed (Fig 2). The only improvement would have been to have the outcomes determined by individuals blinded to the treatment group, which apparently was not done. It does seem that, based on these results, we should be thinking of nonoperative treatment more often with the caveat that pain will improve more slowly than with a surgical solution but end up at the same mean level (Table 2).

M. F. Swiontkowski, MD

Clinical Results of Treatment Using a Clavicular Hook Plate Versus a T-plate in Neer Type II Distal Clavicle Fractures
Tan H-L, Zhao J-K, Qian C, et al (Jiangsu Univ, Changzhou, China)
Orthopedics 35:e1191-e1197, 2012

AO clavicular hook plate fixation provides more rigid fixation and good bony union rates for Neer type II distal clavicular fractures. However, the hook may cause rotator cuff tears and subacromial impingement, which adversely affect the clinical results. T-plate fixation is another surgical method of treatment for unstable clavicle fractures, and its clinical efficacy has been demonstrated. The purpose of this study was to compare the clinical outcomes of AO clavicular hook plate and T-plate fixation for Neer type II distal clavicular fractures.

Forty-two patients with Neer type II fractures were divided into 2 groups. The hook plate group comprised 23 patients who underwent hook plate

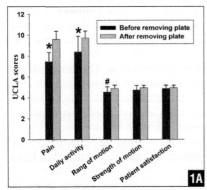
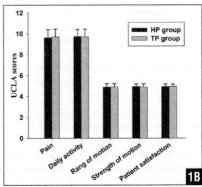

FIGURE 1.—Graph showing University of California, Los Angeles (UCLA) Shoulder rating scale results before and after plate removal in the hook plate group (*$P < .01$; #$P < .05$). No differences in strength or patient satisfaction existed between shoulders before and after plate removal (A). Graph showing UCLA Shoulder rating scale results of the hook plate (HP) group after plate removal compared with the T-plate (TP) group. No differences existed between the 2 groups ($P > .05$) (B). (Reprinted from Tan H-L, Zhao J-K, Qian C, et al. Clinical results of treatment using a clavicular hook plate versus a T-plate in neer type II distal clavicle fractures. *Orthopedics*. 2012;35:e1191-e1197.)

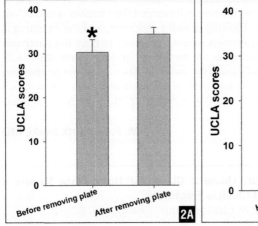
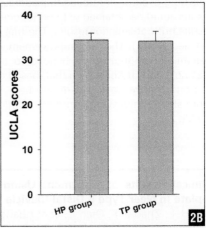

FIGURE 2.—Graph showing University of California, Los Angeles (UCLA) Shoulder rating scale results before and after plate removal in the hook plate group (*$P < .01$) (A). Graph showing comparison of UCLA Shoulder rating scale results between the hook plate (HP) group after plate removal and the T-plate (TP) group. No differences existed between the 2 groups ($P > .05$) (B). (Reprinted from Tan H-L, Zhao J-K, Qian C, et al. Clinical results of treatment using a clavicular hook plate versus a T-plate in neer type II distal clavicle fractures. *Orthopedics*. 2012;35:e1191-e1197, with permission from SLACK Incorporated.)

fixation, and the T-plate group comprised 19 patients who underwent distal radius volar locking T-plate fixation. Hook plates were removed 3 to 14 months postoperatively in 15 patients because of shoulder function limitations. All patients were evaluated postoperatively for shoulder pain, activities of daily living, range of motion, strength, and satisfaction according to the University of California, Los Angeles (UCLA) Shoulder rating scale. All fractures in the 2 groups achieved stable fixation and bony union. Both groups yielded similar outcomes with regard to shoulder strength and patient satisfaction ($P = .207$ and $P = .398$, respectively). Significant differences existed between the 2 groups in the mean scores of shoulder pain, activities of daily living, range of motion, and total UCLA score ($P = .001$, $P = .011$, $P = .038$, and $P = .001$, respectively). More patients (74%) in the hook plate group had mild to severe shoulder pain than in the T-plate group (16%). However, shoulder pain was relieved and function improved significantly after removal of the hook plate ($P = .001$) (Figs 1 and 2).

▶ The hook plate is a novel method for dealing with very distal clavicle fractures without resecting the distal clavicle. The issue is with purchase on a small distal fragment in the face of increased pullout forces because of the disruption of the coracoclavicular ligaments. This well-done comparative cohort functional outcome series confirms that both the hook plate and a locked small fragment T plate can lead to good clinical outcomes. As one would expect, most patients with the hook plate have to have the plate removed to achieve equivalent outcomes because the hook is in the subacromial space and definitely impacts rotator cuff function.

M. F. Swiontkowski, MD

Calcar comminution as prognostic factor of clinical outcome after locking plate fixation of proximal humeral fractures
Osterhoff G, Hoch A, Wanner GA, et al (Univ Hosp Zurich, Switzerland)
Injury 43:1651-1656, 2012

Objective.—In the treatment of proximal humeral fractures, the decision between open fixation and arthroplasty is often difficult. Applicable radiographic prognostic factors would be useful. The purpose of the present study was to investigate the influence of calcar comminution on the clinical and radiologic outcome after locking plate fixation of these fractures.

Methods.—In patients with proximal humeral fractures that were treated by locking plate fixation, fracture morphology and the presence of comminution of the calcar were documented on preoperative radiographs. Follow-up for at least 2 years with radiologic assessment and functional outcome measurements including Constant score, subjective shoulder value (SSV), disabilities of the arm, shoulder and hand score (DASH), visual analogue scale (VAS) and short form (SF)-36 was performed.

Results.—Follow-up examination (50.8 ± 20.6 months) was possible in 74 patients (46 female, 28 male, age 63.0 ± 15.9 years). Mean absolute Constant score (CS abs), CS adapted to age and gender (CS adap), DASH, SSV and VAS were 72.4 ± 14.5, 85.2 ± 17.3%, 15.7 ± 17.3, 80.3 ± 19.6% and 2.1 ± 2.2. Nonunion was present in 1.3%, cut-out in 5.4% and implant failure in 1.3%. Avascular necrosis (AVN) was seen in

TABLE 1.—Revision Surgery

Age	Gender	Neer	Calcar	Complication	Time	Treatment	CS abs	CS adap
69	Male	3	int	Impingement	19 m	Removal	86	100
46	Male	3	int	AVN	10 m	Removal	27	30
50	Female	3	comm	AVN	6 m	Removal, arthrolysis	69	83
41	Female	2	int	Non-union	5 m	Revision, same implant	83	98
53	Male	4	comm	Impingement	18 m	Removal	75	82
77	Male	4	int	Cut-out, omarthrosis	15 m	Arthroplasty	72	84
55	Female	4	comm	Night pain	18 m	Removal	72	87
50	Female	2	int	Impingement	13 m	Removal	79	95
57	Female	3	int	Night pain	19 m	Removal	75	91
29	Male	3	int	Cut-out, omarthrosis	8 m	Arthroplasty	61	65
64	Male	2	comm	Implant failure	7 m	Revision, angled plate	59	66
46	Male	3	int	Impingement	11 m	Removal	89	96
49	Male	4	comm	AVN	13 m	Arthroplasty	31	34
54	Male	3	int	Cut-out	2 m	Change of screws, arthrolysis	45	49

Age in years. Calcar: int: intact, comm: comminuted; AVN: avascular necrosis; Time: time after first intervention; m: months; CS abs: absolute Constant score at follow-up; CS adap: Constant score adapted to age and gender at follow-up.

TABLE 2.—Fracture Morphology and Calcar Integrity

| | Neer Parts | | | |
	2	3	4	Total
Calcar				
Intact	20	23	7	50
Comminuted	6	8	10	24
Total	26	31	17	74

12.2%, in three cases > 24 months after the initial trauma. In the presence of calcar comminution, the clinical outcome (CS abs, CS adap, SSV and several parameters of SF-36) was significantly impaired, the odds ratio for these patients to have an absolute CS < 65 was 4.4 (95% confidence interval (CI): 1.4–13.7).

Conclusions.—The treatment of proximal humeral fractures with locking plate fixation achieves good clinical mid-term results. Calcar comminution is a relevant and easy-to-detect prognostic factor for the functional and subjective outcome in these fractures (Tables 1 and 2).

▶ This retrospective comparative cohort study evaluates the impact of medial humeral metaphyseal comminution on functional outcome as well as complications. The overall combined cohort informs us that truly outstanding functional results are rare indeed. Comminution may well be simply a surrogate for lower bone density. The experimental design is compromised by the issue of detection bias in assigning patients to the comminuted versus simple fracture patterns. The results do add value in informing patients about expectations for functional outcome following proximal humerus fracture. The application of the locked plate remains a technically demanding procedure, as evidenced by the number of subsequent procedures listed in Table 1, which is high in both groups, comminuted and simple fracture patterns.

M. F. Swiontkowski, MD

Intermediate Outcomes Following Percutaneous Fixation of Proximal Humeral Fractures
Harrison AK, Gruson KI, Zmistowski B, et al (Mount Sinai Hosp, NY; Albert Einstein College of Medicine, Bronx, NY; The Rothman Inst, Philadelphia, PA; et al)
J Bone Joint Surg Am 94:1223-1228, 2012

Background.—Mini-open reduction and percutaneous fixation of proximal humeral fractures historically results in good outcomes and a low prevalence of osteonecrosis reported with short-term follow-up. The purpose of this study was to determine the midterm results of our multicenter case series of proximal humeral fractures treated with percutaneous fixation.

Methods.—Between 1999 and 2006, thirty-nine patients were treated with percutaneous reduction and fixation for proximal humeral fractures at three tertiary shoulder referral centers. Twenty-seven of these patients were available for intermediate follow-up at a minimum of three years (mean, eighty-four months; range, thirty-seven to 128 months) after surgery; the follow-up examination included use of subjective outcome measures and radiographic analysis to identify osteonecrosis and posttraumatic osteoarthritis on radiographs.

Results.—Osteonecrosis was detected in seven (26%) of the total group of twenty-seven patients at a mean of fifty months (range, eleven to 101 months) after the date of percutaneous fixation. Osteonecrosis was observed in five (50%) of the ten patients who had four-part fractures, two (17%) of the twelve patients who had three-part fractures, and none (0%) of the five patients who had two-part fractures. Posttraumatic osteoarthritis, including osteonecrosis, was present on radiographs in ten (37%) of the total group of twenty-seven patients. Posttraumatic osteoarthritis was observed in six (60%) of the ten patients who had four-part fractures, four (33%) of the twelve patients who had three-part fractures, and none (0%) of the five patients who had two-part fractures.

Conclusions.—Intermediate follow-up of patients with percutaneously treated proximal humeral fractures demonstrates an increased prevalence of osteonecrosis and posttraumatic osteoarthritis over time, with some patients with these complications presenting as late as eight years postoperatively. Development of osteonecrosis did not have a universally negative impact on subjective outcome scores.

Level of Evidence.—Therapeutic Level IV. See Instructions for Authors for a complete description of levels of evidence (Tables 1 and 2).

▶ Percutaneous pin fixation requires a high level of skill, interest, and attention to reduction detail. It has waned in terms of general interest in the orthopedic

TABLE 1.—Rate of Osteonecrosis and Posttraumatic Osteoarthritis by Fracture Type

Fracture Pattern (No. of Patients)	Osteonecrosis (%)	Posttraumatic Osteoarthritis (%)
Two-part (5)	0	0
Three-part (12)	17	33
Four-part, all valgus-impacted (10)	50	60

TABLE 2.—Comparison of Patients with and Without Osteonecrosis*

	Patients with Osteonecrosis	Patients Without Osteonecrosis	P Value
Average age (yr)	54.4	60.4	0.13
Average ASES[†] score (points)			
At latest follow-up	77	84	0.26
Prior to arthroplasty	65	84	0.02[‡]
Range of motion (deg)			
Forward elevation			
At latest follow-up	129	144	0.08
Prior to arthroplasty	125	144	0.01[‡]
External rotation			
At latest follow-up	33	44	0.32
Prior to arthroplasty	23	44	0.02[‡]
Internal rotation	L2 level	L2 level	0.65

*Comparison data are from the latest follow-up as well as prior to the arthroplasty revision, where variable (i.e., for the patients who had better scores at the time of the latest follow-up as a result of having undergone arthroplasty).
[†]ASES = American Shoulder and Elbow Surgeons.
[‡]Significant value.

community because of the dissemination of locked plate fixation. This longer term study confirms that osteoarthritis and osteonecrosis are prevalent despite the lack of surgical dissection and that in many cases osteonecrosis does not impact functional recovery. Another important take-home point is that radiographic osteonecrosis can occur late in postoperative recovery. I would love to see the results of this study in a matched cohort design with age, sex, and fracture classification patients treated with locked plating. My suspicion is that these results would be at least equivalent and perhaps superior to the results obtained with locked plating.

M. F. Swiontkowski, MD

Acute Compartment Syndrome of the Forearm

Duckworth AD, Mitchell SE, Molyneux SG, et al (Royal Infirmary of Edinburgh, UK)
J Bone Joint Surg Am 94:e63.1-e63.6, 2012

Background.—The aims of this study were to document our experience with acute forearm compartment syndrome and to determine the risk factors for the need for split-thickness skin-grafting and the development of complications after fasciotomy.

TABLE 3.—The Details of the Twenty-nine Patients Who Had Complications After Forearm Fasciotomy

Complication	No (%) of All Patients
Neurological deficit	16 (18)
Contracture	4 (4)
Delayed union	4 (4)
Muscle necrosis with associated weakness	3 (3)
Skin graft tethered to tendon, limiting motion	2 (2)

TABLE 5.—The Effect of Time to Fasciotomy on the Development of Complications in Eighty-One Patients

	No Complications	Complications	P Value*
Total no. (%) of patients	56 (69)	25 (31)	NA
Time to fasciotomy[†] (hr)	15.8 (2-72; 14.7; 12-20)	22.2 (4-55; 16.2; 16-29)	0.044[‡]
Time to fasciotomy of >6 hr[§]	34 (61; 48-72)	22 (88; 69-97)	0.018[‡]

*NA = not applicable.
[†]The values are given as the mean, with the range, standard deviation, and 95% confidence interval in parentheses.
[‡]Mann-Whitney U test.
[§]The values are given as the number of patients, with the percentage and 95% confidence interval in parentheses.

Methods.—We identified from our trauma database all patients who underwent fasciotomy for an acute forearm compartment syndrome over a twenty-two-year period. Diagnosis was made with use of clinical signs in all patients, with compartment pressure monitoring used as a diagnostic adjunct in some patients. Outcome measures were the use of split-thickness skin grafts and the identification of complications following forearm fasciotomy.

Results.—There were ninety patients in the study cohort, with a mean age of thirty-three years (range, thirteen to eighty-one years) and a significant male predominance (eighty-two patients; $p < 0.001$). A fracture of the radius or ulna, or both, was seen in sixty-two patients (69%), with soft-tissue injuries as the causative factor in twenty-eight (31%). The median time to fasciotomy was twelve hours (range, two to seventy-two hours). Risk factors for requiring split-thickness skin-grafting were younger age and a crush injury ($p < 0.05$ for both). Risk factors for the development of complications were a delay in fasciotomy of more than six hours ($p = 0.018$) and preoperative motor symptoms, which approached significance ($p = 0.068$).

Conclusions.—Forearm compartment syndrome requiring fasciotomy predominantly affects males and can occur following either a fracture or soft-tissue injury. Age is an important predictor of undergoing split-thickness skin-grafting for wound closure. Complications occur in a third of patients and are associated with an increasing time from injury to fasciotomy (Tables 3 and 5).

▶ This article is important to review because there are important lessons to learn regarding this relatively rare complication. The take-home message is that compartment syndrome of the forearm can result from injury not related to fracture and that when related to fracture, both bones and distal radius fracture should raise the level of suspicion. Delay to fasciotomy is related to complications; the best way to avoid this is with a high index of suspicion. In an unconscious patient, the threshold for measuring compartment pressures should be very low in order to avoid delay to fasciotomy.

M. F. Swiontkowski, MD

Comparison of Dynamic and Locked Compression Plates for Treating Midshaft Clavicle Fractures

Lai Y-C, Tarng Y-W, Hsu C-J, et al (Kaohsiung Veterans General Hosp, Kaohsiung, Taiwan)
Orthopedics 35:e697-e702, 2012

The purpose of this study was to compare the parameters of perioperative course and cost-effectiveness for patients with midshaft clavicle fractures treated by dynamic compression plates or locked compression plates.

This retrospective, case-controlled study involved 54 patients with midshaft clavicle fractures who received dynamic compression plates (n=21) or locked compression plates (n=33) between January 2002 and December 2008. Indications for surgery included displacement or shortening >2 cm, comminuted fractures, and skin tenting. Patients with previous malunion, nonunion, multiple injuries of the shoulder girdle, or open fractures were excluded. Preoperative demographics showed no statistically significant differences between the 2 groups. Eighteen patients with dynamic compression plates and 28 patients with locked compression plates with postoperative follow-up >1 year were included for comparison. Statistical analyses for operative time, blood loss, complication rate, hospital stay, and union rate demonstrated no statistically significant difference between the 2 groups. The only statistically significant difference was a higher rate of plate removal requests in the dynamic compression plate group. Considering medical expenditure, locked compression plates cost 6 times more than dynamic compression plates in the authors' institution (US $600 vs $100, respectively).

Other than more plate removal requests in the dynamic compression plate group and greater expense in the locked compression plate group, dynamic compression plates and locked compression plates achieved satisfactory operative outcomes in treating midshaft clavicle fractures, with no statistically significant difference between perioperative course and eventual fracture union observed between the 2 groups (Tables 2 and 3).

▶ The multiple well-done randomized clinical trials comparing open reduction, internal fixture with conservative care for significantly displaced clavicle fractures has resulted in a dramatic increase in the operative management of these fractures. Industry has responded with every company developing a form of locked plate that "anatomically" fits the clavicle. This has resulted in a dramatic increase

TABLE 2.—Perioperative Data[a]

Variable	Average		P
	DCP Group	LCP Group	
Operative time, min	82.72	78.95	.7
Blood loss, mL	84.5	41.2	.07
No. of complications	0	0	
Hospital stay,[b] d	3.8	4.4	.325

Abbreviations: DCP, dynamic compression plate; LCP, locked compression plate.
[a]Statistical analysis by Student's *t* test.
[b]Excluding patients with concomitant injuries that may extend hospitalization.

TABLE 3.—Postoperative Follow-up Data[a]

Variable	No. (%)		P
	DCP Group	LCP Group	
Average follow-up, mo	19.9	18.1	
Lost to follow-up	3 (14.3)	5 (15.2)	.929
Cumulative union			
Week 12	11 (61.1)	18 (64.3)	.828
Week 18	16 (88.9)	27 (96.4)	.312
Week 24	17 (94.4)	27 (96.4)	.747
Screw backout	3 (16.7)	1 (3.6)	.124
Loss of reduction	0	1 (3.4)	.417
Implant removal	12 (66.7)	8 (28.6)	.011

Abbreviations: DCP, dynamic compression plate; LCP, locked compression plate.
[a]Statistical analysis by chi-sqaure test.

in the cost of implants. This comparative study provides some evidence that the use of these expensive locking plates is not necessary. Some surgeons have recommended against their use because of the increased rigidity being associated with a higher rate of nonunion, but the documentation is lacking. Implant expense in the face of equivalent clinical outcomes as is demonstrated in this series is enough to prompt return to standard plating.

M. F. Swiontkowski, MD

12 Orthopedic Oncology

Introduction

The Oncology chapter of this YEAR BOOK continues to focus on issues relevant to the practicing orthopedic oncologist. The largest section deals with primary bone tumors (osteosarcoma, in particular). I have selected articles dealing with outcomes and surgical issues (pathologic fracture, local recurrence) that I hope the readership will find interesting. The next largest section involves resection and reconstruction techniques not specific to individual tumor histologies. Pragmatic issues of metastatic disease management follow (what stem length to use, how to address failures). Other areas deal with benign tumors, soft tissue tumors, and other topics of interest in the oncologic field. More articles are incorporated from the general surgical oncology literature this year to cover areas orthopedic oncologists might not be directly exposed to through the classic orthopedic journals alone.

Peter S. Rose, MD

Malignant Bone Tumors

Ultraporous β-Tricalcium Phosphate Alone or Combined with Bone Marrow Aspirate for Benign Cavitary Lesions: Comparison in a Prospective Randomized Clinical Trial

Damron TA, Lisle J, Craig T, et al (SUNY Upstate Med Univ, East Syracuse, NY; Univ of Vermont Med Ctr, Burlington)
J Bone Joint Surg Am 95:158-166, 2013

Background.—Ultraporous β-tricalcium phosphate (TCP) synthetic graft material (Vitoss; Orthovita) persists for a year or longer in some cases. In this study, we prospectively examined healing of cavitary defects filled with TCP versus TCP and bone marrow aspirate (TCP/BM) with the hypothesis that bone-marrow aspirate speeds incorporation of bone graft substitute.

Methods.—Fifty-five patients with a benign bone lesion undergoing surgical curettage were randomized to receive TCP (N = 26; mean duration of follow-up [and standard deviation], 20.2 ± 7.2 months) or TCP/BM (N = 29; mean duration of follow-up, 18.0 ± 7.7 months). There were no significant differences between the groups with regard to demographic or defect parameters. Clinical and radiographic evaluations were done at

1.5, three, six, twelve, eighteen, and twenty-four months, and computed tomography [CT] scans were performed at twelve months. An independent radiographic review was done to evaluate six parameters.

Results.—There was a significant ($p < 0.001$) increase in trabeculation through the defect and graft resorption with decreases in the persistence of the graft in both soft tissue and the defect as well as a decreased radiolucent rim around the graft over time. No significant differences were observed between the TCP and TCP/BM groups in terms of any radiographic parameter. No complications related to the graft material or BM were identified.

Conclusions.—While significant improvements in radiographic parameters were observed in both TCP groups over two years of follow-up, the addition of BM was not found to provide any significant benefit. Results should not be extrapolated to other bone graft substitutes used for this purpose.

▶ These authors present level I evidence, the results of a prospective randomized trial using β-tricalcium phosphate synthetic bone graft material with or without bone marrow aspirate for the treatment of benign cavitary bone defects. Patients were followed with bone plain film radiographs and 12-month CT scans.

In summary, both techniques worked equally well (see Fig 1 in the original article), with healing rates essentially identical in both groups. These results support the use of β-tricalcium phosphate grafts but indicate that the added time, trouble, and expense of bone marrow aspirate is not necessary. The study does not address the use of bone marrow aspirates when combined with other grafts (a common practice) but opens the door to studies of those agents as well.

P. S. Rose, MD

What's New in Primary Bone Tumors

Schwab JH, Springfield DS, Raskin KA, et al (Massachusetts General Hosp, Boston)

J Bone Joint Surg Am 94:1913-1919, 2012

Background.—The current state of knowledge regarding primary bone tumors was assessed via a literature review. The malignant tumors Ewing sarcoma, osteosarcoma, chondrosarsoma, and chordoma were reviewed. New findings were also noted for benign cartilaginous tumors, giant cell tumor of bone, and aneurysmal bone cysts.

Malignant Tumors.—Ewing sarcoma has a characteristic translocation of the eleventh and twenty-second chromosomes. Blocking EWS-FLI1 and RNA helicase A (RHA) interactions indicates that such activities may contribute to Ewing sarcoma pathogenesis. Skeletally based Ewing sarcoma is more likely to occur in younger patients, males, and extremities than non-skeletal disease, Skeletal disease also has a lower 5-year survival. Children's 3-year survival is better than that of adults, perhaps because of lower adult doses of chemotherapy. Local treatment is an important predictor of survival.

Treatments being developed target the insulin-like growth factor (IGF) tyrosine kinase pathway. Zoledronic acid plus lower doses of conventional chemotherapy may be effective with fewer side effects than other approaches.

Low-grade osteosarcomas do not require chemotherapy, but high-grade tumors tend to metastasize and require chemotherapy and surgical resection. Identifying surrogate markers would help predict outcomes for patients with high-grade disease. The histological response to neoadjuvant chemotherapy is the best predictor of survival. Research is looking at imaging modalities, circulating factors, gene expression patterns from tumor cells, and chemokine levels. Pagetic osteosarcoma has a very poor prognosis, but the most aggressive tumors are radiation-induced. The level of radiation associated with disease is much lower than previously thought. Targeted therapies directed at the PI3k pathway are being investigated. Combining carboplatin, ifosfamide, and doxorubicin may be an effective alternative to cisplatin or methotrexate-based chemotherapy. Proton-based radiation offers promising local control and survival benefits for select patients. Dynamic contrast-enhanced magnetic resonance imaging (DCE-MRI) can predict event-free survival and overall survival in pretreated patients, with imaging findings correlating with histologic response to neoadjuvant chemotherapy. Thallium uptake is not an appropriate predictor of necrosis but may predict event-free survival. Procoagulant studies reveal the coagulation cascade may contribute to the pathogenesis of osteosarcoma and offer a treatment target. Adding pamidronate may improve the durability of limb reconstruction.

The prognosis for chondrosarcomas usually correlates with histologic grade. Decreased expression of von Hippel-Lindau (VHL) tumor-suppressor gene correlates with lower apoptosis rates and higher histologic grade but not survival. The treatment of low-grade cartilage lesions has generated considerable research. Wide resection appears better than intralesional resection. Curettage plus cryosurgery is a reasonable alternative to wide resection for low-grade cartilage lesions. Imatinib mesylate has not proved useful for disseminated or unresectable chondrosarcoma. Resection with negative margins is the standard of care, but radiation may be a useful adjuvant.

Most chordomas occur in the sacrum or skull base, so they are difficult to treat and tend to recur. Staged sacral resections are associated with improved outcomes, better resource management, and lower hospital costs. Posterior-only approaches and radiation therapy may also be efficacious. Systemic therapy is still experimental.

Tumor Reconstruction.—For malignant bone sarcomas, specifically high-grade lesions, a negative surgical margin with no entry into the tumor or its surrounding reactive zone is the goal of treatment. As a result, surgical resection causes a large osseous defect. Low-grade malignant tumors are approached less aggressively and produce a smaller defect. Reconstructive procedures for large osseous defects vary with the surgeon's preference, the surgical site, the disease process, and the materials available for reconstruction. Options include structural allograft transplantation, endoprosthetic replacement, and composite reconstruction with allografts and metal prostheses. Recently a classification scheme for failure of endoprostheses has detailed both mechanical and nonmechanical failures. Leaving more bone and soft tissues around a resection can promote better function but higher rates of local recurrence.

Benign Tumors.—Better systemic therapy is needed to manage giant cell tumors, which often affect the spine and sacrum and offer surgical challenges. Recent efforts are focused on monoclonal antibody against RANKL. Bisphosphonates have also been used as an adjuvant for local control. A dose-dependent effect on cellular cytotoxicity is seen with incremental increases in zoledronic acid concentrations. Most of the agent is released in the first 24 hours, with a plateau occurring after 4 days. The cytotoxic effects of zoledronic acid are not mitigated by cement polymerization. Local recurrence is less likely when polymethylmethacrylate (PMMA) filling of bone defects is used instead of allograft chips. Intralesional curettage and PMMA packing allow good local control even with recurrent tumor cases, and local failures are more amenable to additional surgery.

Aneurysmal bone cysts express a TRE17/USP6 translocation, but the cause of these tumors remains unknown. Matrix metalloproteinase (MMP)-9 and MMP-10 activity are associated with degradation and remodeling of bone matrix and may contribute to the etiology of aneurysmal bone cysts. Repetitive sclerotherapy, an outpatient treatment achieves pain relief immediately after the injection and may be a safe, effective means of treating these bone cysts. Results with sclerotherapy are comparable to those using curettage, high-speed burs, and argon beam coagulation, and the argon beam was associated with a higher risk for fractures.

Female gender, having fewer than five sites with exostoses, presence of EXT2 mutations, and absence of EXT1/2 mutations are more commonly seen in mild forms of benign cartilaginous tumors. Male gender, EXT1 mutations, and having more than 20 sites with exostoses are associated with more severe forms. Malignancy is more likely to occur in exostoses from the pelvis, scapula, and proximal femur, as well as patients with a family history of multiple hereditary exostoses rather than sporadic disease. Further study is focused on microRNAs and loss-of-function mutations in PTPN11 in patients with metachondromatosis.

▶ This is a nice specialty update article that reviews recent developments in the care of patients with primary bone tumors. The article reviews common malignant tumors, reconstruction, and benign tumors. Although published in a surgical journal, this article incorporates the use of adjuvant treatment modalities in a very readable form.

P. S. Rose, MD

Low-Grade Central Osteosarcoma: A Difficult Condition to Diagnose

Malhas AM, Sumathi VP, James SL, et al (Royal Orthopaedic Hosp, Birmingham, UK)
Sarcoma 2012:1-7, 2012

Low-grade central osteosarcoma (LGCO) is a rare variant of osteosarcoma which is difficult to diagnose. If not treated appropriately, the tumour can recur with higher-grade disease. We reviewed our experience of this condition to try and identify factors that could improve both diagnosis and outcome. 18 patients out of 1540 osteosarcoma cases (over 25 years) had LGCO (1.2%). Only 11 patients (61%) were direct primary referrals. Almost 40% (7 of 18) cases were referred after treatment elsewhere when the diagnosis had not been made initially and all presented with local recurrence. Of the 11 who presented primarily, the first biopsy was diagnostic in only 6 (55%) cases. Of the remaining cases, up to three separate biopsies were required before a definitive diagnosis was made. Overall survivorship at 5 years was 90%. 17 patients were treated with limb salvage procedures, and one patient had an amputation. The diagnosis of LGCO remains challenging due to the relatively nonspecific radiological and histological findings. Since treatment of LGCO is so different to a benign lesion, accurate diagnosis is essential. Any difficult or nondiagnostic biopsies of solitary bone lesions should be referred to specialist tumour units for a second opinion.

▶ Low-grade central osteosarcoma is a rare variant of osteosarcoma—1.2% of the osteosarcoma experience in this report from Birmingham—that has an excellent prognosis when recognized and treated well from its index presentation. Malhas and colleagues add a modest series to the literature but focus on the diagnosis of this condition. More than one third of their patients did not come to attention until after nononcologic treatment of their condition. This is a good article to remind surgeons of this entity, how to diagnose it properly, and how to differentiate it from other more commonly encountered lesions.

P. S. Rose, MD

Poor Survival for Osteosarcoma of the Pelvis: A Report from the Children's Oncology Group

Isakoff MS, Barkauskas DA, Ebb D, et al (Connecticut Children's Med Ctr, Hartford; Univ of Southern California, Los Angeles, CA; Massachusetts General Hosp, Boston; et al)
Clin Orthop Relat Res 470:2007-2013, 2012

Background.—The pelvis is an infrequent site of osteosarcoma and treatment requires surgery plus systemic chemotherapy. Poor survival has been reported, but has not been confirmed previously by the Children's Oncology Group (COG). In addition, survival of patients with pelvic osteosarcomas has not been compared directly with that of patients with nonpelvic disease treated on the same clinical trials.

Questions/Purposes.—First, we assessed the event-free (EFS) and overall survival (OS) of patients with pelvic osteosarcoma treated on COG clinical trials. We then asked whether patient survival compared with that of patients treated on the same clinical trials with nonpelvic disease. Finally, we asked whether patients with metastatic disease at initial diagnosis had worse survival.

Methods.—We retrospectively reviewed data from 1054 patients with osteosarcoma treated in four studies between 1993 and 2005. Twenty-six of the 1054 patients (2.5%) had a primary tumor of the pelvis. At diagnosis, nine patients had metastatic disease. The minimum followup was 2 months (mean, 34 months; range, 2−102 months).

Results.—Two of the nine patients with metastatic disease at diagnosis and five of the 17 with localized disease were alive at last contact. Estimates of the 5-year EFS for localized versus metastatic disease of the pelvis were 22% versus 23%. OS for patients with localized versus metastatic disease was 47% versus 22%. Patients with osteosarcoma in all other locations had a 5-year EFS of 57% and OS of 69%.

Conclusions.—Our analysis confirms poor survival for patients with pelvic osteosarcoma. Survival with metastatic disease in the absence of a pelvic primary tumor is similar to that for localized or metastatic pelvic osteosarcoma. Improved surgical or medical therapy is needed, and patients with pelvic osteosarcoma may warrant alternate or experimental therapy.

Level of Evidence.—Level II, prognostic study. See Guidelines for Authors for a complete description of levels of evidence.

▶ Clinical experience has shown that pelvic osteosarcoma has a very poor prognosis, but this has been poorly quantified to date in pediatric patients. These authors review patients from four recent Children's Oncology Group trials to determine the outcome of pelvic osteosarcoma and compare it with extremity osteosarcoma.

Event-free and overall survival rates were 23% and 38%. In contrast, extremity tumor patients in these studies had event-free survival of 57% and overall survival of 69%. Only a small fraction of pelvic tumor patients (< 25%) had documented negative margin resections, and these patients appeared to do better.

The oncologic outcome of pelvic osteosarcoma most closely matched that of patients with metastatic extremity tumors (Fig 3 in the original article). This poor prognosis and the rarity of achieving clear surgical margins highlights the need for these patients to be considered for innovative treatments and referral to experienced pelvic tumor centers to allow the best chance of tumor control.

P. S. Rose, MD

Survival Trends and Long-Term Toxicity in Pediatric Patients with Osteosarcoma

Hagleitner MM, de Bont ESJM, te Loo DMWM (Radboud Univ Nijmegen Med Centre, The Netherlands; Univ of Groningen, The Netherlands)
Sarcoma 2012:1-5, 2012

Background.—This study was conducted to investigate the clinical characteristics and treatment results of osteosarcoma in pediatric patients during the past 30 years. Trends in survival rates and long-term toxicity were analyzed.

Procedure.—130 pediatric patients under the age of 20 years with primary localized or metastatic high-grade osteosarcoma were analyzed regarding demographic, treatment-related variables, long-term toxicity, and survival data.

Results.—Comparison of the different time periods of treatment showed that the 5-year OS improved from 58.6% for children diagnosed during 1979–1983 to 78.6% for those diagnosed during 2003–2008 ($P = 0.13$). Interestingly, the basic treatment agents including cisplatin, doxorubicin, and methotrexate remained the same. Treatment reduction due to acute toxicity was less frequent in patients treated in the last era (7.1% versus 24.1% in patients treated in 1979–1983; $P = 0.04$). Furthermore, late cardiac effects and secondary malignancies can become evident many years after treatment.

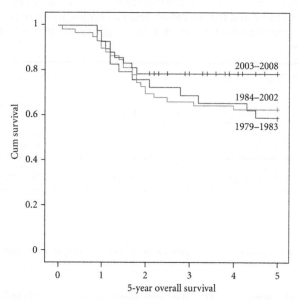

FIGURE 1.—5-year overall survival in pediatric patients with osteosarcoma over three decades. (Reprinted from Hagleitner MM, de Bont ESJM, te Loo DMWM. Survival trends and long-term toxicity in pediatric patients with osteosarcoma. *Sarcoma*. 2012;2012:1-5, with permission from Melanie M. Hagleitner et al.)

Conclusion.—We elucidate the prevalence of toxicity to therapy of patients with osteosarcoma over the past 30 years. The overall improvement in survival may in part be attributed to improved supportive care allowing regimens to be administered to best advantage with higher tolerance of chemotherapy and therefore less chemotherapy-related toxicity (Fig 1).

▶ Are we getting any better at treating osteosarcoma? The answer appears to be yes (Fig 1). Despite using much the same chemotherapy agents, overall survival trends show clear improvement for pediatric osteosarcoma patients. What I found most interesting about this study was the authors' ability to quantify the change in chemotherapy toxicities over time, with more than a 3-fold decrease in the need for treatment reduction because of acute toxicity. Our improvements in survival are likely in large part because of our ability to anticipate and manage chemotherapy better, thus highlighting the importance of maximizing the dose intensity of treatments our patients receive.

P. S. Rose, MD

Outcome of Surgical Treatment of Pelvic Osteosarcoma
Guo W, Sun X, Ji T, et al (Peking Univ, Beijing, China)
J Surg Oncol 106:406-410, 2012

Background and Objectives.—Surgical treatment of pelvic osteosarcoma is often challenging. The objective of this study was to assess the oncologic and functional outcome and the operation-related complications of patients with pelvic osteosarcoma who were treated in a single center in the past decade.

TABLE 2.—Summary of Publications Concerning Pelvic Osteosarcoma

Reference	Author	Country	Number of Patients	Period	Resection	Conservative	Adjunctive Therapy	Recurrence
1	Fahey M	USA	25	1967–1990	18 (72%)	7 (28%)	11 (44%)	13
2	Ozaki T	European	67	1979–1998	50 (74.6%)	17 (25.4%)	67 (100%)	47
3	Ham SJ	Netherlands	40	1978–1995	20 (50%)	20 (50%)	27 (67.5%)	7
4	Donati D	Italy	60	1978–1998	30 (50%)	30 (50%)	25 (41.7%)	8
5	Fuchs B	Switzerland	43	1983–2003	43 (100%)		36 (84%)	15
6	Kawai A	USA	40	1977–1994	30 (75%)	10 (25%)	10 (25%)	9
7	Saab R	Australia	19	1970–2004	9 (47.4%)	10 (52.6%)	19 (100%)	7
8	Grimer RJ	England	36	1971–1996	18 (50%)	18 (50%)	26 (72.2%)	2
9	Current series	China	19	2000–2009	19 (100%)		19 (100%)	5

NED, no evidence of disease; DOD, die of disease; AWD, alive with disease.

Methods.—Nineteen patients underwent surgical procedures between June 2000 and June 2009. There were 11 males and 8 females with a mean age of 30 years. According to Enneking and Dunham pelvic classification system, there were: Type I-3, Type I + IV-3, Type I + II-2, Type II + III-4, Type I + II + III-1, Type III-1, and type I + II + IV-5. All patients received chemotherapy.

Results.—Local recurrence rate was 26.3% (5/19). The 5-year overall survival rate was 44.9%. Seventeen patients received reconstruction after tumor resection. The average MSTS 93 score was 18 (10–23) for the 11 patients with hemipelvic endoprosthetic reconstruction and 23 (20–25) for 6 patients with rod-screw reconstruction. Complication was found in 7 of 19 patients (36.8%).

Conclusion.—The oncological results of pelvic osteosarcoma are poor at best. Even with a higher complication rate, we believe restoration of pelvic ring continuity and hip joint mobility is reasonable option to achieve favorable functional outcomes in selected patients (Table 2).

▶ The outcome of patients with pelvic osteosarcoma has lagged behind that of patients with extremity osteosarcoma. These tumors are rare and often present in advanced stages. Guo and colleagues report a series of 19 patients treated surgically between 2000 and 2009 with this condition. Although a modest number, this presents a modern cohort of patients treated in the era of current chemotherapy protocols, magnetic resonance and computed tomography imaging, and current reconstruction techniques. This distinguishes this report from other series that date back 2 or 3 decades to present reasonable patient numbers.

Unfortunately, even with a modern series in expert hands, the outcome of these tumors remains poor. Local recurrence occurred in 26% of patients, complications

Margin			Surgical Treatment		Prognosis				5-Year Survival Rate
Wide	Marginal	Intralesional	Amputation	Internal Hemipelvectomy	NED	AWD	DOD	Metastasis	
6 (33.3%)	4 (22.2%)	8 (44.4%)	9 (50%)	9 (50%)	1	0	24	16	
25 (50%)	10 (20%)	13 (26%)	12 (24%)	38 (76%)	12	4	51	34	27%
8 (20%)	5 (12.5%)	7 (17.5%)	4 (20%)	16 (80%)	5	0	35	26	21%
18 (30%)	7 (23.3%)	5 (16.7%)	16 (53.3%)	14 (46.7%)	8	0	52	25	16%
30 (70%)		13 (30%)	14 (33%)	29 (67%)	13	0	30	21	38%
16 (53%)	9 (30%)	5 (17%)	14 (46.7%)	16 (53.3%)	23	2	15	18	34% (with surgery: 41%; without surgery: 10%)
5 (55.6%)		4 (44.4%)	2 (22.52)	7 (77.8%)	3	1	15	10	26.3%
7 (38.9%)	4 (22.2%)	7 (38.9%)	6 (33.3%)	10 (66.7%)	7	1	28	26	18% (with surgery: 41%)
10 (52.6%)	4 (21.1%)	5 (26.3%)		19 (100%)	7	5	7	10	44.9%

in 37%, and 5-year overall survival was 45%. Although low, this 5-year survival number exceeds that of other major published series (Table 2).

Where to place this study in current clinical care? This article provides a nice data point for the outcome of patients with this disease using modern treatment paradigms and improves modestly over the results previously seen in the literature. Although the overall prognosis with aggressive treatment lags that of extremity tumors, survival remains reasonable and supports aggressive curative treatment in this patient population.

P. S. Rose, MD

Pathologic Fracture Does Not Influence Local Recurrence and Survival in High-Grade Extremity Osteosarcoma With Adequate Surgical Margins
Xie L, Guo W, Li Y, et al (Peking Univ People's Hosp, Beijing, China)
J Surg Oncol 106:820-825, 2012

Background and Objectives.—The purpose of this study was to estimate the risk factors having relationships with pathologic fracture of osteosarcoma of extremities and to evaluate the role of limb salvage surgery in this group of patients.

Methods.—We retrospectively analyzed 28 consecutive cases of pathologic fracture of primary high-grade localized osteosarcoma of extremities between June 1, 2001 and June 30, 2009. All patients underwent limb salvage surgery and neo-adjuvant chemotherapy. They had a median age of 14 years (range, 6–30 years). The average follow-up time was 40.7 months (range, 9–108 months). Clinicopathological factors were analyzed in relation to pathologic fracture. Their recurrence and survival rates were compared to those in cohort of 171 osteosarcoma patients without pathologic fracture who underwent limb salvage surgery during the same period at the same institution.

Results.—Less than 15 years, telangiectatic histological subtype, tumor located at the proximal humerus, and radiographical manifested as osteolytic features were risk factors in relation to pathologic fracture. The overall 3- and 5-year survival rates were 50.5% and 45.4%, respectively, in the fracture group, and were not significantly different from those in the control group (71.0% and 61.9%, respectively). Of all 28 fracture patients, 4 experienced local recurrences (14.2%) and 14 developed distant metastasis (50%), which were not significantly different from the rates in the control group (8.8% and 37.4%, respectively).

Conclusion.—Limb salvage surgery with adequate margins combined with neo-adjuvant chemotherapy for pathologic fracture of osteosarcoma did not seem to significantly increase the risk of local recurrence or distal metastasis.

▶ The role of limb salvage surgery following pathologic fracture is very nuanced. Xie and colleagues report the outcomes of 28 patients with pathologic fractures and find the oncologic outcomes statistically similar to a companion group of 171 patients treated without pathologic fracture concurrently.

This study confirms other series and clinical experience that patients with pathologic fractures may undergo limb salvage procedures provided wide resection can still be obtained. Although this study did not show a survival decrease in patients with pathologic fracture, this remains controversial, because tumor characteristics that lead to fracture may also portend more aggressive oncologic behavior.

P. S. Rose, MD

Surgical Resection of Relapse May Improve Postrelapse Survival of Patients With Localized Osteosarcoma

Wong KC, Lee V, Shing MMK, et al (The Chinese Univ of Hong Kong, China)
Clin Orthop Relat Res 471:814-819, 2013

Background.—Despite neoadjuvant chemotherapy and wide surgical ablation, 15% to 25% of patients with primary osteosarcoma will relapse (local recurrence or metastases). Neither chemotherapy nor radiation therapy alone will render a patient disease-free without concomitant surgical ablation of relapse. We prefer excision of relapse when possible. However, it is unclear whether excision enhances survival.

Questions/Purposes.—We therefore determined (1) onset, location, and treatments for relapse; (2) postrelapse disease-free survival of patients who underwent surgical ablation and those who did not; and (3) relapse-free interval between initial diagnosis and first relapse in survivors and in those who died of their disease.

Methods.—We retrospectively reviewed 15 children who initially presented with localized, nonmetastatic extremity osteosarcoma and attained initial complete remission after neoadjuvant chemotherapy, wide local resection, postoperative chemotherapy, and subsequently developed disease relapse. Relapse occurred at a median of 28 months, although late relapse after 5 years occurred in three. We resected the recurrent tumor in nine patients and treated six nonoperatively.

Results.—Seven of nine surgically treated patients had a postrelapse disease-free survival ranging from 3 to 14 years and an overall survival ranging from 7 to 16 years. Patients not surgically treated all died within 40 months of their relapse. The median relapse-free interval in patients who survived was longer 34 months (range, 17—152 months) as compared with 17 months (range, 7—40 months) in those who died of their disease.

Conclusions.—Our data confirm the importance of surgery in patients with relapsed osteosarcoma. Disease-free survival in patients with relapsed osteosarcoma is only possible if complete remission is attained. Patients with late relapse may have a better chance of survival.

TABLE 2.—Comparison of Relapse Intervals and Postrelapse and Overall Survival From Published Studies

Author	RFI after Treatment of Primary Disease	Patients Undergoing Surgery for Relapse	Postrelapse Status PRDFS or OS Patient Who Were not Operated
Ferrari et al. [5] 1997 N = 69	<24 months 7% 8-year survival >24 months 40% 8-year survival	N = 24, 9 attained CR and remained alive, 10-year probability of postrelapse survival 30%	N = 26, none attained CR, all died within 40 months of first relapse
Chou et al. [4] 2005 N = 43	<24 months 23% 3-year survival >24 months 53% 3-year survival	N = 35, 26 attained second CR, 3 died of chemotherapy toxicity, 9 remained alive at 3 years	N = 8, none attained CR, all died within
Bacci et al. [1] 2005 N = 235		N = 173, 30% attained CR and remain disease-free at 85 months	N = 62, none attained CR, all died at median of 10 months
Beate Kempf-Bielack et al. [2] 2005 N = 568	<18 months 11% 5-year survival >18 months 34% 5-year survival	N = 339, 148 attained CR and remained alive, median survival 2.2 years (range, 5 days to 18.4 years), 5-year overall survival 39%	N = 229, none attained CR, all died within 44 months
Bielack et al. [3] 2009 N = 249		N = 119, 5-year overall survival 32%	N = 130, none attained CR, 5-year OS 2%
Present study N = 15	Nonsurvivors, median RFI 17 months (range, 7 –40 months) Survivors, median RFI 34 months (range, 17–152 months)	N = 9, 7 attained CR and remain alive, PRDFS (3–14 years), 77% 10-year postrelapse disease-free survival	N = 6, all died within 40 months of relapse

Editor's Note: Please refer to original journal article for full references.
RFI = relapse-free interval; PRDFS = postrelapse disease-free survival; OS = overall survival; CR = complete remission.

Level of Evidence.—Level IV, therapeutic study. See Guidelines for Authors for a complete description of levels of evidence (Table 2).

▶ This article reports the oncologic outcomes in 15 patients with local or distant recurrence of osteosarcoma. Those who underwent surgical removal of disease showed better survival.

The sample size is limited, and the populations are not clearly comparable; those not operated on had extensive recurrences (eg, multiple bilateral lung nodules) compared with solitary or limited metastases in those who underwent surgery.

Why did I pick this article to review? The topic remains relevant, and the authors include an excellent review of the literature on the subject spanning a large number of studies and patients (Table 2). This highlights the point of the article: Surgical resection of local or distant recurrence is necessary for any meaningful hope of cure in these patients.

P. S. Rose, MD

Local Recurrence has only a Small Effect on Survival in High-risk Extremity Osteosarcoma
Kong C-B, Song WS, Cho WH, et al (Korea Cancer Ctr Hosp, Nowon-gu, Seoul; et al)
Clin Orthop Relat Res 470:1482-1490, 2012

Background.—Tumor enlargement after chemotherapy is considered one of the high-risk factors for local recurrence and survival in osteosarcoma. We hypothesized patients with this risk factor will have similar survival regardless of the development of local recurrence.

Questions/Purposes.—We asked (1) the prognostic factors for survival in our cohort, (2) how much effect local recurrence has on survival among patients with similar preoperative risk factors, and (3) what prognostic factors are important for survival in these selected patients.

Methods.—We analyzed the prognostic factors for survival in 449 patients with extremity osteosarcoma without metastatic disease at initial diagnosis and treatment (38 with local recurrence, 411 without local recurrence). We compared the survival difference between patients with local recurrence (n = 38) and without local recurrence (control, n = 76) matched for age, location, initial tumor volume, and tumor volume change after chemotherapy, and assessed prognostic factors in this subgroup.

Results.—In a cohort study, multivariate analysis revealed initial tumor volume, tumor enlargement, inadequate margin, and local recurrence predicted poor survival. In the case-control study, the 10-year metastasis-free survival rates of two groups were 13.1 ± 10.7% and 19.3 ± 9%, respectively. In the case-controlled groups, tumor enlargement and initial tumor volume showed multivariate significance.

Conclusions.—Local recurrence has a small impact on survival in patients with high-risk osteosarcoma.

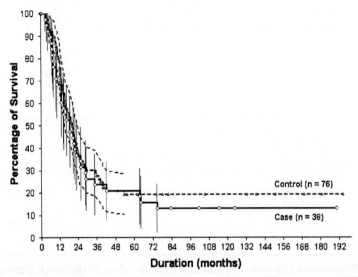

FIGURE 1.—Kaplan-Meier estimated survivorship curves show no differences ($p = 0.511$) between patients in the case (n = 38) and control (n = 76) groups for 10-year metastasis-free survival rates. (Reprinted from Kong C-B, Song WS, Cho WH, et al. Local recurrence has only a small effect on survival in high-risk extremity osteosarcoma. *Clin Orthop Relat Res.* 2012;470:1482-1490, with kind permission from Springer Science+Business Media.)

Level of Evidence.—Level III, prognostic study. See Guidelines for Authors for a complete description of levels of evidence (Fig 1).

▶ Local recurrence in osteosarcoma has traditionally been felt to have a high risk of death from disease; assuming adequate surgery, physicians have speculated whether this represents some unrecognized contamination in surgery or an expression of a biologically aggressive tumor fated to do poorly regardless of local recurrence. This is an excellent article in which the authors report a cohort study of patients with local recurrence of extremity osteosarcoma matched 2:1 with similar patients to investigate this topic.

Patients who had local recurrence were high-risk patients based on tumor size, size change during chemotherapy, and margin status. Their survival was worse but closely paralleled that of patients without local recurrence but who had similar adverse risk factors (13.1 vs 19.3% 10-year metastasis-free survival; Fig 1).

Patients with local recurrence fared worse than those without, but the impact of local recurrence on ultimate survival appears relatively small when these risk factors are accounted for. How best to interpret these results in clinical practice (eg, higher rate of amputation, more aggressive adjuvant chemotherapy) is unclear.

P. S. Rose, MD

Effects of Neoadjuvant Chemotherapy on Image-Directed Planning of Surgical Resection for Distal Femoral Osteosarcoma

Jones KB, Ferguson PC, Lam B, et al (Univ of Utah, Salt Lake City; Mount Sinai Hosp, Toronto, Ontario, Canada; et al)
J Bone Joint Surg Am 94:1399-1405, 2012

Background.—Standard therapy for localized osteosarcoma includes neoadjuvant chemotherapy preceding local control surgery, followed by adjuvant chemotherapy. When limb-salvage procedures were being developed, preoperative chemotherapy allowed a delay in definitive surgery to permit fabrication of custom endoprosthetic reconstruction implants. One rationale for its continuation as the care standard has been the perception that it renders surgery easier and safer. Our objective was to compare surgical procedures planned on the basis of magnetic resonance images (MRIs) of distal femoral osteosarcomas acquired before neoadjuvant chemotherapy with surgical procedures planned on the basis of MRIs acquired after neoadjuvant chemotherapy as a measure of the surgically critical anatomic effects of the chemotherapy.

Methods.—Twenty-four consecutive patients with distal femoral osteosarcoma had available digital MRIs preceding and following neoadjuvant chemotherapy. Thorough questionnaires were used to catalogue surgically critical anatomic details of MRI-directed surgical planning. Four faculty musculoskeletal oncologic surgeons and two musculoskeletal radiologists evaluated the blinded and randomly ordered MRIs. Interrater and intrarater reliabilities were calculated with intraclass correlation coefficients. The Student t test and chi-square test were used to compare pre-chemotherapy and post-chemotherapy continuous and categorical variables on the questionnaire. Mixed-effect regression models were employed to compare surgical procedures planned on the basis of pre-chemotherapy MRIs and with those planned on the basis of post-chemotherapy MRIs.

Results.—The blinded reviews generated strong intraclass correlation coefficients for both interrater (0.772) and mean intrarater (0.778) reliability. The MRI-planned resections for the majority of tumors changed meaningfully after chemotherapy, but in inconsistent directions. On the basis of mixed-effect regression modeling, it appeared that more amputations were planned on the basis of post-chemotherapy MRIs. No other parameters differed in a significant and clinically meaningful fashion. Surgeons demonstrated their expectation that neoadjuvant chemotherapy would improve resectability by planning more radical surgical procedures on the basis of scans that they predicted had been obtained pre-chemotherapy.

Conclusions.—Surgeons can reliably record the anatomic details of a planned resection of an osteosarcoma. Such methods may be useful in future multi-institutional clinical trials or registries. The common belief that neoadjuvant chemotherapy increases the resectability of extremity osteosarcomas remains anecdotally based. Rigorous assessment of this phenomenon in

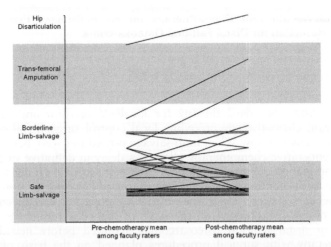

FIGURE 1.—Change in mean surgery-type designation by the four faculty surgeons assessing the blinded pre-chemotherapy and post-chemotherapy MRIs. Surgery-type designations were converted to integers one through four and averaged for each case at each time point. While some remained unchanged, others changed following administration of neoadjuvant chemotherapy toward either more or less radical/risky resections. (Multiple parallel lines are drawn at slight vertical offsets when values overlap, such that a single line represents each case.) (Reprinted from Jones KB, Ferguson PC, Lam B, et al. Effects of neoadjuvant chemotherapy on image-directed planning of surgical resection for distal femoral osteosarcoma. *J Bone Joint Surg Am*. 2012;94:1399-1405, with permission from The Journal of Bone and Joint Surgery, Incorporated.)

larger cohorts and at other anatomic sites as well as re-evaluation of other arguments for neoadjuvant chemotherapy should be considered (Fig 1).

▶ This is an instructive study from the Toronto group evaluating the hypothesis that neoadjuvant chemotherapy improves the resectability (eg, limb salvage) of osteosarcomas. The authors took 25 consecutive cases of osteosarcoma of the distal femur with pre- and postchemotherapy magnetic resonance scans and asked surgeons to plan operations without knowledge of the chemotherapy status of the patients.

Interestingly, the resections changed for the majority of tumors following chemotherapy, but in inconsistent directions and with a trend toward more amputations (Fig 1). Although certainly some patients experienced regression of tumor in critical anatomic areas, others worsened. Overall, more cases had further encroachment on critical structures than regression.

Where to place this in context is difficult. Goorin's often-forgotten prospective randomized trial did not show a benefit to neoadjuvant chemotherapy compared with immediate surgery in an admittedly underpowered trial. The current study reinforces those conclusions and draws into doubt the ability of chemotherapy to salvage limbs with large or otherwise at risk tumors.

P. S. Rose, MD

Results of Surgical Resection in Pelvic Ewing's Sarcoma

Puri A, Gulia A, Jambhekar NA, et al (Tata Memorial Hosp, Mumbai, India)
J Surg Oncol 106:417-422, 2012

Objective.—To evaluate the results of patients with non-metastatic Ewing's sarcoma of the pelvis treated with surgical resection as part of their multimodality treatment.

Methods.—Twenty-six patients treated between September 2000 and September 2009 were evaluated. Thirteen resections included the acetabulum and 13 did not. Thirteen resections excluding the acetabulum had no reconstruction. Arthrodesis was done in two, extracorporeal radiation and reimplantation in two, and pseudarthrosis in nine patients.

Results.—Three patients had involved margins. Seventeen patients had good response to chemotherapy and nine were poor responders. Twenty-one patients were available for follow-up. The follow-up ranged from 4 to 129 months (mean 36 months). Thirteen patients are currently alive. There was one local recurrence. On Kaplan—Meier analysis the overall survival was 72% at 5 years. The 3-year survival in good responders to chemotherapy was 94% compared to 30% in poor responders. The Musculoskeletal Tumor Society Score ranged from 23 to 29, with patients in whom the acetabulum was retained having better function compared to patients in whom acetabulum was resected.

Conclusion.—Surgery provides good local control and oncologic outcomes with acceptable function in these patients.

▶ The role of surgery, radiation, or both for local control of pelvic Ewing's sarcoma remains a controversial and individualized treatment decision. Many centers discount the role of surgery for axial Ewing's sarcoma because of the perceived dismal oncologic prognosis and extreme morbidity. Although it is certainly true that these tumors and their treatment have a tremendous impact on patients, this article from the largest orthopedic tumor center in India gives us actual data to assist in making treatment decisions for pelvic Ewing's sarcoma.

The authors present 26 patients treated surgically between 2000 and 2009; this distinguishes this series from other reports of pelvic Ewing's sarcoma that may go back 2 or 3 decades to accrue patients and span different treatment eras. Treatment was individualized with respect to radiation and surgical reconstruction. Survival was an impressive 72% at 5 years and was closely correlated with chemotherapy response. Three patients died of chemotherapy- or perioperative-related complications, and 7 suffered significant postoperative complications.

Where to place this article in context? Local control of pelvic Ewing's will remain an individualized decision process. This article provides guidance on modern treatment outcomes and morbidity to inform the decisions of surgeons caring for these patients.

P. S. Rose, MD

Clinical Outcome of Central Conventional Chondrosarcoma

Angelini A, Guerra G, Mavrogenis AF, et al (Univ of Bologna, Italy)
J Surg Oncol 106:929-937, 2012

Introduction.—Aim of this study was to analyze (1) survival, local recurrence (LR), and metastasis rates between the three histological tumor grades; (2) whether type of treatment and tumor site influenced prognosis for each histologic grade.

Methods.—We retrospectively studied 296 patients with central conventional chondrosarcomas (CS) (87 grade 1, 162 grade 2, and 47 grade 3). The femur was the most common site (91 cases), followed by the pelvis (82) and other less frequent sites. Type of surgery was related with histologic grade. Margins were wide in 222 cases, marginal in 23, and intralesional in 51 cases.

Results.—At a mean of 7 years, 201 patients remained continuously NED, 33 were NED after treatment of relapse, 15 were AWD, 35 were died of disease, and 12 of other causes. Survival was 92% at 5 years and 84% at 10 years, significantly influenced by histological grading. In grade 3 CS, two factors influenced survival: type of surgery (resection vs. amputation, $P = 0.051$) and site ($P = 0.039$). The two significant factors lost their significance at multivariate analysis.

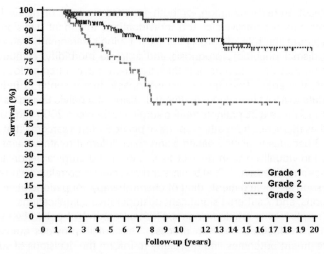

FIGURE 2.—Kaplan—Meier curves illustrating the overall survival for patients with histological grade 1–3 tumors. There is a statistical significant difference between grade 1 and 2 ($P = 0.074$), between grade 1 and 3 ($P < 0.0001$) and between grade 2 and 3 ($P = 0.0005$). (Reprinted from Angelini A, Guerra G, Mavrogenis AF, et al. Clinical outcome of central conventional chondrosarcoma. *J Surg Oncol.* 2012;106:929-937, reprinted by permission of Taylor & Francis Ltd, http://www.informaworld.com.)

Conclusion.—Central conventional CS with low/intermediate grade has a good prognosis, while high-grade tumors have poor outcome. Tumor relapses are strictly related with histologic grade (Fig 2).

▶ These authors retrospectively review the Rizzoli series of patients with central conventional chondrosarcoma, studying 296 patients treated over 28 years. As expected, survival was closely tied to histologic grade (Fig 2). These results mirror those seen in other studies of chondrosarcoma.

Curettage was successful in extremity grade I lesions, although this must be interpreted in light of the fact that the surgical selection was made by an expert group of surgeons. As virtually every study to examine it has shown, wide resection of all pelvic and more aggressive extremity lesions is critical for hope of cure. Because virtually every study on the subject was indicated, wide resection of pelvic and more aggressive extremity lesions is critical.

P. S. Rose, MD

Low-Grade Chondrosarcoma of Long Bones Treated with Intralesional Curettage Followed by Application of Phenol, Ethanol, and Bone-Grafting
Verdegaal SHM, Brouwers HFG, van Zwet EW, et al (Leiden Univ Med Ctr, The Netherlands)
J Bone Joint Surg Am 94:1201-1207, 2012

Background.—A common treatment of low-grade cartilaginous lesions of bone is intralesional curettage with local adjuvant therapy. Because of the wide variety of different diagnoses and treatments, there is still a lack of knowledge about the effectiveness of the use of phenol as local adjuvant therapy in patients with grade-I central chondrosarcoma of a long bone.

Methods.—A retrospective study was done to assess the clinical and oncological outcomes after intralesional curettage, application of phenol and ethanol, and bone-grafting in eighty-five patients treated between 1994 and 2005. Inclusion criteria were histologically proven grade-I central chondrosarcoma and location of the lesion in a long bone. The average age at surgery was 47.5 years (range, 15.6 to 72.3 years). The average duration of follow-up was 6.8 years (range, 0.2 to 14.1 years). Patients were evaluated periodically with conventional radiographs and gadolinium-enhanced magnetic resonance imaging (Gd-MRI) scans. When a lesion was suspected on the basis of the MRI, the patient underwent repeat intervention. Depending on the size of the recurrent lesion, biopsy followed by radiofrequency ablation (for lesions of <10 mm) or repeat curettage (for those of ≥10 mm) was performed.

Results.—Of the eighty-five patients, eleven underwent repeat surgery because a lesion was suspected on the basis of the Gd-MRI studies during follow-up. Of these eleven, five had a histologically proven local recurrence (a recurrence rate of 5.9% [95% confidence interval, 0.9% to 10.9%]), and all were grade-I chondrosarcomas. General complications consisted of one superficial infection, and two femoral fractures within six weeks after surgery.

Conclusions.—This retrospective case series without controls has limitations, but the use of phenol as an adjuvant after intralesional curettage of low-grade chondrosarcoma of a long bone was safe and effective, with a recurrence rate of <6% at a mean of 6.8 years after treatment.

Level of Evidence.—Therapeutic <u>Level IV</u>. See Instructions for Authors for a complete description of levels of evidence.

▶ Treatment of extremity low-grade chondrosarcoma remains in flux; wide resection offers excellent oncologic outcome but may be "overtreatment" of many central, indolent lesions. This series expounds on thoughtful intralesional treatment combined with phenol for low-grade tumors on long bones.

It is emphasized that this technique is not applicable to central (eg, pelvic) chondrosarcoma, where intralesional treatment has predictably poor results.

The authors present 85 patients treated and followed by magnetic resonance for local recurrence (the use of magnetic resonance distinguishes this series from most others on this topic). Local recurrence was suspected in 11 patients but only histologically confirmed in 5; of these, the authors state that in hindsight 2 were cases of residual rather than recurrent tumor. Recurrence-free survival was very good (Fig 5 in the original article).

This article continues our understanding of the acceptability of intralesional treatment of low-grade extremity chondrosarcoma; the adjuvant used (phenol as in this series, or cryosurgery or the argon beam coagulator) is likely less important than careful patient selection and meticulous surgical technique.

P. S. Rose, MD

The 'other' bone sarcomas: prognostic factors and outcomes of spindle cell sarcomas of bone

Pakos EE, Grimer RJ, Peake D, et al (Royal Orthopaedic Hosp, Birmingham, UK)
J Bone Joint Surg Br 93-B:1271-1278, 2011

We aimed to identify the incidence, outcome and prognostic factors associated with spindle cell sarcomas of bone (SCSB). We studied 196 patients with a primary non-metastatic tumour treated with the intent to cure. The results were compared with those of osteosarcoma patients treated at our hospital during the same period. The overall incidence of SCSB was 7.8% of all patients with a primary bone sarcoma. The five- and ten-year survival rates were 67.0% and 60.0%, respectively, which were better than those of patients with osteosarcoma treated over the same period. All histological subtypes had similar outcomes. On univariate analysis, factors that were significantly associated with decreased survival were age > 40 years, size > 8 cm, the presence of a pathological fracture, amputation, involved margins and a poor response to pre-operative chemotherapy.

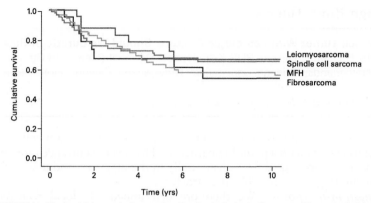

Time (yrs)

FIGURE 4.—Kaplan-Meier survival curve showing the similarity in disease-specific survival of the four main types of spindle cell sarcoma of bone (MFH, malignant fibrous histiocytoma). (Reprinted from Pakos EE, Grimer RJ, Peake D, et al. The 'other' bone sarcomas: prognostic factors and outcomes of spindle cell sarcomas of bone. *J Bone Joint Surg Br.* 2011;93-B:1271-1278, with permission from British Editorial Society of Bone and Joint Surgery.)

Multivariate analyses showed that age > 65 years, amputation and involved margins were all statistically significant prognostic factors. Involved margins and poor response to pre-operative chemotherapy were associated with an increased risk of local recurrence. SCSB has a better prognosis than osteosarcoma when matched for age. Most prognostic factors for osteosarcoma also seem to apply to SCSB. Patients with SCSB should be treated in the same way as patients of the same age with osteosarcoma (Fig 4).

▶ The terminology for bone sarcomas other than osteosarcomas, Ewings sarcoma, and chondrosarcomas has evolved over the past several decades, but all of these tumors are appropriately described as spindle cell sarcomas of bone. Prior studies from the Mayo, Rizzoli, and Memorial groups had reported on reasonable patient cohorts but suffered from broad time ranges spanning diagnostic and treatment advances.

Pakos and colleagues from the Birmingham group report here on 196 patients with spindle cell sarcomas of bone diagnosed between 1970 and 2006. They identify a better net prognosis for these tumors than other reports suggested, with an outcome similar to osteosarcoma. Risk factors for poor outcome included large size, age > 40, pathologic fractures, inadequate margins, and poor chemotherapy response.

Although rare, these tumors are certainly encountered in an oncology practice. This article improves our understanding of the prognosis of such lesions.

P. S. Rose, MD

Benign Bone Tumors

Giant Cell Tumor With Pathologic Fracture: Should We Curette or Resect?

van der Heijden L, Dijkstra PDS, Campanacci DA, et al (Univ Med Ctr, Leiden, The Netherlands; Azienda Ospedaliero-Universitaria Careggi, Florence, Italy; et al)
Clin Orthop Relat Res 471:820-829, 2013

Background.—Approximately one in five patients with giant cell tumor of bone presents with a pathologic fracture. However, recurrence rates after resection or curettage differ substantially in the literature and it is unclear when curettage is reasonable after fracture.

Questions/Purposes.—We therefore determined: (1) local recurrence rates after curettage with adjuvants or en bloc resection; (2) complication rates after both surgical techniques and whether fracture healing occurred after curettage with adjuvants; and (3) function after both treatment modalities for giant cell tumor of bone with a pathologic fracture.

Methods.—We retrospectively reviewed 48 patients with fracture from among 422 patients treated between 1981 and 2009. The primary treatment was resection in 25 and curettage with adjuvants in 23 patients. Minimum followup was 27 months (mean, 101 months; range, 27–293 months).

Results.—Recurrence rate was higher after curettage with adjuvants when compared with resection (30% versus 0%). Recurrence risk appears higher with soft tissue extension. The complication rate was lower after curettage with adjuvants when compared with resection (4% versus 16%) and included aseptic loosening of prosthesis, allograft failure, and pseudoarthrosis. Tumor and fracture characteristics did not increase complication risk. Fracture healing occurred in 24 of 25 patients. Mean Musculoskeletal Tumor Society score was higher after curettage with adjuvants (mean, 28; range, 23–30; n = 18) when compared with resection (mean, 25; range, 13–30; n = 25).

Conclusions.—Our observations suggest curettage with adjuvants is a reasonable option for giant cell tumor of bone with pathologic fractures. Resection should be considered with soft tissue extension, fracture through a local recurrence, or when structural integrity cannot be regained after reconstruction.

Level of Evidence.—Level III, therapeutic study. See Guidelines for Authors for a complete description of levels of evidence.

▶ This article from the Leiden group was presented and well received at the 2011 International Society of Limb Salvage meeting in Berlin. The authors analyzed 48 patients treated for pathologic fracture of giant cell tumors (GCTs) with resection or extended curettage.

The results have few surprises; curetted lesions recurred more frequently but had fewer complications and improved Musculoskeletal Tumor Society outcome scores. Readers should be cautioned that the study took patients from 3 centers with different local treatment criteria (decreasing the generalizability of the results).

The study is as notable for what it lacks—a comparison of the outcome of GCTs with pathologic fracture to those without. Unfortunately, the authors' dataset did not allow investigation of this clinically relevant issue.

P. S. Rose, MD

Which Treatment is the Best for Giant Cell Tumors of the Distal Radius? A Meta-analysis

Liu Y-p, Li K-h, Sun B-h (Central South Univ, Changsha, Hunan, PR China)
Clin Orthop Relat Res 470:2886-2894, 2012

Background.—Intralesional excision and en bloc resection are used to treat giant cell tumors (GCTs) of the distal radius. However, it is unclear whether one provides lower rates of recurrences and fewer complications, and whether the use of polymethylmethacrylate (PMMA) after curettage reduces the risk of recurrence.

Questions/Purposes.—We examined whether curettage was associated with lower rates of recurrence and fewer major complications compared with en bloc excision, and whether PMMA resulted in lower rates of recurrence compared with a bone graft.

Methods.—We systematically searched the literature using the criteria, "giant cell tumor" AND "curettage" OR "intralesional excision" OR "resection". Six relevant articles were identified that reported data for 80 curettage cases (PMMA, n = 49; bone graft, n = 26; no PMMA or bone grafts, n = 5) and 59 involving en bloc excision. A meta-analysis was performed using these data.

Results.—Overall, patients in the intralesional excision group had a higher recurrence rate (relative risk [RR], 2.80; 95% CI, 1.17—6.71), especially for Campanacci Grade 3 GCTs (RR, 4.90; 95% CI, 1.36—17.66), yet fewer major complications (RR, 0.21; 95% CI, 0.09—0.54) than the en bloc resection group. The use of PMMA versus bone graft did not affect the recurrence rate (RR, 0.98; 95% CI, 0.44—2.17).

Conclusions.—Based on data obtained from the limited number of studies available, intralesional excision appears to be more appropriate for the treatment of local lesions (eg, Grades 1 and 2) than Grade 3 GCTs of the distal radius. Moreover, PMMA was not additionally effective as an adjuvant.

Level of Evidence.—Level III, therapeutic study (systematic review). See Guidelines for Authors for a complete description of levels of evidence.

▶ Approximately 10% of giant cell tumors arise in the distal radius, and the high functional demands and complex local anatomy make selecting the best treatment option challenging. Liu and colleagues performed a meta-analysis to investigate whether resection or curettage provided the best treatment option.

The results are difficult to interpret because of the heterogeneity of the data set (in spite of great efforts by the authors to address a focused question). The results likely come as no surprise to surgeons who care for these patients; extensive Campanacci grade 3 lesions did best with resection, whereas lesser lesions were often well treated with curettage. Other expected results followed (eg, lower recurrence with resection).

Clearly, there is no superior treatment. Rather than a prescription for treatment, I find this article (with its analysis, nuances, and limitations) to be confirmation of the need to continue to individualize treatment options in this anatomic location.

P. S. Rose, MD

Evaluation of volume and solitary bone cyst remodeling using conventional radiological examination
Glowacki M, Ignys-O'Byrne A, Ignys I, et al (Karol Marcinkowski Univ of Med Sciences, Poznan, Poland; J. Strus City Hosp, Poznan, Poland)
Skelet Radiol 39:251-259, 2010

Objective.—To evaluate cyst remodeling, including complete healing and recurrence, and its relation to the cyst volume in two groups of patients, using curettage and bone grafting or methylprednisolone injection.

Materials and Methods.—A retrospective analysis was carried out on data from 132 patients with solitary bone cyst, where 79 (59.9%) had undergone curettage and bone grafting and 53 (40.1%) had been administered methylprednisolone injection, with a mean time to follow up of 12 years. The cyst volume was evaluated from conventional radiographs and the method originally reported by Göbel et al. to evaluate the volume of Ewing's sarcoma. The results were analyzed using the criteria of Neer et al. and Capanna et al.

Results.—The mean cyst volume was 36.8 cm^3. Recurrence was noted in 16 (20.2%) patients treated with curettage and in nine (17.0%) treated with methylprednisolone. Cyst volume in patients treated with curettage and bone grafting ranged from 8.3 cm^3 to 100.0 cm^3 and with methylprednisolone from 14.0 cm^3 to 50.6 cm^3. In neither group was the cyst volume related to recurrence. Volumes from 1.3 cm^3 to 81.9 cm^3 were stated for patients treated with curettage and bone grafting, when complete healing was observed; they were significantly lower than for those of the total group of patients who underwent curettage and bone grafting.

Conclusions.—1. An association between solitary cyst volume and recurrence in patients treated with either bone curettage and grafting or methylprednisolone was not found. 2. The frequency of complete healing in patients treated with bone curettage and grafting decreased with an increase in the cyst volume.

▶ This article was previously presented at the European Society of Musculoskeletal Radiology meeting. The authors retrospectively review 132 patients treated for unicameral bone cysts with either curettage and grafting or methylprednisolone. Healing rates were similar between both groups; recurrence was not related to cyst volume, but larger cysts had less complete healing.

Where to place this study in the context of orthopedic oncology? A large number of treatment options exist for these benign bony cysts that can be individualized for patient presentations and surgeon preference. Both options appear to offer good chance of healing for patients; as expected, larger cysts are less likely to completely fill in but can still have good outcome.

P. S. Rose, MD

Resection and Reconstruction Techniques

Computer-generated Custom Jigs Improve Accuracy of Wide Resection of Bone Tumors
Khan FA, Lipman JD, Pearle AD, et al (Stony Brook Univ School of Medicine, NY; Hosp for Special Surgery, NY; et al)
Clin Orthop Relat Res 2013 [Epub ahead of print]

Background.—Manual techniques of reproducing a preoperative plan for primary bone tumor resection using rudimentary devices and imprecise localization techniques can result in compromised margins or unnecessary removal of unaffected tissue. We examined whether a novel technique using computer-generated custom jigs more accurately reproduces a preoperative resection plan than a standard manual technique.

Description of Technique.—Using CT images and advanced imaging, reverse engineering, and computer-assisted design software, custom jigs were designed to precisely conform to a specific location on the surface of partially skeletonized cadaveric femurs. The jigs were used to perform a hemimetaphyseal resection.

Methods.—We performed CT scans on six matched pairs of cadaveric femurs. Based on a primary bone sarcoma model, a joint-sparing, hemimetaphyseal wide resection was precisely outlined on each femur. For each pair, the resection was performed using the standard manual technique on one specimen and the custom jig-assisted technique on the other. Superimposition of preoperative and postresection images enabled quantitative analysis of resection accuracy.

Results.—The mean maximum deviation from the preoperative plan was 9.0 mm for the manual group and 2.0 mm for the custom-jig group. The percentages of times the maximum deviation was greater than 3 mm and greater than 4 mm was 100% and 72% for the manual group and 5.6% and 0.0% for the custom-jig group, respectively.

Conclusions.—Our findings suggest that custom-jig technology substantially improves the accuracy of primary bone tumor resection, enabling a surgeon to reproduce a given preoperative plan reliably and consistently.

▶ In this surgical technique article, the authors explore a different twist on navigation: Rather than using a computer navigation system (with its expense and cumbersome nature), they use computer-generated cutting jigs to perform resections. This article is a proof-of-concept test of this innovative way of approaching this problem.

Although not yet commercially available, I have included this article because it may provide a practical method for centers that lack the resources to purchase sophisticated equipment but still wish to develop navigation capabilities.

P. S. Rose, MD

Aseptic Failure: How Does the Compress® Implant Compare to Cemented Stems?
Pedtke AC, Wustrack RL, Fang AS, et al (Univ of California San Francisco; The Permanente Med Group, South San Francisco, CA; et al)
Clin Orthop Relat Res 470:735-742, 2012

Background.—Failure of endoprosthetic reconstruction with conventional stems due to aseptic loosening remains a challenge for maintenance of limb integrity and function. The Compress® implant (Biomet Inc, Warsaw, IN, USA) attempts to avoid aseptic failure by means of a unique technologic innovation. Though the existing literature suggests survivorship of Compress® and stemmed implants is similar in the short term, studies are limited by population size and followup duration.

Questions/Purposes.—We therefore compared (1) the rate of aseptic failure between Compress® and cemented intramedullary stems and (2) evaluated the overall intermediate- term implant survivorship.

Methods.—We reviewed 26 patients with Compress® implants and 26 matched patients with cemented intramedullary stems. The patients were operated on over a 3-year period. Analysis focused on factors related to implant survival, including age, sex, diagnosis, infection, aseptic loosening, local recurrence, and fracture. Minimum followup was 0.32 years (average, 6.2 years; range, 0.32–9.2 years).

Results.—Aseptic failure occurred in one (3.8%) patient with a Compress® implant and three (11.5%) patients with cemented intramedullary stems. The 5-year implant survival rate was 83.5% in the Compress® group and 66.6% in the cemented intramedullary stem group.

Conclusions.—The Compress® implant continues to be a reliable option for distal femoral limb salvage surgery. Data regarding aseptic failure is encouraging, with equivalent survivorship against cemented endoprosthetic replacement at intermediate-term followup.

Level of Evidence.—Level III, therapeutic study. See Guidelines for Authors for a complete description of levels of evidence (Fig 2).

▶ Despite its early introduction in the 1990s, relatively little has been reported on the outcome of the Compress® implant, a unique form of osseointegration for endoprosthetic limb salvage. This article reports the risk of aseptic failure of the first 26 prostheses used in the US Food and Drug Administration approval study and compares them with a cohort of cemented endoprostheses in a

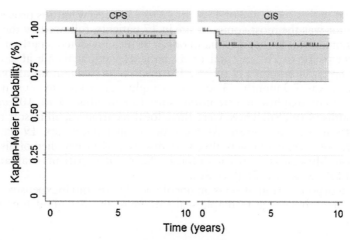

FIGURE 2.—A Kaplan-Meier survival curve shows no difference ($p = 0.22$) in the 5-year implant survival rates using aseptic loosening as the end point between the CPS and CIS implants: 95.7% and 91.3%, respectively. Hash marks = censored data. Gray lines = 95% CIs. (Reprinted from Pedtke AC, Wustrack RL, Fang AS, et al. Aseptic failure: how does the compress® implant compare to cemented stems? *Clin Orthop Relat Res*. 2012;470:735-742, with kind permission from Springer Science+Business Media.)

collaborative effort between the University of California San Francisco and Birmingham groups.

Given the small numbers involved, there was no difference in aseptic failure between the 2 groups (Fig 2). The authors also report a higher implant survival rate in the Compress group, but this is more nuanced in interpretation, as it mixes in septic failure and local recurrences, which are likely independent of implant design and hard to interpret in a small cohort.

The Compress implant is a unique advance in endoprosthetic design; this article provides refreshing evidence of its equivalency to conventional implants.

P. S. Rose, MD

The outcome of the treatment of diaphyseal primary bone sarcoma by resection, irradiation and re-implantation of the host bone: extracorporeal irradiation as an option for reconstruction in diaphyseal bone sarcomas

Puri A, Gulia A, Jambhekar N, et al (Tata Memorial Hosp, Mumbai, India)
J Bone Joint Surg Br 94-B:982-988, 2012

We analysed the outcome of patients with primary non-metastatic diaphyseal sarcomas who had *en bloc* resection with preservation of the adjoining joints and reconstruction with re-implantation of sterilised tumour bone after extracorporeal radiation (50 Gy). Between March 2005 and September 2009, 32 patients (16 Ewing's sarcoma and 16 osteogenic sarcoma) with a mean age of 15 years (2 to 35) underwent this procedure. The femur was the most common site in 17 patients, followed by the tibia in 11, humerus in three and ulna in one. The mean resected length of bone was 19 cm (10 to 26). A total of 31 patients were available at a mean follow-up of 34 months (12 to 74). The mean time to union for all osteotomy sites was 7.3 months (3 to 28): metaphyseal osteotomy sites united quicker than diaphyseal osteotomy sites (5.8 months (3 to 10) *versus* 9.5 months (4 to 28)). There were three local recurrences, all in soft-tissue away from irradiated graft. At the time of final follow-up, 19 patients were free of disease, one was alive with disease and 11 had died of disease. The mean Musculoskeletal Tumor Society Score for 29 patients evaluated at the last follow-up was 26 (9 to 30).

Extracorporeal irradiation is an oncologically safe and inexpensive technique for limb salvage in diaphyseal sarcomas and has good functional results.

▶ A number of options exist for the reconstruction of diaphyseal bone tumor resections, and this variety of options reminds us that no clear optimal method has yet been identified. In this report, Puri and colleagues describe the outcome of resection, extracorporal irradiation, and reimplantation of 31 patients with diaphyseal primary bone tumors. Although allografts, vascularized autografts, and endoprostheses are more commonly used in North American centers, this remains a valid technique that the authors report in a contemporary series.

Specimens were irradiated to 50 Gy in a single session (with an anticipated biologic effective dose much greater than a typical 50 Gy fractionated dose). Three recurrences occurred within the soft-tissue envelope in conjunction with metastatic disease; reoperation rate was 45%. Ultimate function in surviving patients was good.

This is a valuable article for surgeons interested in incorporating this technique into their own clinical practice. The complication rate is high but probably similar to that of other techniques.

P. S. Rose, MD

Does Limb Salvage Surgery Offer Patients Better Quality of Life and Functional Capacity Than Amputation?
Malek F, Somerson JS, Mitchel S, et al (Univ of Texas Health Science Ctr San Antonio)
Clin Orthop Relat Res 470:2000-2006, 2012

Introduction.—Patients with aggressive lower extremity musculoskeletal tumors may be candidates for either above-knee amputation or limb-salvage surgery. Patients with amputations and access to modern prostheses had similar Short Form-36 and Toronto Extremity Salvage Scores compared to limb salvage patients. However, the subjective and objective benefits of limb-salvage surgery compared with amputation are not fully clear.

Questions/Purposes.—We therefore compared functional status and quality of life for patients treated with above-knee amputation versus limb-salvage surgery.

Methods.—We reviewed 20 of 51 patients aged 15 years and older treated with above-knee amputation or limb-salvage surgery for aggressive musculoskeletal tumors around the knee between 1994 and 2004 as a retrospective cohort study. At last followup we obtained the Physiological Cost Index, the Reintegration to Normal Living Index, SF-36, and the Toronto Extremity Salvage Score questionnaires. The minimum followup was 12 months (median, 56 months; range, 12—108 months).

Results.—Compared with patients having above-knee amputation, patients undergoing limb-salvage surgery had superior Physiological Cost Index scores and Reintegration to Normal Living Index. The Toronto Extremity Salvage scores and SF-36 scores were similar in the two groups.

Conclusion.—These data suggest that limb-salvage surgery offers better gait efficiency and return to normal living compared with above-knee amputation, but does not improve the patient's perception of quality of life.

▶ As a principle of preserving function in orthopedic oncology resections, our standard of care is to offer patients limb salvage surgery whenever possible; most surgeons and nearly all patients maintain a belief that this will provide superior clinical outcomes.

These authors retrospectively reviewed a group of patients treated with lower extremity amputation or limb salvage surgery. Despite no amputation, patients having access to current advanced prostheses (eg, C-leg and similar devices), similar Short Form-36 and Toronto Extremity Salvage Scores were seen in both groups. Limb salvage patients had less physiologic strain (measured by heart rate change while ambulating and a higher "Reintegration to Normal Living Index") (see Fig 1 in the original article).

Where do we place this article in context? Despite many limitations and potential selection biases, amputation patients equaled limb salvage patients in major clinical outcomes. These results reinforce the excellent expected outcome for patients after either treatment modality.

P. S. Rose, MD

Functional Outcomes and Gait Analysis of Patients After Periacetabular Sarcoma Resection With and Without Ischiofemoral Arthrodesis
Carmody Soni EE, Miller BJ, Scarborough MT, et al (Washington Hosp Ctr, DC; Univ of Iowa; Univ of Florida, Gainesville)
J Surg Oncol 106:844-849, 2012

Background.—Treatment of periacetabular sarcomas remains a difficult challenge. Many reconstruction options are fraught with high complication and failure rates. Little is known about patients' functional outcomes, and there have been no studies that examine how these reconstructions affect patients' gait parameters. The purpose of this study is to evaluate gait parameters and functional outcome in patients whom have undergone periacetabular resections with either an ischiofemoral pseudoarthrodesis or soft tissue reconstruction only.

Methods.—Ten patients with sarcoma of the periacetabular region were identified from our database. Functional outcome was assessed using the Musculoskeletal Tumor Society Scores (MSTS) and Toronto Extremity Salvage Score (TESS) scoring systems. Gait analysis was performed on all subjects.

Results.—Patients in both surgical groups had average functional scores. All patients were ambulatory. Cadence and velocity in the surgical group were significantly slower than the control group, however, the remainder of the gait parameters examined were similar to controls.

Conclusion.—Patients who underwent minimal reconstruction following periacetabular resections demonstrated average functional scores, comparable to those undergoing more extensive reconstructions. With the exception of speed, gait parameters were not significantly different than controls. Complication rates were low. Pseudoarthrodesis or even no bone reconstruction following periacetabular resection is reasonable and functional options for many of these patients.

▶ Surgeons continue to debate the role of anatomic reconstruction versus lesser or minimal reconstruction following periacetabular resections. Authors at the University of Florida analyzed outcome scores and gait laboratory parameters on 10 patients who either had a flail reconstruction or an ischiofemoral arthrodesis attempt and compared these with reported series and other controls.

Results were quite favorable, with all patients ambulatory and with similar gait parameters to controls except for slower gait cadence and velocity. This article gives quantitative support to the generally favorable results from limited reconstruction after periacetabular resections. Given the high complication rates of extensive reconstructive procedures, these data are important in selecting procedures for patients who may need to rapidly resume chemotherapy.

P. S. Rose, MD

Poor Long-term Clinical Results of Saddle Prosthesis After Resection of Periacetabular Tumors
Jansen JA, van de Sande MAJ, Dijkstra PDS (Leiden Univ Med Ctr, The Netherlands)
Clin Orthop Relat Res 471:324-331, 2013

Background.—The saddle prosthesis originally was developed to reconstruct large acetabular defects in revision hip arthroplasty and was used primarily for hip reconstruction after periacetabular tumor resections. The long-term survival of these reconstructions is unclear.

Questions/Purpose.—We therefore examined the long-term function, complications, and survival in patients treated with saddle prostheses after periacetabular tumor resection.

Patients and Methods.—Between 1987 and 2003 we treated 17 patients with a saddle prosthesis after periacetabular tumor resection (12 chondrosarcomas, three osteosarcomas, one malignant fibrous histiocytoma, one metastasis). During followup, 11 patients died, resulting in a median overall survival of 49 months (95% CI, 30—68 months). The remaining six patients were alive without disease (mean followup, 12.1 years; range, 8.3—16.8 years). In one patient the saddle prosthesis was removed after 3 months owing to dislocation and infection. We obtained SF-36 questionnaires, Toronto Extremity Salvage Scores (TESS), and Musculoskeletal Tumor Society (MSTS) scores.

Results.—Thirteen of 17 patients used walking assists for mobilization at last followup: eight patients required two crutches, five needed one crutch, and one did not use any walking aids. The other three patients were not able to mobilize independently and only made bed to chair transfers. The mean hip flexion in the six surviving patients was 60° (range, 40°—100°) at last followup. Local complications were seen in 14 of the 17 patients: nine wound infections, seven dislocations, and two leg-length discrepancies requiring additional surgery. In the five surviving patients with their index prosthesis still in situ, the mean MSTS score at long-term followup was 47% (range, 20%—77%), the mean TESS score was 53% (range, 41%—67%), and the mean composite SF-36 physical and mental component summaries were 43.9 and 50.6, respectively.

Conclusion.—Reconstruction with saddle prostheses after periacetabular tumor surgery has a high risk of complications and poor long-term function with limited hip flexion; therefore, we no longer use the saddle prosthesis for reconstruction after periacetabular tumor resections.

Level of Evidence.—Level IV, retrospective case series. See the Guideline for Authors for a complete description of levels of evidence.

▶ Reliable reconstruction after periacetabular resection remains elusive; this article from the 2011 International Society of Limb Salvage symposium published in *Clinical Orthopaedics and Related Research* reports long-term followup on a group of 17 patients treated with saddle prostheses at the Leiden center, including Toronto Extremity Salvage Scores (TESS) and Musculoskeletal Tumor Society (MSTS) scores on surviving patients.

The results were disappointing, and the authors state they have abandoned this technique. Although the long-term function is poor, function after acetabular resection is expected to be unpredictable and compromised. What is most striking about this report is the very high complication rate (14 of 17 patients). Although pelvic tumor reconstruction is always individualized and the saddle may continue to be an option for some patients, its use is probably best avoided in patients requiring rapid resumption of chemotherapy postoperatively (in whom complications would delay resumption of adjuvant therapy).

P. S. Rose, MD

Extensor Function After Medial Gastrocnemius Flap Reconstruction of the Proximal Tibia

Jentzsch T, Erschbamer M, Seeli F, et al (Balgrist Univ Hosp, Zurich, Switzerland)
Clin Orthop Relat Res 2013 [Epub ahead of print]

Background.—Reconstruction of the extensor mechanism after resection of the proximal tibia is challenging, and several methods are available. A medial gastrocnemius flap commonly is used, although it may be associated with an extensor lag. This problem also is encountered, although perhaps to a lesser extent, with other techniques for reconstruction of the extensor apparatus. It is not known how such lag develops with time and how it correlates with functional outcome.

Questions/Purposes.—We therefore (1) assessed patellar height with time, (2) correlated patellar height with function using the Musculoskeletal Tumor Society (MSTS) score, and (3) correlated patellar height with range of motion (ROM) after medial gastrocnemius flap reconstruction.

Methods.—Sixteen patients underwent tumor endoprosthesis implantation and extensor apparatus reconstruction between 1997 and 2009 using a medial gastrocnemius flap after sarcoma resection of the proximal tibia. These patients represented 100% of the population for whom we performed extensor mechanism reconstructions during that time. The minimum followup was 2 years (mean, 5 years; range, 2–11 years). Fourteen patients were alive at the time of this study. We used the Blackburne-Peel Index to follow patellar height radiographically with time. Functional outcomes were assessed retrospectively using the MSTS, and ROM was evaluated through active extensor lag and flexion.

Results.—Eleven patients had patella alta develop, whereby the maximal patellar height was reached after a mean of 2 years and then stabilized. More normal patellar height was associated with better functional scores, a smaller extensor lag, but less flexion; the mean extensor lag (and flexion) of patients with patella alta was 17° (and 94°) compared with only 4° (and 77°) without.

Conclusions.—In our patients patella alta evolved during the first 2 postoperative years. Patella alta is associated with extensor lag, greater flexion, and worse MSTS scores. Surgical fixation of the patellar tendon more distally to its anatomic position or strict postoperative bracing may be advisable.

Level of Evidence.—Level IV, clinical cohort study. See the Guidelines for Authors for a complete description of levels of evidence.

▶ Although retrospective in nature, this is an excellent evaluation of a group of 16 extensor mechanism reconstructions after proximal tibia tumor resections. The authors thoughtfully analyze how these reconstructions evolve (more bluntly, stretch out) over time and how this influences range of motion and Musculoskeletal Tumor Society (MSTS) outcome scores.

The results are notable for patella alta developing with time but largely stabilizing by 2 years and correlating with worse MSTS scores. I have selected this study for inclusion in the YEAR BOOK because it is a clinically relevant problem for surgeons who treat tibial tumors and includes a thoughtful analysis and literature-based discussion.

P. S. Rose, MD

Vascularized fibula transfer for lower limb reconstruction
Beris AE, Lykissas MG, Korompilias AV, et al (Univ of Ioannina School of Medicine, Greece; et al)
Microsurgery 31:205-211, 2011

Massive bony defects of the lower extremity are usually the result of high-energy trauma, tumor resection, or severe sepsis. Vascularized fibular grafts are useful in the reconstruction of large skeletal defects, especially in cases of scarred and avascular recipient sites, or in patients with combined bone and soft-tissue defects. Microvascular free fibula transfer is considered the most suitable autograft for reconstruction of the middle tibia because of its long cylindrical straight shape, mechanical strength, predictable vascular pedicle, and hypertrophy potential. The ability to fold the free fibula into two segments or to combine it with massive allografts is a useful technique for reconstruction of massive bone defects of the femur or proximal tibia. It can also be transferred with skin, fascia, or muscle as a composite flap. Proximal epiphyseal fibula transfer has the potential for longitudinal growth and can be used in the hip joint remodeling procedures. Complications can be minimized by careful preoperative planning of the procedure, meticulous intraoperative microsurgical techniques, and strict postoperative rehabilitation protocols. This literature review highlights the different surgical techniques, indications, results, factors influencing the outcome, and major complications of free vascularized fibular graft for management of skeletal or composite defects of the lower limb.

▶ Rather than a research study, this is a review article in the microsurgery literature. I have selected it for inclusion in the YEAR BOOK article because it provides an accessible review of vascularized reconstructive options for lower extremity oncologic surgeons. Although some of the information provided deals with other clinical scenarios (eg, posttraumatic bony defects), the techniques and principles included are valuable for the oncologic surgeon.

P. S. Rose, MD

The current role of the vascularized-fibular osteocutaneous graft in the treatment of segmental defects of the upper extremity
Hollenbeck ST, Komatsu I, Woo S, et al (Duke Univ Hosp, Durham, NC)
Microsurgery 31:183-189, 2011

Large osseous defects of the upper extremity can be a challenging problem for the reconstructive surgeon. There are numerous treatment options reported in the literature with variable results. We review our experience with the vascularized-fibular osteocutaneous graft for these complex defects with a focus on surgical techniques and outcomes.

▶ Upper extremity defects can be difficult to treat in orthopedic oncology given the high functional demands of the upper extremity and the relatively less-advanced nature of our prosthetic options. All tumor surgeons have experience using vascularized fibula grafts in this setting. I have chosen this article as a well-written review of the use of free fibula grafts in this setting; although not confined to strictly oncologic indications, it reports well the relevant literature as well as union and complication rates for tumor surgeons to refer to and become familiar with.

P. S. Rose, MD

Allograft Reconstruction for the Treatment of Musculoskeletal Tumors of the Upper Extremity
Aponte-Tinao LA, Ayerza MA, Muscolo DL, et al (Italian Hosp of Buenos Aires, Argentina)
Sarcoma 2013:1-6, 2013

In comparison with the lower extremity, there is relatively paucity literature reporting survival and clinical results of allograft reconstructions after excision of a bone tumor of the upper extremity. We analyze the survival of allograft reconstructions in the upper extremity and analyze the final functional score according to anatomical site and type of reconstruction. A consecutive series of 70 allograft reconstruction in the upper limb with a mean followup of 5 years was analyzed, 38 osteoarticular allografts, 24 allograft-prosthetic composites, and 8 intercalary allografts. Kaplan-Meier survival analysis of the allografts was performed, with implant revision for any cause and amputation used as the end points. The function evaluation was performed using MSTS functional score. Sixteen patients (23%) had revision surgery for 5 factures, 2 infections, 5 allograft resorptions, and 2 local recurrences. Allograft survival at five years was 79% and 69% at ten years. In the group of patients treated with an osteoarticular allograft the articular surface survival was 90% at five years and 54% at ten years. The limb salvage rate was 98% at five and 10 years. We conclude that articular deterioration and fracture were the most frequent mode of failure in proximal humeral osteoarticular reconstructions and allograft resorption in elbow reconstructions. The best functional score was observed in the intercalary humeral allograft (Fig 5).

▶ In contrast to the nearby article reviewing free fibula options in the treatment of upper extremity defects, Aponte and colleagues present 70 consecutive allograft reconstructions of the upper extremity. Readers should know that this group enjoys unparalleled experience with the use of allografts in limb salvage surgery.

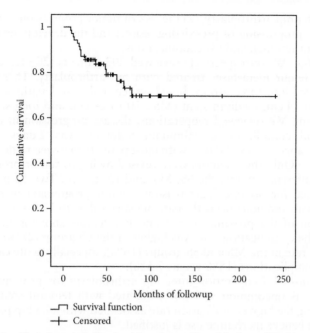

Months of followup

⌐ Survival function

─┼─ Censored

FIGURE 5.—Allograft survival. (Reprinted from Aponte-Tinao LA, Ayerza MA, Muscolo DL, et al. Allograft reconstruction for the treatment of musculoskeletal tumors of the upper extremity. *Sarcoma.* 2013;2013:1-6, with permission from Luis A. Aponte-Tinao et al.)

This article provides a review of techniques and outcomes possible for upper extremity reconstruction. Even in these experienced hands, revision surgery was seen in 23% of patients (primarily for fracture or resorption). Allograft survival was ~70% at 10 years, similar to most prosthetic series (Fig 5). This article can inform treatment options, just as surgeon preference and local resources will determine different clinical decisions.

P. S. Rose, MD

Metastatic Disease

A Long Femoral Stem Is Not Always Required in Hip Arthroplasty for Patients With Proximal Femur Metastases

Xing Z, Moon BS, Satcher RL, et al (Univ of South Alabama College of Medicine, Mobile, AL; Univ of Texas MD Anderson Cancer Ctr, Houston)
Clin Orthop Relat Res 2013 [Epub ahead of print]

Background.—During hip arthroplasties for treating proximal femur metastases, a long femoral stem frequently is used, presumably protecting the entire femur against progression of the existing lesions or development of new lesions. However, it is unclear whether a long stem is really required.

Questions/Purposes.—We therefore determined in patients with proximal femur metastases (1) the reoperation rate related to different stem lengths after hip arthroplasty, (2) the risk of tumor progression in the same femur (the progression of preexisting lesions and the development of new distal femur lesions), and (3) complications.

Methods.—We retrospectively reviewed 203 patients (206 femurs) with proximal femur metastases treated with hip arthroplasty. These femurs were divided into three groups based on femoral stem length: short stem (SS), 12 to 14 cm; medium stem (MS), 20 to 24 cm; and long stem (LS), 25 to 35 cm. We reviewed reoperations, disease progression in the same femur, and complications. Minimum followup was 2 days (median, 487 days; range, 2–4853 days), with most patients followed to their death.

Results.—Only three femurs were revised owing to tumor progression, with no difference among the SS, MS, and LS groups. Two SS prostheses were revised for nononcologic reasons. Tumor progression in the same femur was uncommon during the patient's survival, with 11 femurs showing progression of the proximal lesion and five femurs showing new distal lesions. The complication rate was higher in the LS group (28%) than the combined rate in the MS and SS groups (16%), especially acute cardiopulmonary complications (18% versus 7.5%).

Conclusions.—Reoperation after hip arthroplasty for proximal femur metastases is uncommon and not correlated with femoral stem length. Considering the high complication rate associated with a LS hip prosthesis, we do not believe its routine use is justified.

Level of Evidence.—Level III, therapeutic study. See Instructions for Authors for a complete description of levels of evidence (Table 2).

▶ Similar to the article by Alvi and Damron below, these authors report on the MD Anderson experience with different length femoral stems for proximal femoral metastases. The results show similar rates of reoperation for oncologic failure for

TABLE 2.—Postoperative Data of the Three Groups with Different Stem Lengths

Variable	SS	MS	LS	p Value
Number of femurs	35	99	72	
Reoperation (all reasons)	3	1	1	0.034
Reoperation (oncologic reasons)	1	1	1	0.734
Progression of proximal lesions	1	3	7	0.145
New distal lesions	1	2	2	1.0
Overall complications	4	17	20	0.038 (LS versus MS + SS)
Cardiovascular complications	2	8	13	0.020 (LS versus MS + SS)

*Values are expressed as number of femurs; SS = short stem; MS = medium stem; LS = long stem.

short-stem, medium-stem, and long-stem devices. However, the complication rate was significantly higher in the long-stem group (Table 2).

As with the Alvi and Damron article, which can also be found in this section, this article alone may not justify a change in clinical practice. However, it does in particular call into question the reflexive use of a long cemented stem in the absence of identifiable distal lesions. Nononcologic failure was surprisingly high in the short-stem group, and when presented at the podium the authors expressed a preference for medium-stem implants based on these data. This seems a very reasonable starting point for clinical decision making.

P. S. Rose, MD

Prophylactic Stabilization for Bone Metastases, Myeloma, or Lymphoma: Do We Need to Protect the Entire Bone?
Alvi HM, Damron TA (Northwestern Univ Feinberg School of Medicine, Chicago, IL; Upstate Med Univ, East Syracuse, NY)
Clin Orthop Relat Res 471:706-714, 2013

Background.—The current operative standard of care for disseminated malignant bone disease suggests stabilizing the entire bone to avoid the need for subsequent operative intervention but risks of doing so include complications related to embolic phenomena.

Questions/Purposes.—We questioned whether progression and reoperation occur with enough frequency to justify additional risks of longer intramedullary devices.

Methods.—A retrospective chart review was done for 96 patients with metastases, myeloma, or lymphoma who had undergone stabilization or arthroplasty of impending or actual femoral or humeral pathologic fractures using an approach favoring intramedullary fixation devices and long-stem arthroplasty. Incidence of progressive bone disease, reoperation, and complications associated with fixation and arthroplasty devices in instrumented femurs or humeri was determined.

Results.—At minimum 0 months followup (mean, 11 months; range, 0–72 months), 80% of patients had died. Eleven of 96 patients (12%) experienced local bony disease progression; eight had local progression at the original site, two had progression at originally recognized discretely separate lesions, and one had a new lesion develop in the bone that originally was surgically treated. Six subjects (6.3%) required repeat operative intervention for symptomatic failure. Twelve (12.5%) patients experienced physiologic nonfatal complications potentially attributable to embolic phenomena from long intramedullary implants.

Conclusions.—Because most patients in this series were treated with the intent to protect the bone with long intramedullary implants when possible, the reoperation rate may be lower than if the entire bone had not been protected. However, the low incidence of disease progression apart from originally identified lesions (one of 96) was considerably lower than the physiologic complication rate (12 of 96) potentially attributable to long intramedullary implants.

Level of Evidence.—Level IV, therapeutic study. See Guidelines for Authors for a complete description of levels of evidence.

▶ This is a provocative retrospective review article that questions the standard approach of placing long-stem implants when treating metastatic disease in the femur. These authors reviewed 96 patients treated for metastatic or systemic malignancies and found only one case of disease progression at a new site not previously recognized in the bone. In contrast, 12 patients suffered complications potentially attributable to the use of long stem devices. The clear implication is that many could have undergone lesser surgeries.

The article suffers from the well-recognized flaws of a retrospective analysis and has a large number of potentially eligible patients lost to follow-up. Although I do not think this article can or should necessarily change our standard of care, it is an interesting analysis that reinforces the need to critically select the best treatment for individual patients rather than use a single long stem protocol for all patients with metastatic disease.

P. S. Rose, MD

Which Implant Is Best After Failed Treatment for Pathologic Femur Fractures?

Forsberg JA, Wedin R, Bauer H (Naval Med Res Ctr, Silver Spring, MD; Karolinska Univ Hosp, Stockholm, Sweden)
Clin Orthop Relat Res 471:735-740, 2013

Background.—Successful treatment of pathologic femur fractures can preserve a patient's independence and quality of life. The choice of implant depends on several disease and patient-specific variables; however, its durability must generally match the patient's estimated life expectancy. Failures do occur, however, it is unclear which implants are associated with greater risk of failure.

Questions/Purposes.—We evaluated patients with femoral metastases in whom implants failed to determine (1) the rate of reoperation; (2) the timing of and most common causes for failure; and (3) incidence of perioperative complications and death.

Methods.—From a prospectively collected registry, we identified 93 patients operated on for failed treatment of femoral metastases from 1990 to 2010. We excluded five patients who subsequently underwent amputations leaving 88 who underwent salvage procedures. These included intramedullary nails (n = 11), endoprostheses (n = 61), and plate fixation (n = 16). The primary outcome was reoperation after salvage treatment.

Results.—Seventeen of the 88 patients (19%) required subsequent reoperation a median of 10 months (interquartile range, 4–14) from the time of salvage surgery: 15 for material failure, one for local progression of tumor, and one for a combination of these. Five patients died within 4 weeks of surgery. Although perioperative complications were higher in the endoprosthesis group and dislocations occurred, overall treatment failures after salvage surgery were lower in the that group (four of 61) compared the group with plate fixation (eight of 16) and intramedullary nail groups (five of 11).

Conclusions.—Despite relatively common perioperative complications, salvage using endoprostheses may be associated with fewer treatment failures as compared with internal fixation.

Level of Evidence.—Level III, therapeutic study. See Guidelines for Authors for a complete description of levels of evidence.

▶ Forsberg and colleagues have taken a mundane but clinically relevant topic—salvage treatment for pathologic femur fractures—and lent scientific validity to established practice patterns at many centers around the world. In short, revision of pathologic fracture constructs was most reliably performed using arthroplasty. These larger procedures came with a modest complication rate.

This article confirms the clinical experience of many surgeons; it also highlights the manner in which these fractures differ from nononcologic fractures. As such, its value is probably greatest to the nononcologic surgeon who is treating these patients as a quantitative reminder of the need to manage these fractures differently from standard traumatic injuries.

P. S. Rose, MD

Minimally invasive surgery of humeral metastasis using flexible nails and cement in high-risk patients with advanced cancer
Kim JH, Kang HG, Kim JR, et al (Natl Cancer Ctr, Gyeonggi-do, Republic of Korea; Chonbuk Natl Univ Med School, Jeonju, Republic of Korea; et al)
Surg Oncol 20:e32-e37, 2011

This study was conducted to evaluate the preliminary outcome of palliative minimally invasive surgery for humeral metastasis in patients who have multiple advanced cancers with short life expectancy. Percutaneous Ender nailing and direct transcortical intramedullary cementing were performed on a total of 15 patients with metastatic disease of the humerus. The origins of the cancers were the lung ($n = 9$), breast ($n = 3$), colon ($n = 2$) and liver ($n = 1$). Each patient had multiple unresectable organic metastases and proved to be at high risk for anesthesia and bloody surgery. All procedures were performed under regional anesthesia and fluoroscopic guidance. The mean amount of intramedullary cement injection after Ender nailing was 13.4 ml. The mean of the numeric rating scale (NRS) score for pain decreased from 9.6 points before surgery to 3.6 points after surgery ($P < 0.001$). The mean of the Musculoskeletal Tumor Society (MSTS) functional score increased from 10.6 points before surgery to 19.9 points after surgery ($P < 0.001$). Seven patients died within 7 months. There were no complications associated with cement leakage, fixation failure and surgical wound even in cases of early postoperative radiation or chemotherapy. Percutaneous flexible nailing along with intramedullary cementing could be a useful minimally invasive surgical method for the palliation of humeral metastasis in selective terminal cancer patients by providing immediate reliable fixation and effective pain relief (Fig 1).

▶ This is a well-documented series of 15 patients with advanced metastatic malignancy and present or impending pathologic fractures of the humerus treated with a very limited surgical procedure: percutaneous insertion of an Ender's nail

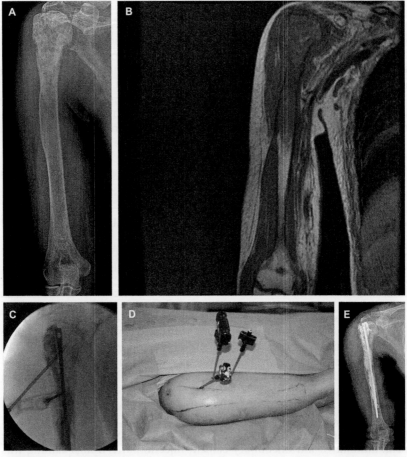

FIGURE 1.—A 49-year-old female patient with lung cancer (case 7). Plain radiograph (A) and MR image (B) taken after radiation therapy show the extent of metastatic lesion in the right proximal humerus with a linear pathologic fracture. Intraoperative fluoroscopy (C) exhibits an Ender nail and bone cement injected into the intramedullary metastatic lesion through the 3 PV needles. Photograph shows the operative field (D). Postoperative plain radiograph (E) shows bone cement filling in the intramedullary space along the Ender nail. (Reprinted from Kim JH, Kang HG, Kim JR, et al. Minimally invasive surgery of humeral metastasis using flexible nails and cement in high-risk patients with advanced cancer. *Surg Oncol.* 2011;20:e32-e37, with permission from Elsevier.)

and subsequent cementoplasty around the nail. Although the procedure may seem inadequate compared with other more robust treatment options, the authors present it as a treatment option for patients with painful lesions who are poor medical candidates for more aggressive procedures (Fig 1).

This is a useful technique for orthopedic oncologists to consider in select patients, and I have personally used a similar method in a modest number of cases. Although I do not think this will replace our more traditional surgical methods, I have included it in the YEAR BOOK as an alternative treatment for surgeons to be familiar with in the care of metastatic patients.

P. S. Rose, MD

Treatment and Survival of Osseous Renal Cell Carcinoma Metastases

Evenski A, Ramasunder S, Fox W, et al (Univ of Pennsylvania, Philadelphia; Duke Univ, Durham, NC; Naval Postgraduate School, Monterey; CA; et al)
J Surg Oncol 106:850-855, 2012

Background.—Renal cell carcinoma is the seventh leading cause of cancer deaths. Studies have shown patients with solitary osseous metastases have a better prognosis; however, methods of resection are not well defined. The purpose of this study was to review factors associated with survival and assess the impact of wide versus intralesional management on function and disease-specific outcomes in patients with renal cell carcinoma metastases.

Methods.—Sixty-nine patients with 86 osseous renal cell metastases were reviewed. Potential factors associated with survival were evaluated with Kaplan—Meier curves. ANOVA was performed to compare means between groups.

Results.—One year survival for the group was 77% and 32.5% at 5 years. The absence of metastatic disease at presentation, nephrectomy, and pre-operative status were associated with improved survival. There was a lower rate of local recurrence with wide resection (5%) versus intralesional procedures (27%).

Conclusions.—Improved pre-operative status, nephrectomy, and metachronous lesions had better overall survival. Wide resection results in decreased local recurrence and revision surgeries. However, it did not reliably predict improved survival. Our recommendation is for individual evaluation of each patient with osseous renal cell carcinoma metastases. Wide excision may be used for resectable lesions to prevent local progression and subsequent surgeries (Fig 1).

▶ Metastatic renal cell carcinoma continues to present a challenge to orthopedic oncologists in selecting appropriate surgical treatments for patients. These authors present the University of Miami experience with this type of tumor.

Although past small series had suggested patients with solitary metastases from renal cell carcinoma could be "cured" with en bloc resection, this study (in addition to others) calls that assertion into question (Fig 1). However, wide resection in this series was more durable with less local recurrence and need for revision.

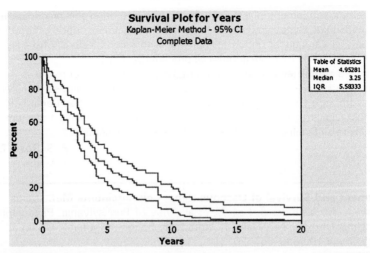

FIGURE 1.—Kaplan–Meier curve shows the overall survival rate (in years) of patients with 95% confidence intervals. [Color figure can be seen in the online version of this article, available at http://wileyonlinelibrary.com/journal/jso]. (Reprinted from Evenski A, Ramasunder S, Fox W, et al. Treatment and survival of osseous renal cell carcinoma metastases. *J Surg Oncol.* 2012;106:850-855, reprinted by permission of Taylor & Francis Ltd, http://www.informaworld.com.)

Although intuitive, this is the first study to document Eastern Cooperative Oncology Group performance status as a prognostic factor for survival in this patient population.

Interested readers are also referred to the MD Anderson series by Lin et al[1] published in the *Journal of Bone Joint Surgery* in 2007. There is certainly a role for aggressive resections in these patients to achieve durable functional outcome in a disease with the potential for prolonged survival, with this article giving more support and information toward this goal.

P. S. Rose, MD

Reference

1. Lin PP, Mirza AN, Lewis VO, et al. Patient survival after surgery for osseous metastases from renal cell carcinoma. *J Bone Joint Surg Am.* 2007;89:1794-1801.

Metabolic and clinical assessment of efficacy of cryoablation therapy on skeletal masses by ^{18}F-FDG positron emission tomography/computed tomography (PET/CT) and visual analogue scale (VAS): initial experience
Masala S, Schillaci O, Bartolucci AD, et al (Univ Hosp Tor Vergata, Rome, Italy)
Skeletal Radiol 40:159-165, 2011

Various therapy modalities have been proposed as standard treatments in management of bone metastases. Radiation therapy remains the standard of care for patients with localized bone pain, but up to 30% of them do not experience notable pain relief. Percutaneous cryoablation is a minimally invasive technique that induces necrosis by alternately freezing and thawing a target tissue. This technique is successfully used to treat a variety of malignant and benign diseases in different sites. ^{18}F-FDG positron emission tomography/computed tomography (^{18}F-FDG PET/CT) is a single technique of imaging that provides in a "single step" both morphological and metabolic features of neoplastic lesions of the bone. The aim of this study was to evaluate the efficacy of the cryosurgical technique on secondary musculoskeletal masses according to semi-quantitative PET analysis and clinical-test evaluation with the visual analogue scale (VAS). We enrolled 20 patients with painful bone lesions (score pain that exceeded 4 on the VAS) that were non-responsive to treatment; one lesion per patient was treated. All patients underwent a PET-CT evaluation before and 8 weeks after cryotherapy; maximum standardized uptake value (SUV$_{max}$) was measured before and after treatment for metabolic assessment of response to therapy. After treatment, 18 patients (90%) showed considerable reduction in SUV$_{max}$ value (>50%) suggestive of response to treatment; only 2 patients did not show meaningful reduction in metabolic activity. Our preliminary study demonstrates that quantitative analysis provided by PET correlates with response to cryoablation therapy as assessed by CT data and clinical VAS evaluation.

▶ Percutaneous cryoablation is an increasingly common method of treatment of benign and metastatic skeletal lesions. Relatively few data are published on this topic. Masala and colleagues report the results and correlation of F-18 deoxyglucose (FDG) positron emission tomography scan activity and patient visual analogue scores following cryoablation of skeletal metastases. Patients generally improved symptomatically, and a modest correlation was seen between FDG avidity of lesions and patient visual analog scale scores (Figs 1 and 2 in the original article).

Radiotherapy is and will remain the standard of care and default treatment modality for symptomatic metastases. However, this is a good technique for physicians who care for cancer patients to be aware of, particularly for those patients who have failed radiation or those for whom local considerations make further radiation a poor option. It will be interesting to see how this method evolves in the treatment of patients.

P. S. Rose, MD

Soft Tissue Tumors

Ionizing Radiation Exposure and the Development of Soft-Tissue Sarcomas in Atomic Bomb Survivors

Samartzis D, Nishi N, Cologne J, et al (Radiation Effects Res Foundation, Hiroshima and Nagasaki, Japan)
J Bone Joint Surg Am 95:222-229, 2013

Background.—Very high levels of ionizing radiation exposure have been associated with the development of soft-tissue sarcoma. The effects of lower levels of ionizing radiation on sarcoma development are unknown. This study addressed the role of low to moderately high levels of ionizing radiation exposure in the development of soft-tissue sarcoma.

Methods.—Based on the Life Span Study cohort of Japanese atomic-bomb survivors, 80,180 individuals were prospectively assessed for the development of primary soft-tissue sarcoma. Colon dose in gray (Gy), the excess relative risk, and the excess absolute rate per Gy absorbed ionizing radiation dose were assessed. Subject demographic, age-specific, and survival parameters were evaluated.

Results.—One hundred and four soft-tissue sarcomas were identified (mean colon dose = 0.18 Gy), associated with a 39% five-year survival rate. Mean ages at the time of the bombings and sarcoma diagnosis were 26.8 and 63.6 years, respectively. A linear dose-response model with an excess relative risk of 1.01 per Gy (95% confidence interval [CI]: 0.13 to 2.46; $p = 0.019$) and an excess absolute risk per Gy of 4.3 per 100,000 persons per year (95% CI: 1.1 to 8.9; $p = 0.001$) were noted in the development of soft-tissue sarcoma.

Conclusions.—This is one of the largest and longest studies (fifty-six years from the time of exposure to the time of followup) to assess ionizing radiation effects on the development of soft-tissue sarcoma. This is the first study to suggest that lower levels of ionizing radiation may be associated with the development of soft-tissue sarcoma, with exposure of 1 Gy doubling the risk of soft-tissue sarcoma development (linear dose-response). The five-year survival rate of patients with soft-tissue sarcoma in this population was much lower than that reported elsewhere.

Level of Evidence.—Prognostic Level I. See Instructions for Authors for a complete description of levels of evidence.

▶ This is a fascinating and unique study that prospectively evaluated the risk of developing soft-tissue sarcomas in a cohort of > 80 000 individuals exposed to radiation from the Hiroshima and Nagasaki atomic bomb blasts over 56 years. Although the study suffers from the risk of missing data and heterogeneous follow-up inherent in a study that spans a half-century, it provides a unique look into the long-term oncologic effects of radiation exposure in a large cohort.

The authors noted a small but linear dose-response model for development of sarcoma after radiation exposure. Survival was poor.

How to interpret these results? The patients in this study received a single bolus dose, so it is not clear exactly how this might apply to persons exposed to chronic, low levels in occupational settings. However, it is clear that even modest doses of radiation exposure may increase the risk of sarcoma development.

P. S. Rose, MD

FDG PET/CT in Initial Staging of Adult Soft-Tissue Sarcoma

Roberge D, Vakilian S, Alabed YZ, et al (McGill Univ Health Centre, Montreal, Quebec, Canada)
Sarcoma 2012:1-7, 2012

Soft-tissue sarcomas spread predominantly to the lung and it is unclear how often FDG-PET scans will detect metastases not already obvious by chest CT scan or clinical examination. Adult limb and body wall soft-tissue sarcoma cases were identified retrospectively. Ewing's sarcoma, rhab-domyosarcoma, GIST, desmoid tumors, visceral tumors, bone tumors, and retroperitoneal sarcomas were excluded as were patients imaged for fol-lowup, response assessment, or recurrence. All patients had a diagnostic chest CT scan. 109 patients met these criteria, 87% of which had interme-diate or high-grade tumors. The most common pathological diagnoses were leiomyosarcoma (17%), liposarcoma (17%), and undifferentiated or pleomorphic sarcoma (16%). 98% of previously unresected primary tumors were FDG avid. PET scans were negative for distant disease in 91/109 cases. The negative predictive value was 89%. Fourteen PET scans were positive. Of these, 6 patients were already known to have metastases, 3 were false positives, and 5 represented new findings of metastasis (positive predictive value 79%). In total, 5 patients were upstaged by FDG-PET (4.5%). Although PET scans may be of use in specific circumstances, routine use of FDG PET imaging as part of the initial staging of soft-tissue sarcomas was unlikely to alter management in our series (Table 2).

▶ "But, doctor, I would feel a lot better if I had a PET (positron emission tomog-raphy) scan." All oncologic caregivers frequently hear this or a variant of it in routine clinical practice. Roberge and colleagues help us define the value of these expensive scans in the evaluation of adults newly diagnosed with soft-tissue sarcoma: very little. In a series of 109 patients, 4.5% were upstaged by PET compared with standard chest computed tomography scans. However, more patients had false-negative results than informative new positive data (Table 2). As health expenditures become increasingly scrutinized, it is hard to justify these scans as a part of routine practice on unselected patients.

P. S. Rose, MD

TABLE 2.—PET Results

True negative	81 (74%)
False negative	10 (9%)
True positive	
Known	6 (5.5%)
New	5 (4.5%)
False positive	3 (3%)
Indeterminate	4 (4%)

Follow-up After Primary Treatment of Soft Tissue Sarcoma of Extremities: Impact of Frequency of Follow-Up Imaging on Disease-Specific Survival

Chou Y-S, Liu C-Y, Chen W-M, et al (Taipei Veterans General Hosp, Taiwan; Natl Yang-Ming Univ School of Medicine, Taipei, Taiwan)
J Surg Oncol 106:155-161, 2012

Background and Objectives.—We explored the impact of frequency of surveillance imaging on disease-specific survival (DSS) in patients with extremity soft tissue sarcoma (STS).

Methods.—Locoregional imaging (LRI) and chest imaging (CI) were used to detect local recurrence (LR) and distant metastasis (DM), respectively. Relapsing patients were retrospectively assigned to more frequent surveillance (MFS) or less frequent surveillance (LFS) groups, according to the median interval for each follow-up modality. Outcome measures included overall DSS (O-DSS), post-LR DSS, and post-DM DSS.

Results.—We assigned 165 patients to three distinct risk groups according to tumor size ($\leq$5 vs. >5 cm), depth (superficial- vs. deep-seated), grade (I vs. II or III), and surgical margin ($\geq$10 vs. <10 mm). Data for 80 patients who relapsed were analyzed. Among 50 high-risk (with all four risk factors) relapsing patients, those in the MFS group for either LRI or CI had better O-DSS (LRI, median 44.07 vs. 27.43 months, $P = 0.008$; CI, median 43.60 vs. 36.93 months, $P = 0.036$), post-LR DSS (median 27.20 vs. 10.63 months, $P = 0.028$) and post-DM DSS (median 13.20 vs. 6.24 months, $P = 0.031$).

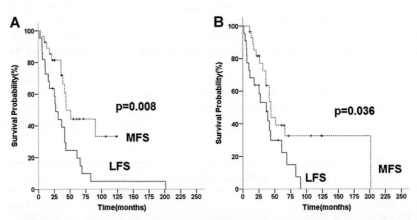

FIGURE 2.—O-DSS in all relapsing patients with high-risk features (n = 50). Patients in the high-frequency follow-up group (MFS, dotted line) had a better O-DSS than patients in the low-frequency follow-up group (LFS, solid line) for both (A) LRI and (B) CI. (Reprinted from Chou Y-S, Liu C-Y, Chen W-M, et al. Follow-up after primary treatment of soft tissue sarcoma of extremities: impact of frequency of follow-up imaging on disease-specific survival. *J Surg Oncol.* 2012;106:155-161, reprinted by permission of Taylor & Francis Ltd, http://www.informaworld.com.)

Conclusion.—More frequent follow-up were associated with improved survival in high-risk relapsing patients with extremity STS by providing greater opportunities for adequate reoperation (Fig 2).

▶ This is an intriguing study that analyzes the oncologic benefit of more versus less frequent posttreatment surveillance for local and distant recurrence on disease-specific survival from soft-tissue sarcoma. The authors found that more frequent imaging was associated with improved survival, presumably by earlier detection and treatment of tumor recurrence (Fig 2).

This is not a perfect study in that patients were retrospectively assigned to the more or less frequent imaging groups. However, this certainly suggests a benefit for high-risk patients in undergoing intensive imaging to improve their disease-specific survival.

P. S. Rose, MD

Surgery Quality and Tumor Status Impact on Survival and Local Control of Resectable Liposarcomas of Extremities or the Trunk Wall
Rutkowski P, Trepka S, Ptaszynski K, et al (Maria Sklodowska-Curie Memorial Cancer Ctr and Inst of Oncology, Roentgena, Warsaw, Poland; HolyCross Oncological Ctr, Kielce, Poland)
Clin Orthop Relat Res 471:860-870, 2013

Background.—The 5-year survival rates for localized liposarcomas reportedly vary from 75% to 91% with histologic grade as the most important prognostic factor. However, it is unclear which other factors, including the initial surgery quality and recurrent tumors, influence survival in localized liposarcomas (LPS).

Questions/Purposes.—We analyzed factors (including AJCC staging system) influencing survival and local control of resectable LPS of the extremities/trunk wall and the impact of surgery quality and tumor status and type of disease recurrences according to pathological subtype.

Methods.—We retrospectively reviewed 181 patients with localized LPS: 110 were treated for primary tumors, 50 for recurrent tumors, and 21 for wide scar resection after unplanned nonradical resection. We determined survival rates and examined factors influencing survival. The minimum followup was 4 months (median, 52 months; range, 4—168 months).

Results.—Five-year disease-specific (DSS), disease-free (DFS), and local relapse-free survival (LRFS) rates were: 80%, 58%, and 75%, respectively. Five-year local relapse-free survival rates for primary versus clinically recurrent tumor versus scar after nonradical resection were: 86.1%, 52.1%, and 73.3%, respectively. The following were independent negative prognostic factors for DSS (AJCC Stage ≥ IIb), DFS (Grade 3; clinical recurrence; skin infiltration), and LRFS (clinical recurrence; R1 resection). An unplanned excision, although influencing local relapse-free survival, had no impact on disease-specific survival (calculated from date of first excision

5-year rate of 80%, considering impact of combined treatment of clinical recurrence/scar).

Conclusions.—We confirmed the value of AJCC staging for predicting disease-specific survival in extremity/trunk wall LPS. Radical reresection of scar after nonradical primary tumor resection (+ radiotherapy) seems to improve disease-free and local relapse-free survival in liposarcomas. Patients with unplanned excision can be cured when referred to a sarcoma unit.

Level of Evidence.—Level IV, prognostic study. See the Guidelines for Authors for a complete description of levels of evidence.

▶ This article represents a presentation at the 2011 International Society Of Limb Salvage (ISOLS) meeting; the authors attempt to validate the American Joint Committee on Cancer (AJCC) staging system for its prognostic value in liposarcomas and to look at tumor characteristics at presentation (primary, recurrent, or after unplanned excision) in survival.

The article includes well-differentiated liposarcomas in its analysis, whereas many centers are moving toward treating these as premalignant lesions rather than sarcomas (with marginal resection, observation, and the terminology of atypical lipomatous tumor). Readers should be aware that this article includes these, as it may be felt to dilute the results.

I have selected this article for its role as part of the ISOLS symposium, its inclusion and validation of the AJCC staging system, and its continued message about aggressively treating patients who have undergone unplanned sarcoma resections.

P. S. Rose, MD

The Use of Radiation Therapy in the Management of Selected Patients with Atypical Lipomas

Kang J, Botros M, Goldberg S, et al (Harvard Radiation Oncology Program, Boston, MA; Med College of Wisconsin, Milwaukee; Massachusetts General Hosp, Boston)
Sarcoma 2013:1-5, 2013

Background and Objectives.—Atypical lipomas are uncommon, slow-growing benign tumors. While surgery has been the primary treatment modality, we have managed some patients with radiation (RT) as a component of the treatment and have reported their outcomes in this study.

Methods.—A retrospective review of all cases of extremity and trunk atypical lipomas in The Sarcoma Database at the study institution was conducted.

Results.—Thirteen patients were identified. All patients underwent surgical resection at initial presentation and received pre- or postoperative radiation for subtotal resection ($n = 2$), local recurrence ($n = 8$), or progressive disease ($n = 3$). The median total radiation dose was 50 Gy. Median followup was 65.1 months. All patients treated with RT remained free of disease at the last followup. No grade 3 or higher late toxicity from radiation was observed. No cases of tumor dedifferentiation occurred.

Conclusion.—For recurrent or residual atypical lipomas, a combination of reexcision and RT can provide long-term local control with acceptable morbidity. For recurrent tumors, pre-op RT of 50 Gy appears to be an effective and well-tolerated management approach.

▶ Recurrent atypical lipomatous tumors are a frustrating clinical problem that often arises after incomplete resection elsewhere. Kang and colleagues report the Massachusetts General Hospital experience with radiotherapy for these tumors after incomplete resection, recurrence, or local progression. Stable tumor outcomes were seen. Although there is little current literature on this topic, this modest series can help guide treatment in an otherwise ambiguous situation. Although few if any surgeons would advocate frequent radiation of these tumors at index presentation, and most recurrences can still be handled surgically, this provides an option for select recurrent tumors with poor presentations (eg, multifocal recurrences).

P. S. Rose, MD

Extra-Abdominal Desmoid Tumours: A Review of the Literature
Molloy AP, Hutchinson B, O'Toole GC (St Vincent's Univ Hosp, Dublin, Ireland)
Sarcoma 2012:1-9, 2012

Extra-abdominal desmoid lesions, otherwise known as aggressive fibromatosis, are slow-growing benign lesions which may be encountered in clinical practice. Recent controversies exist regarding their optimal treatment. Given their benign nature, is major debulking surgery justified, or is it worth administering chemotherapy for a disease process which unusually defies common teaching and responds to such medications? We present a literature review of this particular pathology discussing the aetiology, clinical presentation, and various current controversies in the treatment options.

▶ Desmoid tumors remain a controversial clinical topic with treatments ranging from benign neglect to aggressive surgery, chemotherapy, or radiation. I have chosen to include this review article on the subject because of its discussion of recently discovered genetic aspects of these tumors as well as its discussion of novel chemotherapy approaches (eg, tyrosine kinase inhibitor—based therapy) and cryotherapy. Although not directly surgical, these are topics that surgeons caring for these patients need to be familiar with.

P. S. Rose, MD

Does Combined Open and Arthroscopic Synovectomy for Diffuse PVNS of the Knee Improve Recurrence Rates?

Colman MW, Ye J, Weiss KR, et al (The Univ of Pittsburgh, PA)
Clin Orthop Relat Res 471:883-890, 2013

Background.—Diffuse-type pigmented villonodular synovitis (PVNS) has a high local recurrence rate and as such can lead to erosive destruction of the involved joint. Multiple surgical modalities exist, but it is unknown which technique best minimizes local recurrence and surgical morbidity.

Questions/Purposes.—We compared recurrence rates, arthritis progression, and complications between arthroscopic and open modalities for diffuse PVNS of the knee.

Methods.—We retrospectively identified 103 patients with PVNS treated between 1993 and 2011. Of these, 48 had diffuse-type PVNS of the knee treated by all-arthroscopic, open posterior with arthroscopic anterior, or open anterior and open posterior synovectomy. We recorded patient demographics, treatment profiles, recurrence rates, and arthritic progression. Minimum followup was 3 months (median, 40 months; range, 3−187 months).

Results.—Recurrence rates were lower in the open/arthroscopic group compared with the arthroscopic or open/open groups: 9% versus 62% versus 64%, respectively. Arthritic progression occurred in 17% of the total study group with 8% going onto total knee arthroplasty within the followup period. We detected no difference between groups with regard to arthritic progression or progression to arthroplasty. The most common complication was hemarthrosis, which we drained in three patients (6% of the total study group), but there were no detectable differences between groups.

Conclusion.—Open posterior with arthroscopic anterior synovectomy is a viable, comprehensive approach to diffuse PVNS of the knee and provides both low recurrence rates and a low postoperative complication profile. Greater numbers of recurrences may be partially explained in the arthroscopic group by technical challenges associated with posterior arthroscopic synovectomy and in the open/open group by selection bias toward more aggressive disease.

Level of Evidence.—Level III, therapeutic study. See Guidelines for Authors for a complete description of levels of evidence.

▶ Like desmoid tumors, diffuse pigmented villonodular synovitis (PVNS) provides a real challenge in local control of a benign process. This article shows a striking difference in recurrence-free survival favoring open posterior and arthroscopic anterior surgery for diffuse PVNS of the knee (see Fig 4 in the original article) by a wide margin (9% vs > 60% for other modalities).

No difference was seen in arthritic progression or need for arthroplasty among the different treatment groups, true functional outcome measures are lacking, and the sample size was modest at 48 with subsequent low power. That said, these results highlight the need to achieve a thorough synovectomy in these patients and the role of a combined (and potentially team-based) surgical approach; they confirm the intuitions of many surgeons by a surprisingly wide margin.

P. S. Rose, MD

Sentinel Lymph Node Biopsy for Melanoma: American Society of Clinical Oncology and Society of Surgical Oncology Joint Clinical Practice Guideline
Wong SL, Balch CM, Hurley P, et al (Univ of Michigan, Ann Arbor; Univ of Texas Southwestern, Dallas; American Society of Clinical Oncology, Alexandria, VA; et al)
J Clin Oncol 30:2912-2918, 2012

Purpose.—The American Society of Clinical Oncology (ASCO) and Society of Surgical Oncology (SSO) sought to provide an evidence-based guideline on the use of lymphatic mapping and sentinel lymph node (SLN) biopsy in staging patients with newly diagnosed melanoma.

Methods.—A comprehensive systematic review of the literature published from January 1990 through August 2011 was completed using MED-LINE and EMBASE. Abstracts from ASCO and SSO annual meetings were included in the evidence review. An Expert Panel was convened to review the evidence and develop guideline recommendations.

Results.—Seventy-three studies met full eligibility criteria. The evidence review demonstrated that SLN biopsy is an acceptable method for lymph node staging of most patients with newly diagnosed melanoma.

Recommendations.—SLN biopsy is recommended for patients with intermediate-thickness melanomas (Breslow thickness, 1 to 4 mm) of any anatomic site; use of SLN biopsy in this population provides accurate staging. Although there are few studies focusing on patients with thick melanomas (T4; Breslow thickness, > 4 mm), SLN biopsy may be recommended for staging purposes and to facilitate regional disease control. There is insufficient evidence to support routine SLN biopsy for patients with thin melanomas (T1; Breslow thickness, < 1 mm), although it may be considered in selected patients with high-risk features when staging benefits outweigh risks of the procedure. Completion lymph node dissection (CLND) is recommended for all patients with a positive SLN biopsy and achieves good regional disease control. Whether CLND after a positive SLN biopsy improves survival is the subject of the ongoing Multicenter Selective Lymphadenectomy Trial II (Table 1).

▶ I have included this article on current sentinel lymph node biopsy recommendations for the subset of orthopedic oncologists who treat melanoma as a part of their practice. The role of sentinel lymph node biopsy for melanoma is an evolving field, and this article (a joint statement from the American Society of Clinical Oncology and the Society of Surgical Oncology groups) succinctly outlines evidence-based practical guidelines for the use of sentinel lymph node biopsy in patients with newly diagnosed melanoma.

TABLE 1.—Summary of Clinical Practice Guideline Recommendations

Clinical Question	Recommendation
What are the indications for SLN biopsy?	
Intermediate-thickness melanomas	SLN biopsy is recommended for patients with intermediate-thickness cutaneous melanomas (Breslow thickness, 1 to 4 mm) of any anatomic site. Routine use of SLN biopsy in this population provides accurate staging, with high estimates for PSM and acceptable estimates for FNR, PTPN, and PVP
Thick melanomas	Although there are few studies focusing specifically on patients with thick melanomas (T4; Breslow thickness, > 4 mm), use of SLN biopsy in this population may be recommended for staging purposes and to facilitate regional disease control
Thin melanomas	There is insufficient evidence to support routine SLN biopsy for patients with thin melanomas (T1; Breslow thickness, < 1 mm), although it may be considered in selected patients with high-risk features when the benefits of pathologic staging may outweigh the potential risks of the procedure. Such risk factors may include ulceration or mitotic rate $\geq 1/mm^2$, especially in the subgroup of patients with melanomas 0.75 to 0.99 mm in Breslow thickness
What is the role of CLND?	CLND is recommended for all patients with positive SLN biopsy. CLND achieves regional disease control, although whether CLND after a positive SLN biopsy improves survival is the subject of the ongoing MSLT II

Abbreviations: CLND, completion lymph node dissection; FNR, false-negative rate; MSLT II, Multicenter Selective Lymphadenectomy Trial II; PSM, proportion successfully mapped; PTPN, post-test probability negative; PVP, positive predictive value; SLN, sentinel lymph node.

A summary of recommendations is included in Table 1. Additionally, the guideline includes a nice discussion of the role of sentinel node biopsy and complete lymph node dissection in this setting.

P. S. Rose, MD

Tumor Science

RT-PCR Analysis for FGF23 Using Paraffin Sections in the Diagnosis of Phosphaturic Mesenchymal Tumors With and Without Known Tumor Induced Osteomalacia

Bahrami A, Weiss SW, Montgomery E, et al (Mayo Clinic, Rochester, MN; Emory Univ, Atlanta, GA; Johns Hopkins Med Institutions, Baltimore, MD; et al)
Am J Surg Pathol 33:1348-1354, 2009

Phosphaturic mesenchymal tumors of the mixed connective tissue type (PMTMCT) are extremely rare, histologically distinctive neoplasms, which cause tumor-induced osteomalacia (TIO) in most cases through the elaboration of a phosphaturic hormone, fibroblast growth factor-23 (FGF23). Rarely, identical tumors without known TIO may be observed. We studied a large group of PMTMCT for expression of FGF23, using a novel reverse transcription polymerase chain reaction (RT-PCR) assay for FGF23 in formalin-fixed, paraffin-embedded tissues. Twenty-nine PMTMCT (17 with and 12 without TIO) and 23 non-PMTMCT (16 various mesenchymal tumors, including 5 chondromyxoid fibroma, 8 chondroblastoma, 1 hemangiopericytoma, 1 aneurysmal bone cyst, and 1 high grade sarcoma; 5 carcinomas; and 2 non-neoplastic tissues) were retrieved. Total RNA was extracted from formalin-fixed, paraffin-embedded sections for RT-PCR analysis. FGF23 was amplified using 3 sets of primers that spanned the intron/exon boundaries to amplify the 3 exons of FGF23 gene (140, 125, and 175 bp). The housekeeping gene phosphoglycerokinase (189 bp) was coamplified to check the RNA quality. Sixteen of 17 (94%) PMTMCT with TIO were FGF23-positive. Nine of 12 (75%) PMTMCT without TIO were FGF23-positive. Two chondromyxoid fibroma and 1 aneurysmal bone cyst were positive; all other non-PMTMCT were negative. We conclude that RT-PCR for FGF23 is a sensitive and specific means of confirming the diagnosis of PMTMCT both in patients with and without TIO. FGF23 gene expression was present in more than 90% of PMTMCT with known TIO, confirming the role of FGF23 in this syndrome. Rare FGF23-negative PMTMCT with known TIO likely express other phosphaturic hormones (eg, frizzled-related protein 4). Our finding of expression of FGF23 in 75% of histologically identical tumors without known TIO confirms the reproducibility of the diagnosis of PMTMCT, even in the absence of known phosphaturia.

▶ This article reports the results of an reverse transcription polymerase chain reaction assay for the diagnosis of phosphaturic mesenchymal tumors. These are rare tumors, and I have included this article for 2 reasons: First, it may aid in the diagnosis of a rare and sometimes vexing neoplasm. Second, and importantly, results of this nature are likely to impact the science of musculoskeletal oncology as more diagnoses become ascertained (or excluded) via molecular means.

The results are encouraging but not perfect; the test identifies tumors in 90% of patients with tumor-induced osteomalacia and 75% of those without, albeit with a modest sample size of patients. Methods and reports like this are likely to continue to be refined as an adjunct to classical pathologic analysis.

P. S. Rose, MD

Miscellaneous

2011 Mid-America Orthopaedic Association Dallas B. Phemister Physician in Training Award: Can Musculoskeletal Tumors be Diagnosed with Ultrasound Fusion-Guided Biopsy?
Khalil JG, Mott MP, Parsons TW III, et al (Henry Ford Hosp, Detroit, MI; et al)
Clin Orthop Relat Res 470:2280-2287, 2012

Background.—Percutaneous biopsy for musculoskeletal tumors commonly relies on imaging adjuncts including ultrasound (US), CT, or MRI. These modalities however have disadvantages (US) or are cumbersome, not universally available, and costly (CT and MRI). US fusion is a novel technique that fuses previously obtained CT or MRI data with real-time US, which allows biopsies to be performed in an US suite. It has proven useful in various body systems but musculoskeletal applications remain scarce. Our goal is to evaluate the fusion technology and determine its ability to diagnose musculoskeletal tumors.

Questions/Purposes.—We determined whether biopsies performed via US fusion compared with CT guidance provide equivalent diagnostic yield and accuracy and allow quicker biopsy scheduling and procedure times.

Methods.—Forty-seven patients were assigned to undergo either US fusion (with MR, n = 16 or CT, n = 15) or CT-guided biopsies (n = 16). We evaluated adequacy of the histologic specimen (diagnostic yield) and correlation with surgical pathology (diagnostic accuracy). We determined scheduling times and lengths of the biopsy.

Results.—US fusion and CT-guided biopsy groups had comparable diagnostic yields (CT = 94%; US/MRI = 94%; US/CT = 93%) and accuracy (CT = 83%; US/MRI = 90%; US/CT = 100%). US fusion biopsies were faster to schedule and perform. All procedures were safe with minimal complications.

Conclusions.—US fusion provides a high diagnostic yield and accuracy comparable to CT-guided biopsy while performed in the convenience of an US suite. This may have resulted in the observed faster scheduling and biopsy times.

Level of Evidence.—Level II, diagnostic study. See Guidelines for Authors for a complete description of levels of evidence.

▶ This article won the 2011 Mid America Orthopaedic Association Dallas B. Phemister Physician in Training Award. In it, Khalil and colleagues describe applying the technique of ultrasound fusion to guide biopsies of musculoskeletal tumors. This involves electronically fusing the previously obtained computed tomography (CT) or magnetic resonance (MR) images of a tumor with real-time ultrasound (US); it allows US-guided biopsies of deep soft tissue or intra-osseous lesions that would not normally be suitable for US-guided biopsy.

Equivalent diagnostic accuracy was seen between patients nonrandomly assigned to US-fusion biopsy from CT images, MR images, or standard CT-guided biopsy. The authors note faster scheduling times for the US fusion procedure, but that would be a characteristic of their local radiology access protocols.

This is an interesting article; time will tell if it will bear clinical relevance. The authors speculate that this technology could be used in the office setting to allow surgeons to rapidly perform biopsies without delay. A more intriguing use would be for intraoperative localization of small tumors (the technique is currently often applied in this manner in hepatic surgery).

P. S. Rose, MD

High Infection Rate Outcomes in Long-bone Tumor Surgery with Endoprosthetic Reconstruction in Adults: A Systematic Review

Racano A, Pazionis T, Farrokhyar F, et al (McMaster Univ, Hamilton, Ontario, Canada)
Clin Orthop Relat Res 2013 [Epub ahead of print]

Background.—Limb salvage surgery (LSS) with endoprosthetic replacement is the most common method of reconstruction following bone tumor resection in the adult population. The risk of a postoperative infection developing is high when compared with conventional arthroplasty and there are no appropriate guidelines for antibiotic prophylaxis.

Questions/Purposes.—We sought to answer the following questions: (1) What is the overall risk of deep infection and the causative organism in lower-extremity long-bone tumor surgery with endoprosthetic reconstruction? (2) What antibiotic regimens are used with endoprosthetic reconstruction? (3) Is there a correlation between infection and either duration of postoperative antibiotics or sample size?

Methods.—We conducted a systematic review of the literature for clinical studies that reported infection rates in adults with primary bony malignancies of the lower extremity treated with surgery and endoprosthetic reconstruction. The search included articles published in English between 1980 and July 2011.

Results.—The systematic literature review yielded 48 studies reporting on a total of 4838 patients. The overall pooled weighted infection rate for lower-extremity LSS with endoprosthetic reconstruction was approximately 10% (95% CI, 8%−11%), with the most common causative organism reported to be Gram-positive bacteria in the majority of cases. The pooled weighted infection rate was 13% after short-term postoperative antibiotics and 8% after long-term postoperative antibiotics. There was no correlation between sample size and infection rate.

Conclusions.—Infection rates of 10% are high when compared with rates for conventional arthroplasty. Our results suggest that long-term antibiotic prophylaxis decreases the risk of deep infection. However, the data should be interpreted with caution owing to the retrospective nature of the studies.

▶ Infection after endoprosthetic tumor reconstruction remains a significant clinical problem. Racano and colleagues performed a systematic review of the literature to identify the pooled risk of infection and to investigate any effect of antibiotic duration on risk.

The overall infection risk was 10%, which is surprisingly high in light of the rates with more common orthopedic procedures. The authors then conclude that current data suggest a benefit to prolonged antibiotic administration postoperatively.

This article certainly does a service to the field by quantifying the infection rate after these procedures. The conclusions regarding the value of different antibiotic regimens must be tempered against the retrospective nature and heterogeneous data that formed the study. A prospective, randomized trial has been initiated (in large part by the senior author of this study) to rigorously evaluate the benefit of different antibiotic regimens in this setting and will hopefully provide level I evidence to guide future practice in this area.

P. S. Rose, MD

Article Index

Chapter 1: Basic Science

Chapter 2: General Orthopedics

Chapter 3: Forearm, Wrist, and Hand

Chapter 4: Elbow

Chapter 5: Shoulder

Chapter 6: Spine

Chapter 7: Total Hip Arthroplasty

Chapter 8: Total Knee Arthroplasty

Chapter 9: Foot and Ankle

Chapter 10: Sports Medicine

Chapter 11: Trauma and Amputation

Chapter 12: Orthopedic Oncology

Author Index

A

Abu Osman NA, 214
Adeli B, 113
Ahmed J, 46
Ahn UM, 92
Ain MC, 225
Åkesson K, 107
Alabed YZ, 349
Albäck A, 171
Aleksyeyenko S, 46
Allema JH, 274, 277
Alonso-Rodriguez N, 239
Altindas M, 174
Alvi HM, 341
Amendola A, 210
Amin AK, 136
Amirfeyz R, 111
Anderson PA, 79
Anderson SE, 20
Angelini A, 322
Anz A, 190
Aponte-Tinao LA, 338
Archdeacon MT, 260
Arnoczky SP, 72
Arnold PM, 98
Asleh K, 115
Atoun E, 289
Attinger CE, 176
Augereau B, 66
Ayerza MA, 338

B

Babu R, 93
Bachmann LM, 32
Bae J-H, 205
Bae S, 167
Bahrami A, 356
Baker PN, 142
Balch CM, 355
Barbour J, 48
Barco R, 279
Barkauskas DA, 309
Barnett AJ, 111
Barrack TN, 134
Barrett DS, 147
Bartolucci AD, 346
Bastrom TP, 161
Bauer H, 342
Baumhauer JF, 155
Behrbalk E, 85
Beitzel K, 7
Beris AE, 337

Berkes MB, 245
Bernasek TL, 150
Bertelsen G, 76
Biancari F, 171
Bilsel K, 198
Bini SA, 141
Bishop JA, 58, 268
Bisset L, 51
Biter LU, 274, 277
Blizzard L, 17
Bohensky MA, 194
Bolder SBT, 120
Boons HW, 292
Botros M, 352
Bozic KJ, 14
Brafman RT, 208
Brannon R, 10
Braun RM, 29
Bray C, 94
Briggs L, 71
Brinckmann P, 82
Brooks P, 51
Broom N, 1
Brouwer KM, 56, 288
Brouwer S, 16
Brouwers HFG, 323
Buchanan TS, 2
Bui CNH, 130
Burston BJ, 111

C

Camathias C, 232
Campagna EJ, 81
Campanacci DA, 326
Carlin B, 87
Carmody Soni EE, 333
Carry P, 281
Casemyr NE, 30
Cason GW, 84
Ceber M, 174
Cevolani L, 191
Cha S-M, 38
Chahal J, 63
Chandrakant V, 166
Chang K, 286
Chémaly O, 117
Chen AF, 90
Chen C-W, 34, 243
Chen CT, 8
Chen L, 119
Chen W-M, 350
Chen Y, 141
Chivukula S, 90
Cho WH, 317

Choi GW, 169
Choi WJ, 169
Chou Y-S, 350
Christensen TM, 170
Colaris JW, 274, 277
Colige A, 5
Collinge C, 260
Collinge CA, 236
Collins JE, 201
Collins RA, 136
Colman MW, 354
Cologne J, 347
Comer GC, 96
Coombes BK, 51
Costa F, 101
Cote MP, 7
Craig T, 305
Crall TS, 58
Cram P, 13
Cunningham P, 157

D

Damron TA, 305, 341
Daniels EW, 92
de Bock GH, 33
de Bont ESJM, 311
de Vries HJ, 16
de wijer A, 186
Dean E, 273
del-Prado G, 239
Delamarter RB, 103
Deng Y, 119
deSteiger R, 194
Di Paola J, 196
Di Schino M, 66
Digas G, 118
Dijkstra PDS, 326, 334
Dikos GD, 268
Dines D, 185
Dines J, 185
Dishkin-Paset JG, 23
Do V, 47
Dolmans GH, 33
Donati D, 191
Donken CCMA, 218, 223
Donnell-Fink LA, 201
Doornberg JN, 56
Dorey FJ, 284
Dragu A, 43
Drion PV, 5
Duckworth AD, 300
Dulaney-Cripe E, 260
Durrani SK, 112
Dwyer T, 200

373

Printed and bound by CPI Group (UK) Ltd, Croydon, CR0 4YY

08/05/2025

01864755-0012